FIRST AID

FOR THE®
Medicine Clerkship

Second Edition

LATHA G. STEAD, MD, FACEP
Assistant Professor
Education Chair and Vice-Chair for Research
Department of Emergency Medicine
Clerkship Director, EM Rotation
Mayo Clinic College of Medicine
Rochester, Minnesota

S. MATTHEW STEAD, MD, PhD
Resident in Pediatric Neurology
Mayo Clinic College of Medicine
Rochester, Minnesota
Class of 2001
State University of New York—Downstate Medical Center
Brooklyn, New York

MATTHEW S. KAUFMAN, MD
Fellow, Department of Hematology/Oncology
Long Island Jewish Medical Center
Albert Einstein College of Medicine
New Hyde Park, New York
Class of 2001
State University of New York—Downstate Medical Center
Brooklyn, New York

SUPERVISING EDITOR AND CONTRIBUTING AUTHOR:

SAMY I. McFARLANE, MD, MPH, FACP, FACE, CCD
Associate Professor of Medicine
Director, Fellowship Program in Endocrinology, Diabetes and Hypertension
Department of Medicine
State University of New York Health Science Center—Brooklyn
Brooklyn, New York

D0209576

McGraw-Hill
MEDICAL PUBLISHING DIVISION

New York / Chicago / San Francisco / Lisbon / London / Madrid / Mexico City
Milan / New Delhi / San Juan / Seoul / Singapore / Sydney / Toronto

The McGraw·Hill Companies

First Aid for the® Medicine Clerkship, Second Edition

Copyright © 2006 by The McGraw-Hill Companies, Inc. All rights reserved. Printed in the United States of America. Except as permitted under the United States Copyright Act of 1976, no part of this publication may be reproduced or distributed in any form or by any means, or stored in a data base or retrieval system, without the prior written permission of the publisher.

5 6 7 8 9 0 QPD/QPD 0 9 8 7

ISBN 978-0-07-144875-8
MHID 0-07-144875-6

NOTICE

Medicine is an ever-changing science. As new research and clinical experience broaden our knowledge, changes in treatment and drug therapy are required. The authors and the publisher of this work have checked with sources believed to be reliable in their efforts to provide information that is complete and generally in accord with the standards accepted at the time of publication. However, in view of the possibility of human error or changes in medical sciences, neither the authors nor the publisher nor any other party who has been involved in the preparation or publication of this work warrants that the information contained herein is in every respect accurate or complete, and they disclaim all responsibility for any errors or omissions or for the results obtained from use of the information contained in this work. Readers are encouraged to confirm the information contained herein with other sources. For example and in particular, readers are advised to check the product information sheet included in the package of each drug they plan to administer to be certain that the information contained in this work is accurate and that changes have not been made in the recommended dose or in the contraindications for administration. This recommendation is of particular importance in connection with new or infrequently used drugs.

This book was set in Electra LH by Rainbow Graphics.
The editor was Catherine A. Johnson.
The production supervisor was Catherine Saggese.
Project management was provided by Rainbow Graphics.
The index was prepared by Rainbow Graphics.
Quebecor World/Dubuque was the printer and binder.

This book is printed on acid-free paper.

Library of Congress Cataloging-in-Publication Data

First aid for the medicine clerkship : the student to student guide / series editors, Latha G. Stead, S. Matthew Stead, Matthew S. Kaufman ; supervising editor and contributing author, Samy I. McFarlane.– 2nd ed.
p. ; cm.
Includes index.
ISBN 0-07-144875-6
1. Clinical clerkship. I. Title: Medicine clerkship. II. Stead, Latha G. III. Stead, S. Matthew. IV. Kaufman. Matthew S.
[DNLM: 1. Clinical Clerkship—Handbooks. 2. Career Choice—Handbooks. 3. Fellowships and Scholarships—Handbooks. 4. Medicine—Handbooks. W 49 F527 2005]
R839.F57 2005
610'.71'1—dc22

2005046302

DEDICATION

To the contributors to this and future editions, who took time to share their experience, advice, and humor for the benefit of students.

and

To our families, friends, and loved ones, who endured and assisted in the task of assembling this guide.

CONTENTS

Introduction ix

Acknowledgments xi

SECTION 1: **HOW TO SUCCEED IN THE MEDICINE CLERKSHIP** 1

SECTION 2: **DATABASE OF HIGH-YIELD FACTS** 13

Cardiology 15

Endocrinology 61

Gastroenterology 99

Hematology–Oncology 147

Infectious Disease 179

Nephrology and Acid–Base Disorders 219

Pulmonology 251

Rheumatology 279

Neurology 305

Dermatology 329

Health Maintenance and Evidence-Based Medicine 363

SECTION 3: **CLASSIFIED** 381

Awards and Opportunities for Students Interested in Medicine 381

General 382

Research 387

Summer Externships 389

Year-Long Fellowships 393

For Minority Students 395
Ethnic 396
For Women 397
Evidence-Based Medicine Links 398
Index 399

CONTRIBUTING AUTHORS

Michelle Weisfelner Bloom, MD
Post-Doctoral Clinical Research Fellow
Clinical Pharmacology Unit
Department of Dermatology
Columbia-Presbyterian University Hospital
New York, New York
Dermatology chapter

Akua Boah, MD
Fellow, Department of Rheumatology
Long Island Jewish Medical Center
New Hyde Park, New York
Infectious Disease chapter and Nephrology chapter

Baaz Mishiev, MD
Resident, Internal Medicine
Long Island Jewish Medical Center
New Hyde Park, New York
Gastroenterology chapter

Peggy Nelson, MD
Attending Physician, Internal Medicine
New York, New York
Health Maintenance and Evidence-Based Medicine chapter

David J. Revere, MD
Resident, Internal Medicine
Long Island Jewish Medical Center
New Hyde Park, New York
Rheumatology chapter

Michael Shanik, MD
Fellow, Department of Endocrinology
Long Island Jewish Medical Center
New Hyde Park, New York
Endocrinology chapter

David Tang, MD
Attending Physician, Internal Medicine
New York, New York
Pulmonary chapter

Joshua Latzman, MD
Resident, Internal Medicine
North Shore University Hospital
Manhasset, New York
Neurology chapter

Rebecca Vanasse, MD
Fellow, Department of Hematology/Oncology
Long Island Jewish Medical Center
New Hyde Park, New York
Hematology/Oncology chapter

Adam Auerbach, MD
Fellow, Department of Cardiology
Long Island Jewish Medical Center
New Hyde Park, New York
Cardiology chapter

Mansoor Khan, MD
Combined Resident in Internal Medicine/Emergency Medicine
Long Island Jewish Medical Center
New Hyde Park, New York
Acid–Base Interpretation

Garry Choy, MD
Albert Einstein College of Medicine Class of 2005
Radiology Residency to begin 2006, Massachusetts General Hospital
Medical Student Reviewer and Contributor

FIRST EDITION CONTRIBUTING AUTHORS

Robin R. Blum, MD
Resident in Dermatology
Mount Sinai School of Medicine
New York
Dermatology

Thomas M. Boyd, MD
Attending in Emergency Medicine
Bronx-Lebanon Hospital
Bronx
Nephrology and Acid–Base, Endocrinology

Eric Michael Fields, DO
Resident in Emergency Medicine
Beth Israel Medical Center
Albert Einstein College of Medicine
New York
Gastroenterology

Barbara G. Lock, MD
Attending Physician in Emergency Medicine
Columbia Presbyterian Medical Center
New York
Cardiology, Pulmonology, Gastroenterology, Health Promotion

R. Anand Narasimhan, MD
Resident in Internal Medicine
Mayo Graduate School of Medicine
Rochester
Neurology, Hematology–Oncology

Jonathan Posner, MD
Resident in Psychiatry
Columbia Presbyterian Medical Center
New York
Rheumatology

INTRODUCTION

This clinical study aid was designed in the tradition of the *First Aid* series of books, formatted in the same way as the other titles in this series. Topics are listed by bold headings to the left, while the "meat" of the topic comprises the middle column. The outside margins contain mnemonics, diagrams, summary or warning statements, "pearls," and other memory aids. These are further classified as "exam tip" noted by the symbol and "ward tip" noted by the symbol.

The content of this book is based on the Committee of Directors in Internal Medicine (www.im.org/cdim/) recommendations for the internal medicine curriculum for third-year medical students. Each of the chapters contain the major topics central to the practice of internal medicine and closely parallel CDIM's medical student learning objectives.

The Medicine clerkship can be an exciting hands-on learning experience. For some medical students, it may be the first opportunity for patient interaction during medical school. There are two keys to doing well in this clerkship: Treat all patients and staff with respect and kindness, and organize your learning. You will find that rather than simply preparing you for success on the clerkship exam, this book will also help guide you in the clinical diagnosis and treatment of the many interesting problems you will see during your medicine rotation.

ACKNOWLEDGMENTS

We would like to thank the following faculty for their help in reviewing the manuscript for the first edition of this book:

Anderson Spickard III, MD
Director of Medical Student Clerkships
Department of Medicine
Vanderbilt University School of Medicine
Nashville, Tennessee

Kevin D. Whittle, MD
Assistant Professor of Internal Medicine
Third-Year Clerkship Director
University of South Dakota School of Medicine
Sioux Falls, South Dakota

We would like to thank the following student for his help reviewing and contributing to the second edition of this book:

Garry Choy, BS, MS
Class of 2005
Albert Einstein College of Medicine
Bronx, New York
(Radiology match at Mass General in 2006)

SECTION I

How to Succeed in the Medicine Clerkship

▶ HOW TO BEHAVE ON THE WARDS

Be on Time

Most medical ward teams begin rounding between 7 and 8 A.M. If you are expected to "pre-round," you should give yourself at least 10 minutes per patient that you are following to see the patient and learn about the events that occurred overnight. Like all working professionals, you will face occasional obstacles to punctuality, but make sure this is occasional. When you first start a rotation, try to show up at least 15 minutes early until you get the routine figured out. If the morning vitals are not yet recorded, take them yourself. Also, look at the chart to update yourself on any developments.

Dress in a Professional Manner

Even if the resident wears scrubs and the attending wears stiletto heels, you must dress in a professional, conservative manner. Wear a *short* white coat over your clothes unless discouraged (as in pediatrics).

Men should wear long pants, with cuffs covering the ankle, a long collared shirt, and a tie. No jeans, no sneakers, no short-sleeved shirts.
Women should wear long pants or knee-length skirt and a blouse or dressy sweater. No jeans, no sneakers, no heels greater than 1½ inches, no open-toed shoes.
Both men and women may wear scrubs occasionally, during overnight call or in the operating room. Do not make this your uniform.

Act in a Pleasant Manner

The medical rotation is often difficult, stressful, and tiring. Smooth out your experience by being nice to be around. Smile a lot and learn everyone's name. Don't be afraid to ask how your resident's weekend was. If you do not understand or disagree with a treatment plan or diagnosis, do not "challenge." Instead, say "I'm sorry, I don't quite understand, could you please explain. . . ." Show kindness and compassion toward your patients. Never participate in callous talk about patients.

Be Aware of the Hierarchy

The way in which this will affect you will vary from hospital to hospital and team to team, but it is always present to some degree. In general, address your questions regarding ward functioning to interns or residents. Address your medical questions to attendings; make an effort to be somewhat informed on your subject prior to asking attendings medical questions. It's always good to make your residents look good on rounds (. . . "Dr. Smith was nice enough to teach me about . . ."). Make sure the resident knows new patient developments ASAP.

Address Patients and Staff in a Respectful Way

Address patients as Sir, Ma'am, or Mr., Mrs., or Miss. Try not to address patients as "honey," "sweetie," and the like. Although you may feel these names are friendly, patients will think you have forgotten their name, that you are being inappropriately familiar, or both. Address all physicians as "doctor," unless told otherwise.

Show Initiative

Often, residents are busy with work and neglect their teaching responsibilities. Read up on your patient's condition, find an article, and offer to summarize in a few minutes what you learned. Give a copy of the article to your resident. This kind of initiative goes a long way in evaluations.

Take Responsibility for Your Patients

Know everything there is to know about your patients: their history, test results, details about their medical problem, and prognosis. Keep your intern or resident informed of new developments that they might not be aware of, and ask them for any updates you might not be aware of. Assist the team in developing a plan; speak to radiology, consultants, and family. Never give bad news to patients or family members without the assistance of your supervising resident or attending.

▶ RESPECT PATIENTS' RIGHTS

1. All patients have the right to have their personal medical information kept private. This means do not discuss the patient's information with family members without that patient's consent, and do not discuss any patient in hallways, elevators, or cafeterias.
2. All patients have the right to refuse treatment. This means they can refuse treatment by a specific individual (you, the medical student) or of a specific type (no nasogastric tube). Patients can even refuse life-saving treatment. The only exceptions to this rule are if the patient is deemed to not have the capacity to make decisions or understand situations, in which case a health care proxy should be sought, or if the patient is suicidal or homicidal.
3. All patients should be informed of the right to seek advanced directives on admission. Often, this is done by the admissions staff, in a booklet. If your patient is chronically ill or has a life-threatening illness, address the subject of advanced directives with the assistance of your attending.

Volunteer

Be self-propelled, self-motivated. Volunteer to help with a procedure or a difficult task. Volunteer to give a 20-minute talk on a topic of your choice. Volunteer to take additional patients. Volunteer to stay late. If the answer is "You don't have to," do it anyway.

Be a Team Player

Help other medical students with their tasks; teach them information you have learned. Support your supervising intern or resident whenever possible. Never steal the spotlight, steal a procedure, or make a fellow medical student look bad. Making other people look good always helps you, too.

Be Honest

If you don't understand, don't know, or didn't do it, make sure you always say that. Never say or document information that is false (a common example: "bowel sounds normal" when you did not listen). This can get you into serious trouble.

Keep Patient Information Handy

Use a clipboard, notebook, index cards, or PDA to keep patient information, including a miniature history and physical, and lab and test results, at hand.

Present Patient Information in an Organized Manner

Here is a template for the "bullet" presentation:

> "This is a [age]-year-old [gender] with a history of [major history such as HTN, DM, coronary artery disease, CA, etc.] who presented on [date] with [major symptoms, such as cough, fever, and chills] and was found to have [working diagnosis]. [Tests done] showed [results]. Yesterday, the patient [state important changes, new plan, new tests, new medications]. This morning the patient feels [state the patient's words], and the physical exam is significant for [state major findings]. Plan is [state plan].

The newly admitted patient generally deserves a longer presentation following the complete history and physical format.

Some patients have extensive histories. The whole history should be present in the admission note, but in ward presentation, it is often too much to absorb. In these cases, it will be very much appreciated by your team if you can generate a **good summary** that maintains an accurate picture of the patient. This usually takes some thought, but it's worth it.

▶ HOW TO PRESENT A CHEST RADIOGRAPH (CXR)

- First, confirm that the CXR belongs to your patient.
- If possible, compare to a previous film.

Then, present in a systematic manner:

1. *Technique:* Rotation, anteroposterior (AP) or posteroanterior (PA), penetration, inspiratory effort.
2. *Bony structures:* Look for rib, clavicle, scapula, and sternum fractures.

3. *Airway:* Look for tracheal deviation, pneumothorax, pneumomediastinum.
4. *Pleural space:* Look for fluid collections, which can represent hemothorax, chylothorax, pleural effusion.
5. *Lung parenchyma:* Look for infiltrates and consolidations: These can represent pneumonia, pulmonary contusions, hematoma, or aspiration. The location of an infiltrate can provide a clue to the location of a pneumonia:
   - Obscured right (R) costophrenic angle = Right lower lobe
   - Obscured left (L) costophrenic angle = Left lower lobe
   - Obscured R heart border = Right middle lobe
   - Obscured L heart border = Left upper lobe
6. *Mediastinum:* Look at size of mediastinum—a widened one (> 8 cm) goes with aortic dissection. Look for enlarged cardiac silhouette (> ½ thoracic width at base of heart), which may represent congestive heart failure (CHF), cardiomyopathy, or pericardial effusion.
7. *Diaphragm:* Look for free air under the right hemidiaphragm (suggests perforation). Look for stomach, bowel, or nasogastric tube (NGT) above diaphragm (suggests diaphragmatic rupture).
8. *Tubes and lines:*
   - Identify all tubes and lines.
   - An endotracheal tube should be 2 cm above the carina. A common mistake is right mainstem bronchus intubation.
   - A chest tube (including the most proximal hole) should be in the pleural space (not in the lung parenchyma).
   - An NGT should be in the stomach and uncoiled.
   - The tip of a central venous catheter (central line) should be in the superior vena cava (not in the right atrium).
   - The tip of a Swan–Ganz catheter should be in the pulmonary artery.
   - The tip of a transvenous pacemaker should be in the right atrium.

A sample CXR presentation may sound like:

> This is the CXR of Mr. Jones. The film is an AP view with good inspiratory effort. There is an isolated fracture of the eighth rib on the right. There is no tracheal deviation or mediastinal shift. There is no pneumo- or hemothorax. The cardiac silhouette appears to be of normal size. The diaphragm and heart borders on both sides are clear; no infiltrates are noted. There is a central venous catheter present, the tip of which is in the superior vena cava.

▶ HOW TO PRESENT AN ELECTROCARDIOGRAM (ECG)

- First, confirm that the ECG belongs to your patient.
- If possible, compare to a previous tracing.

Then, present in a systematic manner:

1. *Rate* (see Figure 1-1): The rate is [number of] beats per minute (bpm):
   - The ECG paper is scored so that one big box is 0.20 seconds. These big boxes consist of five little boxes, each of which is 0.04 seconds.

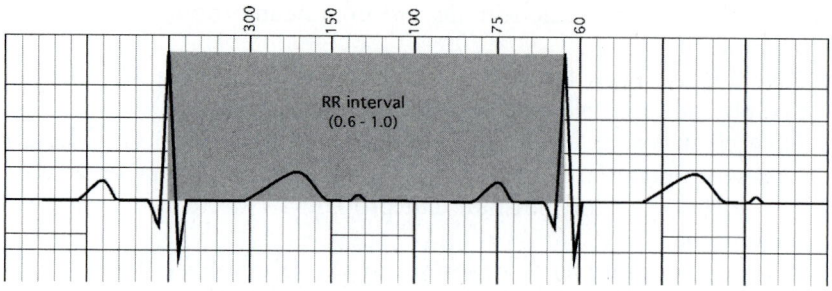

FIGURE 1-1. Calculating rate.

- A quick way to calculate rate when the rhythm is regular is the mantra: **300, 150, 100, 75, 60, 50** (= 300 / # large boxes), which is measured as the number of large boxes between two QRS complexes. Therefore, a distance of one large box between two adjacent QRS complexes would be a rate of 300, while a distance of five large boxes between two adjacent QRS complexes would be a rate of 60.
- For irregular rhythms, count the number of complexes that occur in a 6-second interval (30 large boxes) and multiply by 10 to get a rate in bpm.

2. *Rhythm:* The rhythm is [sinus]/[atrial fibrillation]/[atrial flutter] or other:
   - If p waves are present in all leads and upright in leads I and aVF, then the rhythm is sinus. Lack of p waves suggests a disorganized atrial rhythm, a junctional rhythm, or a ventricular rhythm. A ventricular rhythm (V Fib or V Tach) is an unstable one (could spell imminent death), and you should be getting ready for advanced cardiac life support (ACLS).
   - Normal sinus rhythm is usually a regular narrow-complex rhythm with each QRS complex preceded by a p wave.
3. *Axis* (see Figure 1-2): The axis is [normal]/[deviated to the right]/[deviated to the left]:
   - If I and aVF are both upright or positive, then the axis is normal.
   - If I is upright and aVF is upside down, then there is left axis deviation (LAD).
   - If I is upside down and aVF is upright, then there is right axis deviation (RAD).
   - If I and aVF are both upside down or negative, then there is extreme RAD.
4. *Intervals* (see Figure 1-3): The [PR]/[QRS] intervals are [normal]/[shortened]/[widened]:
   - Normal PR interval = 0.12 to 0.20 seconds:
     - Short PR is associated with Wolff–Parkinson–White syndrome (WPW).
     - WPW syndrome is characterized by a "delta" wave, or slurred upstroke of QRS complex.
     - Long PR interval is associated with heart block of which there are three types:
       - First-degree block: PR interval > 0.20 seconds (one big box)
       - Second-degree (Mobitz type I or Wenckebach) block: PR interval lengthens progressively until a QRS is dropped.

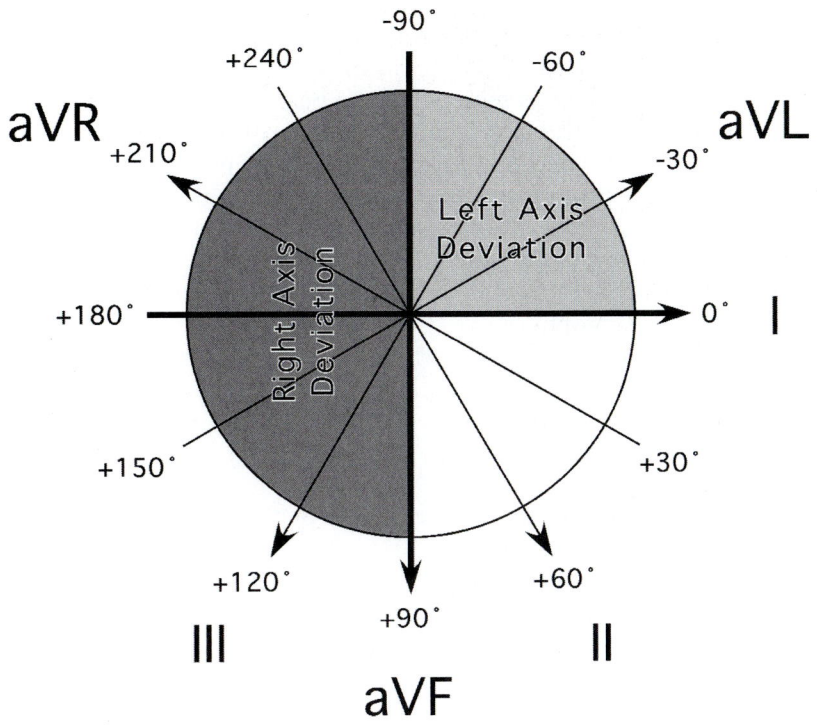

FIGURE 1-2. ECG axes.

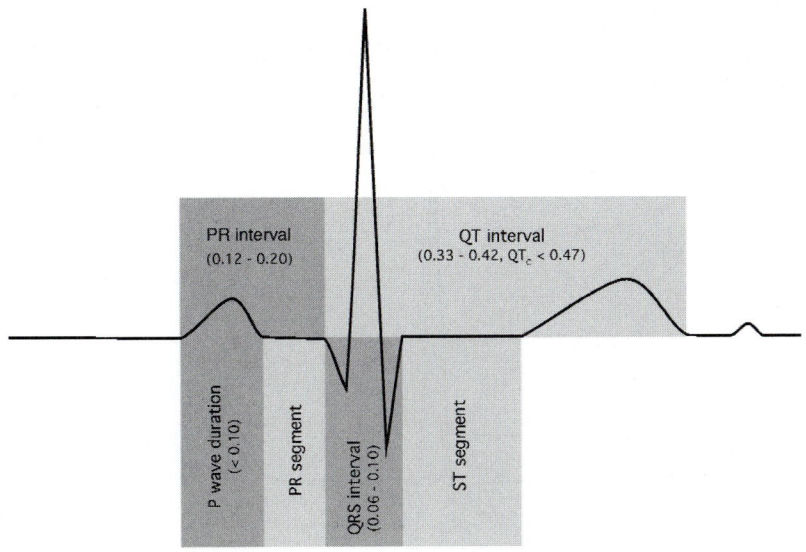

FIGURE 1-3. ECG intervals.

- Second-degree (Mobitz type II) block: PR interval is constant, but one QRS is dropped at a fixed interval.
- Third-degree heart block: Complete AV dissociation
- Normal QRS interval ≤ 0.12 seconds:
  - Prolonged QRS is seen when the beat is initiated in the ventricle rather than the sinoatrial node, when there is a bundle branch block, and when the heart is artificially paced with longer QRS intervals. Prolonged QRS is also noted in tricyclic overdose and Wolfe–Parkinson–White syndrome.

5. *Wave morphology* (see Figure 1-4):
   a. *Ventricular hypertrophy:* There [is/is no] [left/right] [ventricular/atrial] hypertrophy:
   - There are multiple criteria for determining right (RVH) and left ventricular hypertrophy (LVH). A few are listed here:
     - *Clues for LVH:*
       - $R_I > 15$ mm
       - $R_{I, II \text{ or } aVF} > 20$ mm
       - $R_{aVL} > 11$ mm
       - R_{V5} or $R_{V6} > 26$ mm
       - $R_I + S_{III} > 25$ mm
       - R + S in V lead > 45 mm
       - $S_{V1} + R_{V5}$ or $R_{V6} > 35$ mm
     - *Clues for RVH:*
       - $R_{V1} > 7$ mm
       - $S_{V1} < 2$ mm
       - R/S ratio in $V_1 > 1$
       - RAD of 110° or more

   b. *Atrial hypertrophy:*
   - Right atrial hypertrophy: tall or peaked p waves in limb or precordial leads
   - Left atrial hypertrophy: broad or notched p waves in limb leads

   c. *Ischemic changes:* There [are/are no] S-T wave [depressions/elevations] or [flattened/inverted] T waves. Presence of Q wave indicates an old infarct.

   d. *Bundle branch block:* There [is/is no] [left/right] bundle branch block. Clues:

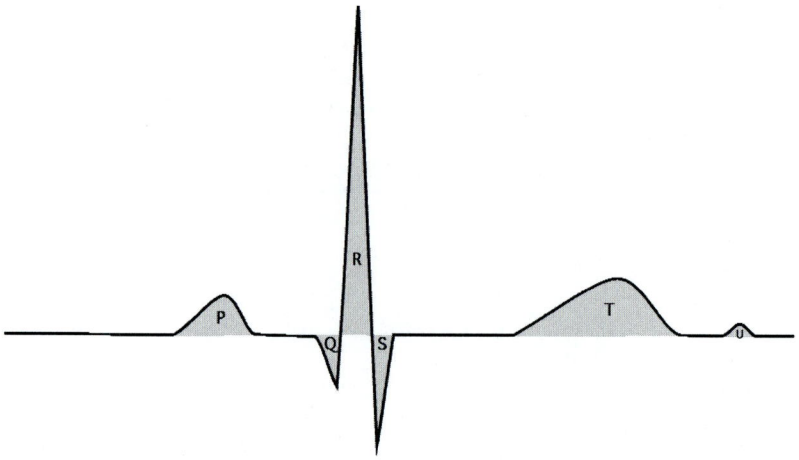

FIGURE 1-4. ECG wave morphology.

- Presence of RSR′ wave in leads V_1–V_3 with ST depression and T wave inversion goes with RBBB.
- Presence of notched R wave in leads I, aVL, and V_4–V_6 goes with LBBB.

Document Information in an Organized Manner

A complete medical student initial History and Physical is neat, legible, organized, and usually two to three pages long. Major topics should include: chief complaint, history of present illness, medical history, surgical history, medications, allergies, sexual history, smoking and alcohol history, occupation, travel, review of systems, vital signs, physical exam, lab results, test results, assessment or problem list, and plan.

▶ HOW TO ORGANIZE YOUR LEARNING

The main advantage to doing the medical clerkship is that you get to see patients. The patient is the key to learning medicine, and the source of most satisfaction and frustration on the wards. Plan your learning before the rotation starts as follows:

Make a List of Core Material to Learn

This list should reflect common symptoms, illnesses, and areas in which you have particular interest, or in which you feel particularly weak. Do not try to learn every possible topic. The Committee of Directors in Internal Medicine (*www.im.org/cdim/*) publishes a list of core content, on which this book is based. The CDIM emphasizes:

Symptoms and Lab Tests
- Abdominal pain
- Altered mental status
- Anemia
- Back pain
- Chest pain
- Cough
- Dysuria
- Fluid, electrolyte, and acid–base disorders

Common Illnesses
- Chronic obstructive pulmonary disease (COPD)
- Congestive heart failure
- Depression
- Diabetes mellitus
- Dyslipidemia
- Human immunodeficiency virus (HIV) infection
- Hypertension
- Smoking cessation
- Substance abuse
- Common cancers

We Also Recommend

- Adult vaccinations
- Domestic violence
- Dysrhythmias
- Nutritional disorders

Select Your Study Material

We recommend:

- This review book, *First Aid for the Clinical Clerkship in Medicine*
- A major medicine textbook such as *Harrison's Principles of Internal Medicine* (costs about $135)
- A full-text online journal database, such as *www.mdconsult.com* (subscription is $99/year for students)
- A small pocket reference book to look up lab values, clinical pathways, and the like, such as *Maxwell Quick Medical Reference* (costs $7)
- A small book to look up drugs, such as *Pocket Pharmacopoeia* (Tarascon Publishers, $9.95)

Make a Schedule to Learn the Illness-Based Topics

This schedule should reflect the rotation you are doing. For example, for the time you are going to be rotating in a clinic or office, make a schedule to study smoking cessation, dyslipidemia, depression, and diabetes. First, read this review book on each topic, then read the major textbook, taking notes. Make sure to include all chosen topics in your schedule, but leave room at least two weeks before the clerkship exam for review.

As You See Patients, Note Their Major Symptoms and Diagnosis for Review

Your reading on the symptom-based topics above should be done with a specific patient in mind. For example, if a patient comes to the office with cough, fever, and night sweats and is thought to have tuberculosis, read about chronic and acute cough, postnasal drip, asthma, gastroesophageal reflux disease (GERD), pneumonia, and tuberculosis in this review book that night.

Prepare a Talk on a Topic

You may be asked to give a small talk once or twice during your rotation. If not, you should volunteer! Feel free to choose a topic that is on your list; however, realize that this may be considered dull by the people who hear the lecture. The ideal topic is slightly uncommon but not rare, for example, cardiomyopathy. To prepare a talk on a topic, read about it in a major textbook and a review article not more than 2 years old, and then search online or in the library for recent developments or changes in treatment.

HOW TO PREPARE FOR THE CLINICAL CLERKSHIP EXAM

If you have read about your core illnesses and core symptoms, you will know a great deal about medicine. To study for the clerkship exam, we recommend:

2 to 3 weeks before exam: Read this entire review book, taking notes.
10 days before exam: Read the notes you took during the rotation on your core content list and the corresponding review book sections.
5 days before exam: Read this entire review book, concentrating on lists and mnemonics.
2 days before exam: Exercise, eat well, skim the book, and go to bed early.
1 day before exam: Exercise, eat well, review your notes and the mnemonics, and go to bed on time. Do not have any caffeine after 2 P.M.

Other helpful studying strategies include:

Study with Friends

Group studying can be very helpful. Other people may point out areas that you have not studied enough and may help you focus on the goal. If you tend to get distracted by other people in the room, limit this to less than half of your study time.

Study in a Bright Room

Find the room in your house or in your library that has the best, brightest light. This will help prevent you from falling asleep. If you don't have a bright light, get a halogen desk lamp or a light that simulates sunlight (not a tanning lamp).

Eat Light, Balanced Meals

Make sure your meals are balanced, with lean protein, fruits and vegetables, and fiber. A high-sugar, high-carbohydrate meal will give you an initial burst of energy for 1 to 2 hours, but then you'll drop.

Take Practice Exams

The point of practice exams is not so much the content that is contained in the questions, but the training of sitting still for 3 hours and trying to pick the best answer for each and every question.

Tips for Answering Questions

All questions are intended to have one best answer. When answering questions, follow these guidelines:

Read the answers first. For all questions longer than two sentences, reading the answers first can help you sift through the question for the key information.

Look for the words "EXCEPT, MOST, LEAST, NOT, BEST, WORST, TRUE, FALSE, CORRECT, INCORRECT, ALWAYS, and NEVER." If you find one of these words, circle or underline it for later comparison with the answer.

Evaluate each answer as being either true or false. Example:

Which of the following is *least* likely to be associated with pulmonary embolism?

A. Tachycardia **T**
B. Tachypnea **T**
C. Chest pain**? F not always**
D. Deep venous thrombosis**? T not always**
E. Back pain **F? aortic dissection**

By comparing the question, noting LEAST, to the answers, "E" is the best answer.

As the Boy Scouts say, "BE PREPARED."

SECTION II

High-Yield Facts

- Cardiology
- Endocrinology
- Gastroenterology
- Hematology–Oncology
- Infectious Disease
- Nephrology and Acid–Base Disorders
- Pulmonology
- Rheumatology
- Neurology
- Dermatology
- Health Maintenance and Evidence-Based Medicine

HIGH-YIELD FACTS IN

Cardiology

Coronary Artery Disease 17

- Causes of Chest Pain 17
- Risk Factors for Coronary Artery Disease 17
- Cardiac Testing 17
- Acute Coronary Syndromes (ACS) 19
- Angina 24

Heart Failure 25

- Overview 25
- Dilated Cardiomyopathy 27
- Restrictive Cardiomyopathy 29
- Hypertrophic Cardiomyopathy 30
- Myocarditis 31

Pericardial Problems 32

- Pericarditis 32
- Pericardial Tamponade 34
- Constrictive Pericarditis 34

Valvular Heart Disease (VHD) 35

- Mitral Stenosis 35
- Mitral Regurgitation 36
- Mitral Valve Prolapse 37
- Aortic Stenosis 37
- Aortic Regurgitation 38
- Tricuspid Stenosis 39
- Tricuspid Regurgitation 40

Dysrhythmias 41

- Ventricular Fibrillation and Pulseless Ventricular Tachycardia 41
- Torsades de Pointes 42
- Atrial Fibrillation 42
- Wolff–Parkinson–White Syndrome 43
- Heart Block 44
- Second-Degree Heart Block 44

Third-Degree Heart Block (Complete Heart Block) 45
Sinus Bradycardia 45
Hypertension 46
Overview 46
Hypertensive Emergency 48
Aortic Dissection 49
Infection-Related Cardiac Conditions 50
Bacterial Endocarditis 50
Rheumatic Fever 53
Dyslipidemia 54
Common Cardiac Medications 57

Coronary Artery Disease

▶ CAUSES OF CHEST PAIN

- **Costochondritis/musculoskeletal:** Sharp, localized pain and reproducible tenderness, often exacerbated by exercise
- **Myocardial infarction/angina:** Chest heaviness, pressure, or pain, typically radiating to left arm, shoulder, or jaw
- **Pericarditis:** Chest pain radiating to shoulder, neck, or back, worse with deep breathing or cough (pleuritic), relieved by sitting up/leaning forward
- **Aortic dissection:** Severe chest pain radiating to the back, can be associated with unequal pulses or unequal blood pressure in right and left arms
- **Abscess/mass:** Often sharp, localized pain, pleuritic
- **Pulmonary embolism:** Often pleuritic. Frequently associated with tachypnea and tachycardia
- **Pneumonia:** Pleuritic, frequently associated with hypoxia
- **GERD/esophageal spasm/tear:** Burning pain, dysphagia, may be similar to pain of myocardial infarction (MI)
- **Other causes:** Peptic ulcer disease, biliary disease, herpes zoster, anxiety, pneumothorax

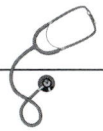

Myocardial infarction can be *silent,* with no symptoms or atypical symptoms, especially in diabetics (due to neuropathy).

▶ RISK FACTORS FOR CORONARY ARTERY DISEASE

Modifiable:
- Smoking
- Hypercholesterol
- Hypertension
- Obesity (apple-shaped)
- Diabetes mellitus
- Physical inactivity

Nonmodifiable:
- Age
- Male
- Family history

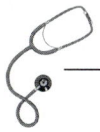

Criteria for **family history** of coronary artery disease:
- MI before age 40 in men
- MI before age 55 in women

▶ CARDIAC TESTING

Exercise Stress Testing

- Patients are asked to walk on a treadmill at increasing levels of difficulty to reach a heart rate that is 85% of predicted maximum for age.
- Alternatively, pharmacologic agents such as dobutamine may be administered IV to stimulate myocardial function in a patient who cannot exercise.
- ECG monitoring during the procedure detects changes.
- A test is considered positive for coronary artery disease if the patient develops:
  - ST elevation
  - ST depression > 1 mm in multiple leads
  - Decreased BP
  - Failure to exercise more than 2 minutes due to symptoms

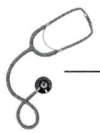

The maximum heart rate is estimated as: [220 – patient's age].

- Failure to complete the test due to reasons other than cardiac symptoms (i.e., arthritis) is not diagnostic.

Stress Myocardial Perfusion Imaging

Patients are injected with a radioisotope (thallium 201 or technetium 99m sestamibi) and stressed (with exercise or pharmacologic agent). Nuclear imaging is obtained immediately after exercise and in 4 hours. The test can detect:

- Myocardial perfusion
- Ventricular volume
- Ejection fraction

Echocardiography

- Echocardiography, or ultrasound of the heart, is used to evaluate many different types of heart disease.
- Transthoracic echo is best done in thin patients. Transesophageal echo is used to see more detail and to assess great vessels.
- For specific uses of echocardiography, see Table 2.1-1.

Cardiac Catheterization

- Cardiac catheterization is used for diagnosis and treatment of many different types of heart disease.
- The right heart is accessed by the femoral or internal jugular vein.
- The left heart is accessed by the femoral or radial artery (from the right heart).
- For specific uses of cardiac catheterization, see Table 2.1-2.

TABLE 2.1-1. Uses of Echocardiography

Myocardial infarction	Assess wall motion abnormalities.
Heart failure	Assess ventricular function, ejection fraction.
Heart murmur	Identify and evaluate valvular disease.
Pericardial effusion	Assess volume and early tamponade.
Aortic dissection	Identify presence of tear.
Pulmonary embolism	Identify saddle emboli or evidence of increased right-sided pressure.
Patent foramen ovale	Assess bubbles traversing PFO (air administered through peripheral IV).
Congenital heart disease	Identify coarctation of the aorta, pulmonary stenosis, tetralogy of Fallot, VSD, ASD.

TABLE 2.1-2. Uses of Cardiac Catheterization

Myocardial infarction and unstable angina	Coronary artery angiography, balloon dilatation of stenoses, stent placement, laser techniques
Valvular heart disease	Balloon valvuloplasty of mitral stenosis, pulmonary stenosis, aortic stenosis
Dysrhythmias	Electrophysiologic mapping of bypass tracts, radiofrequency ablation
Myocardial disease	Biopsy of myocardium for cardiomyopathies, glycogen storage disease
Congenital heart disease	Cardiac and pulmonary angiography to identify abnormality, transcatheter closure of some types of ASDs, VSDs, PFOs

▶ ACUTE CORONARY SYNDROMES (ACS)

Classified as non-ST-elevation and ST-elevation events. Non-ST-elevation events include non-ST-elevation MI and unstable angina (UA). ACS is due to an imbalance of myocardial oxygen demand and supply. The most common cause of decreased oxygen supply is narrowing of coronary artery by thrombus or plaque that has become unstable.

Serum Markers for MI

Enzyme	Onset (hrs)	Peak (hrs)	Duration
Myoglobin	1–4	6–8	24 hrs
Troponin T/I	3–12	18–24	7–10 days
Creatinine kinase	3–12	18–24	3–4 days
Lactate dehydrogenase	6–12	24–48	6–8 days

- Myoglobin: Elevated within 1 hour of MI but is nonspecific
- Creatinine phosphokinase (CPK): Elevated within 4 to 8 hours of MI but is nonspecific
- CK MB isoenzyme: Specific marker for myocardial tissue damage
- Troponin T or I: Very sensitive and specific markers for cardiac muscle injury. Elevated within 3 hours and can stay elevated for more than a week. Renal insufficiency can lead to erroneously high levels depending on the type of troponin and the cutoff value used. For example, > 80% of patients with end-stage renal disease (ESRD) would have an elevated

troponin T if cutoff were ≥ 0.01, but only 1% would if tropinin I cutoff were ≥ 0.5.

- "Serial enzymes": Consists of cardiac biomarkers drawn every 6 to 8 hours for a 24-hour period

Initial Evaluation of ACS

- History and physical
- Typical symptoms:
  - Left-sided/substernal chest pressure with radiation to left shoulder, arm, or jaw
  - Shortness of breath
  - Diaphoresis
  - Nausea or vomiting
  - Unstable angina is associated with increasing frequency and/or severity of symptoms, symptoms at rest or new onset of symptoms.
  - Presentation may be atypical in diabetics and women.
- Initial test:
  - ECG
  - Cardiac enzymes

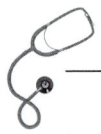

Inferior wall MI:
ST elevation in II, III, aVF (cor pulmonale: ST *depression* in II, III, aVF) (see Figure 2-1.1)
Anteroseptal MI:
ST elevation in V_1, V_2, V_3 (see Figure 2-1.2)
Lateral wall MI:
ST elevation in V_4, V_5, V_6
Posterior wall MI:
ST depression in V_1, V_2

Determining the Type of ACS

- The presence of ACS is based on history, physical, and initial tests; if present, the type of ACS must be determined.

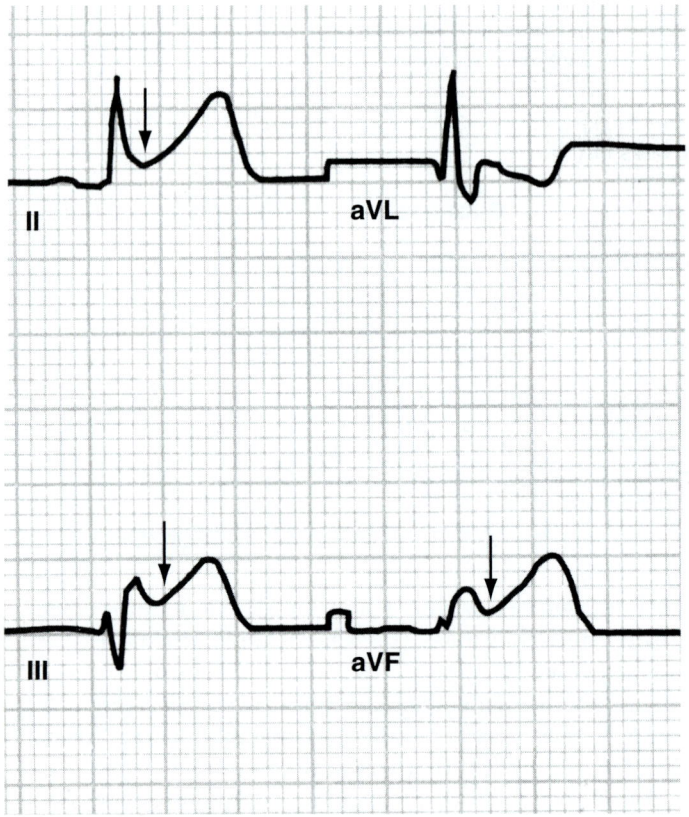

FIGURE 2.1-1. ECG of inferior wall MI demonstrating ST elevation in leads II, III, and aVF.

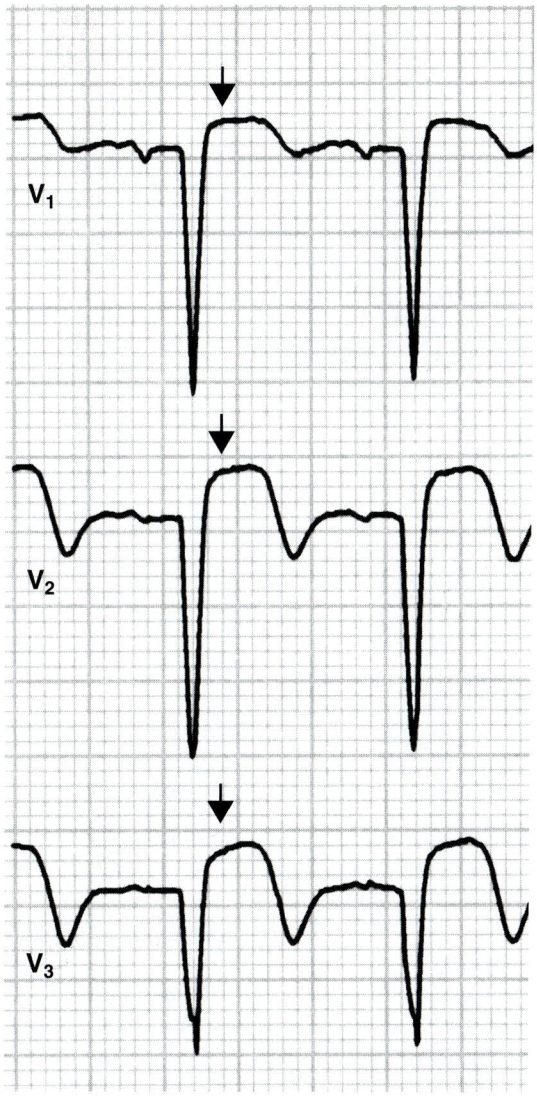

FIGURE 2.1-2. ECG of anteroseptal MI demonstrating ST elevation in leads V_1, V_2, and V_3.

- ST-elevation MI (STEMI) or new left bundle branch block (LBBB) on ECG: These patients are admitted and managed according to guidelines for STEMI.
- Unstable angina/non-ST-elevation MI: These two have similar pathogenesis. Non-ST-elevation MI differs from unstable angina in that the lack of oxygen is severe enough to cause myocardial damage and enzyme leakage (unlike unstable angina, where there is no enzyme leakage).
  - If normal ECG and normal cardiac enzymes and no recurrence of symptoms, patient can have echocardiogram to assess left ventricular function. If either test is abnormal, patient should be managed as acute ischemia.
  - If ST depression, inverted T-waves, positive cardiac enzymes, or recurrence of symptoms (but no ST elevation on ECG), patient should be admitted to the hospital and managed as acute ischemia.

Risk Stratification

TIMI Risk Score

- Age > 65
- Presence of 3 or more CAD risk factors
- Prior coronary stenosis ≥ 50%
- Presence of ST segment deviation on admission ECG
- At least two anginal episodes in last 24 hours
- Elevated serum cardiac biomarkers
- Use of ASA in prior 7 days

Risk of all cause mortality @ 14 days = 0/1 → 4.7%
2 → 8.3%
3 → 13.2 %
4 → 19.9%
5 → 26.2%
6/7 → 40.9%

Initial Treatment for All ACS

- Anti-ischemic treatments:
  - Telemetry monitor
  - Oxygen
  - Nitroglycerin (NTG) for chest pain; can be given sublingually × 3. If pain persists, can be given intravenously.
  - Morphine if pain persists despite NTG
  - Beta blockers decrease cardiac oxygen demand and have been shown to decrease mortality. Aim for a pulse rate of 60.
- Antiplatelet and anticoagulation:
  - Aspirin (chewable preferred). Clopidogrel is an alternative for those with true aspirin allergy.
  - Both unfractionated heparin and low-molecular-weight heparin can be used. The rationale behind using both aspirin and heparin is that they act at different sites.
  - GP IIb/IIa inhibitors have shown to be beneficial for high-risk patients (elevated troponin, TIMI risk score > 4, ongoing ischemia) and patients undergoing percutaneous intervention.
  - *Note:* Thrombolytics are not used in unstable angina or non-ST-elevation MI because in 60 to 80% the infarcted artery is not occluded.

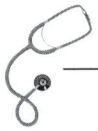

Heparin does not dissolve already-present clots; rather, it prevents future ones from forming.

Treatment for Unstable Angina and Non-ST-Elevation MI

- General ACS anti-ischemic and antiplatelet treatment (as above)
- Decision for early invasive treatment or early conservative treatment:
  - Early invasive treatment (cardiac catheterization) if any of the following are present:
    - Elevated troponin
    - Recurrent chest pain despite medical therapy
    - CHF
    - Positive stress test
    - Left ventricular EF < 40%
    - Sustained ventricular tachycardia
    - Cardiac stent within 6 months

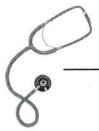

Low-molecular-weight heparin is given sub-Q every 12 hours. PT/PTT does not need to be checked.

- Early conservative therapy with medical management can be considered in patients who respond to medical management without any of the features mentioned above.

Treatment for ST-Elevation MI

- Patients include those with new left bundle branch block.
- Requires early revascularization with thrombolytics and/or cardiac catheterization and stent
- General ACS anti-ischemic and antiplatelet treatment as above

Cardiac Catheterization (aka PTCA or Percutaneous Transluminal Coronary Angioplasty) vs. Thrombolytics

Cardiac Catheterization

- Cardiac catheterization/percutaneous transluminal coronary angioplasty (PTCA): Coronary angiogram can demonstrate the coronary anatomy as well as the specific diseased vessel causing symptoms. The occlusion of the vessel can be reopened by balloon angioplasty and/or coronary stent placement. Success rate as high as 90% compared to 60% with thrombolytics.
- Preferred over thrombolytics if:
  - Skilled lab is available in < 12 hours from onset of symptoms and < 30 minutes from entering the ER
  - High risk of ST-elevation MI (i.e., cardiogenic shock)
  - Late presentation (> 3 hours after symptoms)

Thrombolytics

- Thrombolytics are preferred if patient presents within 12 hours of symptoms, preferably within 3 hours, or if there will be a delay to PTCA or if cardiac catheterization is not an option.
  - Thrombolytics work to break up clots.
  - Examples include streptokinase, urokinase, anistreplase, alteplase, and reteplase.
- Absolute contraindications to thrombolytics:
  - Any prior intracranial hemorrhage
  - Stroke within 1 year
  - Intracranial neoplasm
  - Active internal bleeding
  - Suspected aortic dissection
- Relative contraindications to thrombolytics:
  - Available cath lab within 90 minutes of presentation
  - Systolic blood pressure (sBP) > 180, diastolic blood pressure (DBP) > 110
  - Prior stroke or intracranial lesion other than above
  - Bleeding disorder; warfarin use with international normalized ratio (INR) > 2
  - Major surgery within 3 weeks
  - Age > 75
  - Cardiopulmonary resuscitation (CPR)
  - Peptic ulcer

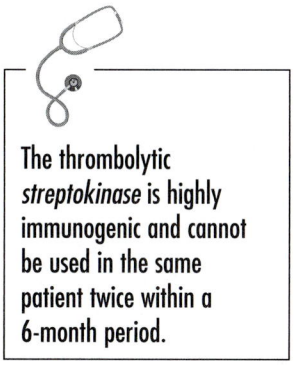

The thrombolytic *streptokinase* is highly immunogenic and cannot be used in the same patient twice within a 6-month period.

Medications at Discharge for Patients with ACS

- Aspirin indefinitely
- Beta blocker indefinitely

Typical scenario:
A 58-year-old man who was discharged from the hospital after MI 2 weeks ago presents with fever, chest pain, and generalized malaise. ECG shows diffuse ST-T wave changes. *Think: Dressler's syndrome.* Treat with nonsteroidal anti-inflammatory drugs (NSAIDs).

- Angiotensin-converting enzyme (ACE) inhibitor indefinitely; initially recommended for patients with ejection fraction (EF) < 40% or anterior wall MI
- Statin (hydroxymethylglutaryl coenzyme A [HMG CoA] reductase inhibitor) to maintain LDL < 70
- Clopidogrel for 1 to 12 months depending on stent placement and type

Postinfarction Complications

- Ruptures (usually occur within 4 to 5 days of a large MI):
  - Free wall rupture
  - Acute ventricular septal perforation
  - Acute mitral regurgitation from papillary muscle rupture
- Arrhythmias:
  - Ventricular tachycardia: If within 48 hours of MI, usually just from reperfusion of myocardium. If it occurs later than 48 hours, consider implantable defibrillator.
  - Bradycardia (usually from inferior wall MI)
  - Atrioventricular (AV) block: If inferior wall MI, this will usually reverse; if anterior wall MI, usually will require pacemaker
- Dressler's syndrome: Usually occurs 1 or 2 weeks after cardiac injury (MI or cardiac surgery). It is associated with fever, pericarditis, and sometimes pericardial or pleural effusions; likely a hypersensitivity process. Treat with NSAIDs.

Secondary Prevention

The following applies to unstable angina/non-ST-elevation MI and ST-elevation MI:

- Smoking cessation
- Aggressive diabetes management
- Aggressive control of hypertension (maintain < 140/90)
- Lipid control with statins as above and dietary modification

▶ ANGINA

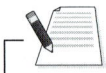

Typical scenario:
A 62-year-old smoker presents complaining of three episodes of severe heavy chest pain this morning. Each episode lasted 3 to 5 minutes, but he has no pain now. He has never had this type of pain before.
Think: Unstable angina.

Definition

Unstable angina (discussed in previous section): An acute coronary syndrome diagnosed by the following history:

- New-onset angina
- Angina that changes or accelerates in pattern, location, or severity
- Angina at rest

Stable angina: A chronic, episodic pain syndrome due to temporary myocardial ischemia. Pattern of pain is similar to that of acute MI, but resolves with rest or medication.

Prinzmetal's angina: Angina due to coronary vasospasm, not linked to exertion. Distinguished from unstable angina by chronic, intermittent nature. Pain usually occurs at a specific hour in the early morning. Coronary vessels are angiographically normal.

Etiology

Temporary myocardial ischemia

Diagnosis

ECG
- ST segment depression or elevation
- T wave inversion
- May be normal

Treatment

For Unstable Angina
- As discussed in previous section

For Stable Angina
- Beta blockade: Reduces myocardial oxygen demand
- Aspirin: Reduces risk of MI in asymptomatic patients
- Morphine: For analgesia, but does not affect outcome
- Modify risk factors for coronary artery disease.
- Sublingual NTG for episodic pain
- Echocardiogram to assess left ventricular function
- Exercise stress test
- Consider coronary revascularization after aforementioned tests: PTCA or coronary artery bypass graft (CABG).

For Prinzmetal's Angina
- Calcium channel blockers and nitrates to reduce vasospasm

Typical scenario:
A 62-year-old man presents with frequent episodes of dull chest pain on and off for 8 months. He says the pain wakes him from sleep. *Think: Prinzmetal's angina.*

Cardiac output is a measure of blood pumped by the left ventricle and is the product of stroke volume and heart rate.

Heart Failure

▶ OVERVIEW

Definition

Congestive heart failure (CHF) is the failure of the heart to pump blood effectively to the tissues. Left heart failure (LHF) causes pulmonary venous congestion (blood flow back-up into the lungs) and compromised systemic circulation. Right heart failure (RHF) causes systemic venous congestion.

Etiology

Can be precipitated by:
- MI/ischemic heart disease (most common)
- Pulmonary embolus (usually right-sided failure)
- Dysrhythmias
- Thyrotoxicosis/wet beriberi (high-output failure)
- Viral (casuses a dilated cardiomyopathy)
- EtOH

Diastolic Dysfunction:
- Accounts for 40 to 60% of heart failure
- Signs/symptoms of heart failure with normal ejection fraction (> 50%)
- More common in women
- Associated with hypertension, left ventricular hypertrophy, dilated cardiomyopathy, and ischemia
- Treat the hypertension, use diuretics for congestion and edema, and control rate if atrial fibrillation.

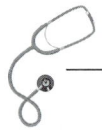

The most common cause of RHF is LHF.

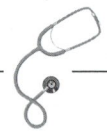

Rule of thirds for viral or pregnancy-induced dilated cardiomyopathy:
- 1/3 get worse
- 1/3 stay the same
- 1/3 get better

Orthopnea is shortness of breath while lying flat.

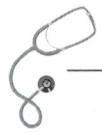

Both preload and afterload reducers may lower blood pressure.

New York Heart Association Functional Class of Heart Failure:
Class I: No limitation
Class II: Slight limitations (symptoms at ordinary efforts)
Class III: Marked limitation (comfortable at rest, symptoms at minimal efforts)
Class IV: Symptomatic at rest

Signs and Symptoms

Left Heart Failure
Orthopnea
Paroxysmal nocturnal dyspnea (PND)
Rales
Dyspnea on exertion (DOE)
Cough
Nocturia
S_3 gallop
Diaphoresis
Tachycardia

Right Heart Failure
RUQ pain (due to hepatic congestion)
Hepatomegaly
Hepatojugular reflex
Jugular venous distention (JVD)
Ascites
Cyanosis
Peripheral edema

Diagnosis

Chest film: Enlargement of cardiac silhouette, pulmonary vascular congestion with redistribution to upper lobes

Echocardiogram: Assess left ventricular function.

Basic natriuretic peptide (BNP): Elevates in CHF.

Treatment

Nonpharmacologic
- Sodium and water restriction, exercise, education, and avoidance of alcohol

Pharmacologic

First-Line Therapy
1. **ACE inhibitors:** Decrease symptoms and mortality in patients with NYHA class II–IV; decrease incidence of heart failure symptoms and decrease hospitalization
2. **Diuretics:** Use in class II–IV for fluid retention.
   Mild: Use thiazide diuretic once daily.
   Significant: Use loop diuretics, twice daily PO (IV in acute exacerbation).
3. **Beta blockers:** For NYHA class II–III (decrease symptoms, improve survival). Use after ACE inhibitors and diuretics.
4. **Digoxin:** Add for NYHA class III–IV (for symptomatic relief only, **does not** improve survival).
5. **Spironolactone:** Low dose, use in NYHA class III–IV.
   - Decreases mortality by 34%
   - Monitor K^+ carefully, especially with concomitant use of ACE inhibitors.

Second-Line Therapy
1. **Angiotensin receptor blockers (ARBs):** If ACE inhibitors are not well tolerated (e.g., cough)
2. **Nitrate–hydralazine combination:**
   - Improve symptoms and survival
   - High rate of intolerance and lower effect on mortality make this therapy a second line to ACE inhibitors.

Acute Pulmonary Edema

Acute pulmonary edema (APE) is caused by rapid decompensation of left ventricular function, due to:

- Dysrhythmias
- MI
- Noncompliance with medications
- Increased dietary or intravenous sodium load
- Drugs that cause decreased inotropy
- Strain

Treatment: NTG, oxygen, morphine, aspirin, diuretic (NOMAD)

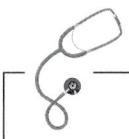

Signs in RHF are similar to those seen in cirrhosis. The clue is that patients with cirrhosis usually do not have trouble lying flat and will not have JVD.

Paroxysmal Nocturnal Dyspnea

- **Definition** (also called cardiac asthma): A brief episode of breathlessness that awakens patient from sleep
- **Etiology:** Due to increased volume load on heart when lying in the horizontal position or sudden decrease in myocardial contractility, which results in pulmonary edema, impairing the exchange of oxygen
- **Diagnosis:** Distinguished from true asthma by improvement with walking a few steps, and lack of improvement with bronchodilators
- **Treatment:** NTG, oxygen, morphine, aspirin, diuretic (NOMAD)

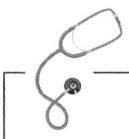

Major reason for CHF exacerbations is noncompliance with medications.

► DILATED CARDIOMYOPATHY

Definition

Left or right ventricular enlargement with loss of contractile function causing congestive heart failure, dysrhythmias, or thrombus formation. Patients typically have symptoms of CHF that is slowly progressive and leads to death in approximately 3 years.

Etiology

Infectious

- Viral myocarditis (one-third improve, one-third stay the same, one-third get worse)

Toxic

- Reversible—prolonged EtOH abuse
- Irreversible—doxorubicin (Adriamycin), cocaine, heavy metals (Pb, Hg, Cb)

Endocrine

- Reversible—thyroid disease (hypo or hyper)
- Irreversible—acromegaly, pheochromocytoma

Metabolic

- Reversible—hypocalcemia, hypophosphatemia, thiamine deficiency (wet beriberi), selenium deficiency
- Genetic: 20% of cases have positive family histories

First-line therapy for APE:
NOMAD
Nitroglycerin
Oxygen
Morphine
Aspirin
Diuretic

Other therapy: **MDDN**

- **M**ilrinone increases inotropy with vasodilation.
- **D**obutamine increases inotropy without vasoconstriction.
- **D**opamine increases inotropy with vasoconstriction.
- **N**esiritide is basic natriuretic peptide—causes smooth muscle to relax and diuresis.

- Pregnancy: Similar prognosis as viral
- Other: Neuromuscular disease (usually irreversible), idiopathic (usually irreversible)

Mechanical
- Dysrhythmias
- Valvular disease

Signs and Symptoms

- Symptoms of heart failure
- Angina due to increased O_2 demands of enlarged ventricles
- Neurologic deficits from thrombus emboli

Diagnosis

- Auscultation—S_3/S_4 gallop murmurs (stiffened ventricular walls), regurgitant valves, rales
- ECG—ventricular hypertrophy, bundle branch blocks (see Figure 2.1-3), nonspecific ST segment/T wave changes, dysrhythmias (atrial fibrillation most common)
- CXR—enlarged cardiac silhouette, pulmonary venous congestion
- Echocardiography—enlarged ventricles/atria, regurgitant valves, low ejection fractions

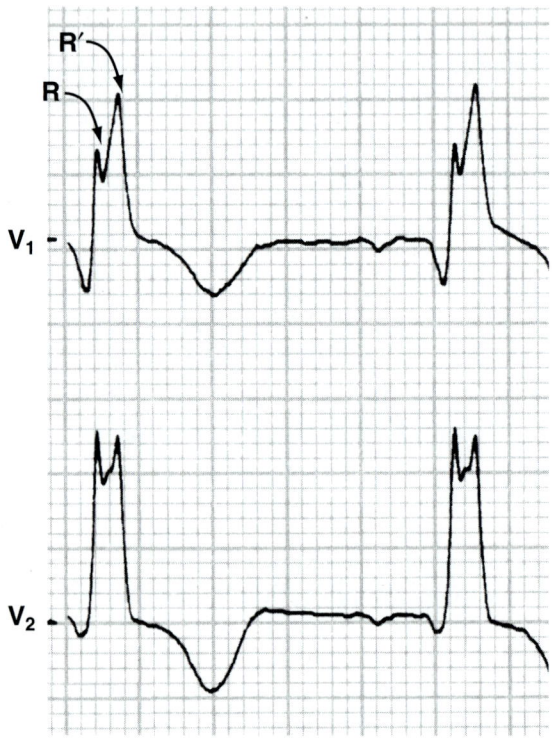

FIGURE 2.1-3. Right bundle branch block.

Treatment

- Address any reversible causes (e.g., discontinue toxic agent)
- Supportive care—medical management of heart failure (ACE inhibitors and diuretics reduce mortality)
- Anticoagulation with Coumadin (even if no evidence of thrombus)
- Implanted automatic defibrillator for patients with life-threatening dysrhythmias
- Heart transplant

▶ RESTRICTIVE CARDIOMYOPATHY

Definition

Scarring and infiltration of the myocardium causing decreased right or left ventricular filling

Etiology

- Amyloidosis
- Endomyocardial fibrosis
- Hemochromatosis
- Sarcoidosis
- Carcinoid heart disease
- Congenital: Gaucher, Hurler, and glycogen storage diseases

Signs and Symptoms

- Signs of left/right heart failure, right failure usually predominates
- Exercise intolerance is a common presenting symptom

Diagnosis

- Auscultation—S_3 and/or S_4 gallop murmurs, occasional mitral or tricuspid regurgitation
- ECG—low voltages, conduction abnormalities, nonspecific ST segment/T wave changes, left bundle branch block
- CXR—normal cardiac silhouette or enlarged atria, pulmonary venous congestion
- Echocardiography—normal-sized ventricles, large atria, thickened ventricular walls, mitral/tricuspid regurgitation; typically has a speckled appearance if amyloid is cause
- Endomyocardial biopsy may detect eosinophilic infiltration or myocardial fibrosis.

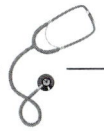

Restrictive cardiomyopathy is often difficult to distinguish from constrictive pericarditis—biopsy can usually confirm.

Treatment

- No specific treatment or cure
- Mainstay is to treat resulting heart failure.
- Anticoagulate and rate control atrial fibrillation if present.
- Treat underlying cause.
- Permanent pacemaker for complete heart block
- Heart transplant for refractory cases

▶ HYPERTROPHIC CARDIOMYOPATHY

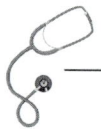

Hypertrophic cardiomyopathy used to be called idiopathic hypertrophic subaortic stenosis, or IHSS.

Definition

Hypertrophy of the interventricular septum narrows the LV outflow tract. High-velocity systolic flow draws the anterior leaflet of the mitral valve into the tract (via the Bernoulli effect) causing a dynamic left ventricular outflow tract obstruction.

Etiology

- ~50% idiopathic, ~50% familial (autosomal dominant, with variable penetrance)
- Conditions that increase the LV end diastolic volume decrease the obstruction (e.g., increased blood volume, negative inotropic drugs, rest, increased peripheral resistance)
- Outflow obstruction can result in left atrial dilatation, atrial fibrillation, CHF, right heart failure, etc.

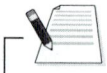

Causes of paradoxical splitting of S_2:
- Hypertrophic cardiomyopathy
- Aortic stenosis
- LBBB

Signs and Symptoms

Angina
- Not well understood in terms of known pathophysiology
- Occurs at rest and during exercise
- Frequently unresponsive to nitroglycerin
- May respond to recumbent position (pathognomonic but rare)

Syncope
- Most often occurs following exercise
- Arrhythmias: Atrial fibrillation, ventricular tachycardia
- Signs of CHF
- Sudden death is usually due to an arrhythmia.

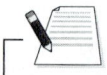

Typical scenario: A 25-year-old man becomes severely dyspneic and collapses while running laps. His father had died suddenly at an early age. *Think: Hypertrophic cardiomyopathy.*

Diagnosis

- Systolic ejection murmur heard best along the left sternal border, decreases with increased LV blood volume (squatting), increases with increased blood velocities (exercise), and decreased LV end-diastolic volume (Valsalva)
- Paradoxical splitting of S_2
- ECG: LVH, PVCs, atrial fibrillation, inferior lateral Q waves, nonspecific ST segment and T wave abnormalities
- Echocardiography: Septal hypertrophy, LVH, small LV

Treatment

- Patient should refrain from vigorous exercise.
- Beta blockers reduce heart rate, increasing LV filling time and decreasing inotropy; calcium channel blockers considered second-line agents.
- The roles of antiarrhythmics, septal myomectomy, pacemaker, and defibrillator are all controversial.
- Avoid anything that decreases preload (nitrates, diuretics, volume depletion) as this will worsen obstruction by allowing left ventricular collapse.

Very few murmurs *decrease* with squatting (HCM does).

▶ MYOCARDITIS

Definition

Inflammation of the myocardium

Etiology

- Viral—coxsackie A or B, echovirus, HIV, cytomegalovirus (CMV), influenza, Epstein–Barr, hepatitis B virus (HBV), adenovirus
- Bacterial—group A beta-hemolytic strep (rheumatic fever), *Corynebacterium*, *Meningococcus*, *B. burgdorferi* (Lyme), *Mycoplasma pneumoniae*
- Parasitic—*Trypanosoma cruzi* (Chagas'), *Toxoplasma*, *Trichinella*, *Echinococcus*
- Systemic disease—Kawasaki's, systemic lupus erythematosus (SLE), sarcoidosis, inflammatory conditions
- Drug allergies—sulfonamides, penicillins
- Cocaine
- Idiopathic—common

Signs and Symptoms

Spectrum of disease ranges from asymptomatic to fulminant cardiac failure and death. Findings may include:

- Retrosternal or precordial chest pain
- Fever, fatigue
- Preceding upper respiratory infection (URI)
- Palpitations, syncope
- Signs of CHF (dyspnea, rales, peripheral edema, JVD)

Diagnosis

- Auscultation—S_3/S_4, mitral or tricuspid regurgitation, friction rub (if pericardium involved)
- ECG—ST segment changes, low voltage, dysrhythmias, conduction disturbances
- CXR—often normal, may see cardiomegaly or pulmonary venous congestion
- Echocardiography—hypokinetic wall movements, dilated ventricles/atria, pericardial effusion
- Labs—leukocytosis, elevated ESR, elevated cardiac enzymes (slower rise and fall than acute MI, troponin I is most sensitive)
- Myocardial biopsy

Treatment

- Primarily supportive—admit to ICU, limit activity
- Treat heart failure, dysrhythmias—ACE inhibitors reduce necrosis and inflammation, digoxin should be used cautiously as its effects may be exaggerated by the inflamed myocardium.
- Address etiology if known/applicable (e.g., antivirals, antibiotics, diptheria—antitoxin).
- Immunosuppressive agents are contraindicated (steroids, cyclosporine, NSAIDs).
- IV immunoglobulin G (IgG) may be of benefit.

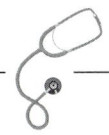

Splitting of S_2:
Normal physiologic:
Aortic before pulmonic valve closure. Split widened by inspiration as increasingly negative intrathoracic pressure augments R heart filling, resulting in longer ventricular emptying times.
Paradoxical:
Pulmonic before aortic valve due to a delay in aortic valve closure. Inspiration still delays pulmonic closure but now brings it closer to aortic closure, *paradoxically* narrowing the split.

Coxsackie B is the most common viral cause of myocarditis.

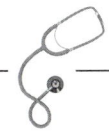

For HCM:
Symptoms prior to 30 years of age correlate with increased risk of sudden death, but severity of symptoms (whenever they occur) does not.

Myocarditis often is associated with acute pericarditis.

Pericardial Problems

▶ PERICARDITIS

Definition

Inflammation of the pericardium

Etiology

Common Causes of Pericarditis

- Viral—pericarditis frequently occurs following a recent viral URI, though a definitive cause is not known.
- Bacterial—TB, streptococci, staphylococci
- Metastases—1° tumors usually breast or lung
- Acute myocardial infarction:
  - Immediate post-MI pericarditis—occurs within 24 hours of a *transmural* infarction due to direct pericardial irritation
  - Dressler's syndrome—pericarditis occurring one week to months after an MI due to an autoimmune response to infarcted myocardium, can progress to chronic condition
- Uremia—chronic renal failure, mental status changes
- Radiation—radiotherapy, occupational/environmental exposure
- Drug reaction—hydralazine, procainamide, isoniazid
- Collagen vascular tissue—SLE, scleroderma
- Myxedema
- Trauma—postpericardiotomy syndrome following CT surgery (usually brief clinical course)
- Idiopathic

Signs and Symptoms

- Chest pain, often pleuritic (inspiratory), radiating to left trapezial ridge
- Pain often relieved by sitting up and leaning forward
- Pain does not respond to nitroglycerin.

Diagnosis

- Auscultation—pericardial friction rub on expiration, pathognomonic but variably present
- ECG—*diffuse* ST elevations and PR depressions, low voltage (see Figure 2.1-4)
- CXR—possibly enlarged cardiac silhouette 2° to pericardial effusion
- Echocardiography—possible pericardial effusion

Treatment

- Address underlying cause if known/applicable.
- NSAIDs to relieve pain and reduce inflammation (ASA, indomethacin, ibuprofen)
- Steroids for intractable cases (e.g., Dressler's)

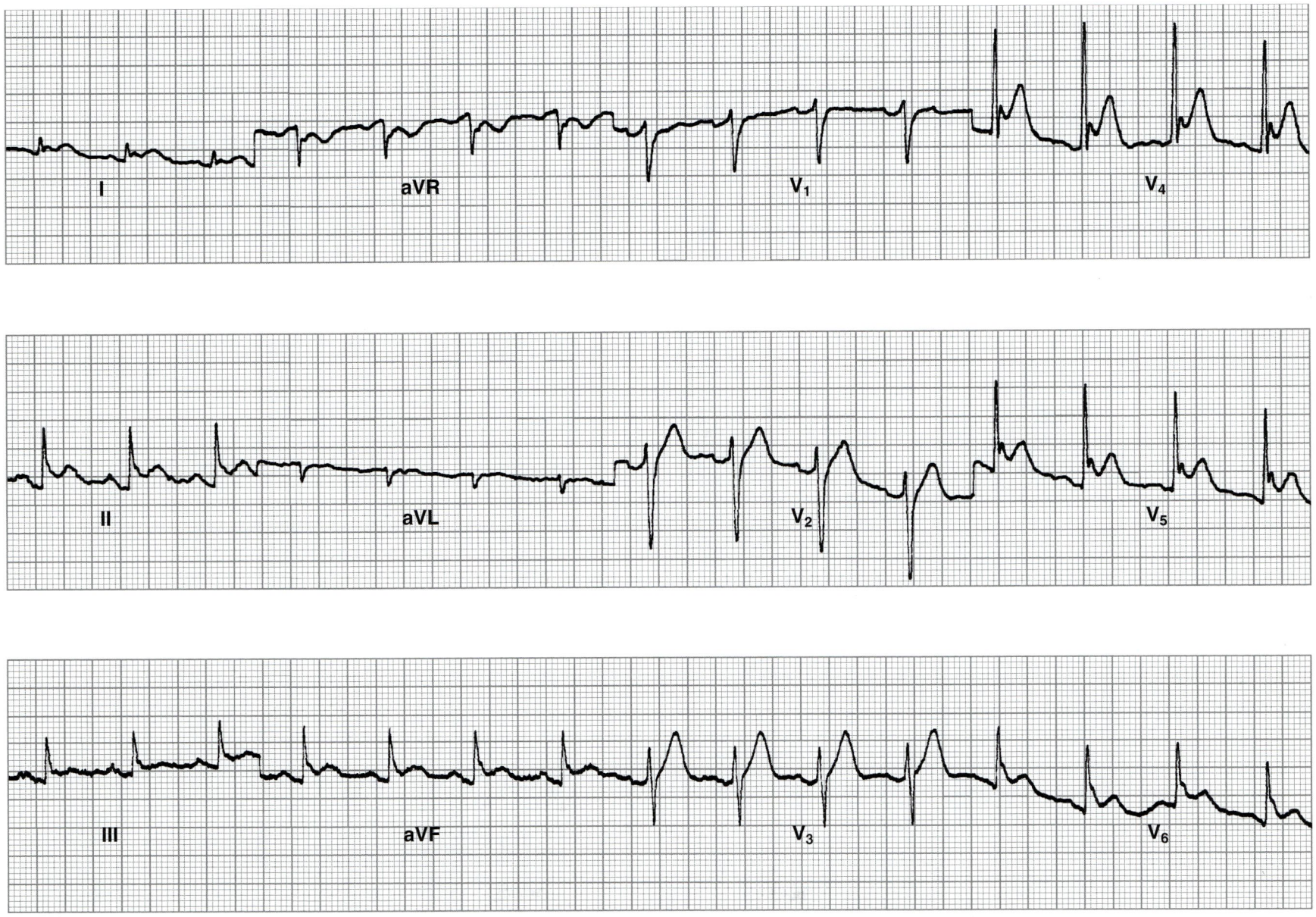

FIGURE 2.1-4. **Pericarditis. Note diffuse ST segment elevation and PR depression.**

▶ PERICARDIAL TAMPONADE

Definition

Tamponade is the physiologic result of rapid accumulation of fluid in the inelastic pericardial sac. Pericardial tamponade impairs cardiac filling and reduces cardiac output.

Etiology

- Pericarditis
- Trauma (accidental or iatrogenic)
- Ruptured ventricular wall (post MI)
- Aortic dissection with rupture into pericardium

Pulsus paradoxus is a transient fall in measured blood pressure > 10 mm Hg associated with inspiration (due to reduced stroke volume during inspiration).

Signs and Symptoms

Beck's Triad
- Hypotension
- Muffled heart sounds
- Jugular vein distention (JVD)

Other Symptoms/Signs
- Dyspnea
- Tachycardia
- **Pulsus paradoxus**—decrease by > 10 mm Hg of sBP with inspiration
- Narrow pulse pressure
- JVD

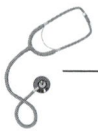

Tamponade physiology: During inspiration, venous return to the right atrium increases. In tamponade, the transiently enlarged right atrium bulges leftward, reducing left ventricular volume and output, causing BP to fall with inspiration.

Diagnosis

- Auscultation may demonstrate distant heart sounds.
- ECG may show low voltage or **electrical alternans.**
- CXR may show enlarged cardiac silhouette.
- Echocardiogram will show large pericardial effusion.

Treatment

- Immediate pericardiocentesis for unstable patients
- Infuse fluids to expand volume.
- Pericardial window (surgery) for meta-stable and stable patients

▶ CONSTRICTIVE PERICARDITIS

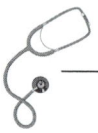

Pericardiocentesis yielding clotting blood probably came from the right ventricle, not the pericardial sac.

Definition

Granulation and scarring of the pericardium due to acute pericarditis. Cardiac output is limited.

Signs and Symptoms

- Dyspnea
- Fatigue
- Tachycardia
- JVD with patient upright

- Kussmaul's sign
- Left ventricular failure
- Peripheral edema

Diagnosis

- Auscultation may demonstrate distant heart sounds.
- CXR may show pericardial calcification.
- ECG may show low voltage, T wave flattening or inversion in V_1 and V_2, notched P waves.
- Echocardiogram may show pericardial thickening.

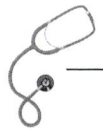

Kussmaul's sign is failure of jugular venous pressure to fall during inspiration.

Treatment

- Pericardiectomy

Valvular Heart Disease (VHD)

▶ MITRAL STENOSIS

Etiology

Rheumatic heart disease (most common), congenital (rare)

Epidemiology

Most cases occur in women.

Signs and Symptoms

- Dyspnea on exertion (DOE)
- Rales
- Cough
- Hemoptysis
- Systemic embolism (due to stagnation of blood in enlarged left atrium)
- Accentuated right ventricle precordial thrust
- Signs of right ventricular failure
- Hoarse voice (due to enlarged left atrium impinging on recurrent laryngeal nerve)

Diagnosis

- Murmur is mid-diastolic with opening snap, low-pitched rumble.
- Best heard over left sternal border between 2nd to 4th interspace (see Figure 2.1-5)
- CXR may show straight left heart border due to enlarged left atrium and Kerley B lines from pulmonary effusion.
- ECG may show left atrial enlargement, right ventricular hypertrophy, atrial fibrillation.
- Echocardiography demonstrates diseased valve.

Remember dilation of the left atrium is a major cause of atrial fibrillation.

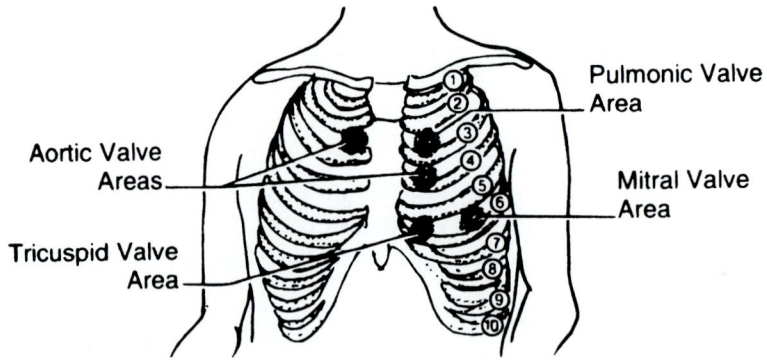

FIGURE 2.1-5. Cardiac auscultation sites.

(Reproduced, with permission, from DeGowin RL. *DeGowin & DeGowin's Diagnostic Examination*, 6th ed. New York: McGraw-Hill, 1994:359.)

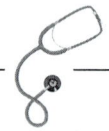

Balloon valvuloplasty in mitral stenosis is an effective intervention; it has a low incidence of restenosis, in contrast to aortic stenosis.

TREATMENT

- Endocarditis prophylaxis
- Treat for heart failure (diuretics, digitalis) and dysrhythmias as needed.
- Anticoagulation for atrial thrombus/fibrillation if present
- Surgical repair or balloon valvuloplasty in symptomatic patients with orifice $\leq 1.2\ cm^2$

▶ MITRAL REGURGITATION

ETIOLOGY

Acute
- MI with papillary muscle rupture
- Endocarditis

Chronic
- Rheumatic fever
- Mitral prolapse
- Left ventricular dilation

SIGNS AND SYMPTOMS

- Dyspnea
- Fatigue
- Weakness
- Cough
- Atrial fibrillation
- Systemic emboli

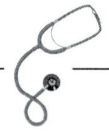

Patient with mitral regurgitation has a good prognosis if LV function is preserved.

DIAGNOSIS/SIGNS

- Murmur is loud, holosystolic, apical radiating to the axilla.
- ECG shows enlarged left atrium.
- Echocardiography demonstrating diseased/prolapsed valve

TREATMENT

- Medical therapy: Not definitive but used until surgery, or in poor surgical candidates

- Diuretics to reduce volume load
- Vasodilators to reduce afterload favoring aortic exit (e.g., ACE inhibitors)
- Anticoagulation for atrial fibrillation
- Surgical therapy: Valve replacement or repair if signs of LV dysfunction
- Acute MR usually results in evere CHF and requires emergent surgery.

▶ MITRAL VALVE PROLAPSE

Etiology

- Most common valvular disorder
- Idiopathic, rheumatic heart disease, ischemic heart disease, ASD, or Marfan's syndrome
- More common in women (90% of cases)
- Genetic predisposition (can be inherited as an autosomal dominant trait)
- Normal variant

Typical scenario:
A young woman presents with atypical chest pain and mid-systolic click. *Think: Mitral valve prolapse.*

Signs and Symptoms

- Mostly asymptomatic
- Atypical chest pain
- Shortness of breath (SOB)
- Fatigue

Diagnosis/Signs

- Mid-systolic click; followed by late-systolic, high-pitched murmur (if mild regurgitation is present also)
- Best heard at apex
- S_3 sometimes present
- Wide splitting of S_2
- Echocardiography demonstrates diseased valve.

Treatment

- Prophylaxis for endocarditis if a murmur is audible or if myxomatous leaflets
- Vigilant follow-up

▶ AORTIC STENOSIS

Etiology

- Degenerative calcific disease (idiopathic, older population)
- Bicuspid aortic valve (most common *congenital* valve abnormality) can result in aortic stenosis around age 40.

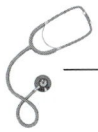

Prognosis:
Mean survival for patients with AS and:
Angina = 5 years
Syncope = 2–3 years
Heart failure = 1–2 years

Symptoms

- Usually asymptomatic early in course
- Dyspnea

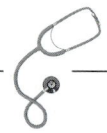

Left ventricular strain pattern is ST segment depression and T wave inversion in I, aVL, and left precordial leads.

Patients with aortic stenosis should be considered for valve replacement for:
- Persistent symptoms
- Aortic orifice < 0.7 cm^2 body surface area
- Gradient > 70 mm Hg

Conditions with wide pulse pressure:
- Aortic regurgitation
- Hyperthyroidism
- Anemia
- Wet beriberi
- Hypertrophic subaortic stenosis
- Hypertension

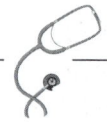

Acute valvular disorders (e.g., acute MR or AR) result in severe decompensation into CHF due to the absence of hemodynamic compensation. Emergent surgery is required.

- Angina and syncope: Particularly during exercise—peripheral resistance falls, LV pressure remains the same due to stenotic valve, CO cannot maintain BP causing syncope, low BP to coronary arteries causes angina
- Heart failure

Diagnosis/Signs

- Forceful apex beat with normally located PMI
- Loud systolic ejection murmur, crescendo–decrescendo, medium pitched loudest at 2nd R interspace, radiates to carotids
- Paradoxical splitting of S_2
- Narrow pulse pressure
- Best heard over right 2nd interspace, transmitted to carotid arteries
- ECG may show left ventricular strain pattern.
- Echocardiography demonstrates diseased valve.
- Calcification of aortic valve may be seen on CXR.

Treatment

- Avoid strenuous activity.
- Avoid afterload reduction.
- Valve replacement is definitive therapy.
- Valvuloplasty produces only temporary improvement as rate of restenosis is very high.

▶ AORTIC REGURGITATION

Etiology

- Aortic root dilatation: Idiopathic (correlates with hypertension [HTN] and age), collagen vascular disease, Marfan's syndrome
- Valvular disease: Rheumatic heart disease, endocarditis
- Proximal aortic root dissection: Cystic medial necrosis (Marfan's syndrome), syphilis, HTN, Ehlers–Danlos, Turner's syndrome, 3rd trimester pregnancy

Signs and Symptoms

- Dyspnea, orthopnea, paroxysmal nocturnal dyspnea
- Angina (due to reduced diastolic coronary blood flow due to low pressure in aortic root)
- Left ventricular failure
- Wide pulse pressure
- Bounding "Corrigan" pulse, "pistol shot" femorals, pulsus bisferiens (dicrotic pulse with two palpable waves in systole)
- Duroziez sign: Presence of diastolic femoral bruit when femoral artery is compressed enough to hear a systolic bruit
- Hill's sign: Systolic pressure in the legs > 20 mm Hg higher than in the arms
- Quincke's sign: Alternating blushing and blanching of the fingernails when gentle pressure is applied
- De Musset's sign: Bobbing of head with heartbeat

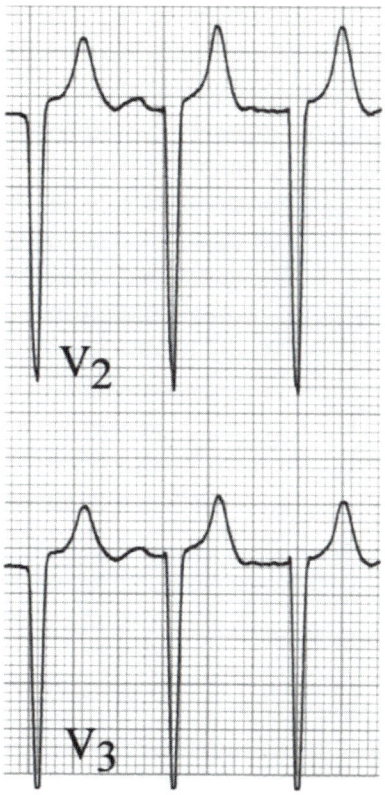

FIGURE 2.1-6. Left ventricular hypertrophy.

Diagnosis/Signs

- High-pitched, blowing, decrescendo diastolic murmur best heard over 2nd right interspace or 3rd left interspace, accentuated by leaning forward
- Austin Flint murmur: Observed in severe regurgitation, low-pitched diastolic rumble due to regurgitated blood striking the anterior mitral leaflet (similar sound to mitral regurgitation)
- Hyperdynamic down and laterally displaced PMI due to LV enlargement
- ECG shows left ventricular hypertrophy (see Figure 2.1-6).
- Echocardiography demonstrates regurgitant valve.

Treatment

- Treat left ventricular failure.
- Endocarditis prophylaxis
- Valve replacement is necessary for severe cases and is the only definitive treatment.

▶ TRICUSPID STENOSIS

Etiology

- Rheumatic heart disease, congenital, carcinoid
- Rare

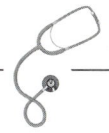

A rumbling diastolic murmur can be due to mitral stenosis (MS) or tricuspid stenosis (TS). TS will increase with inspiration.

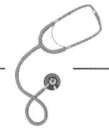

The Murmurs

Mitral stenosis—diastolic rumble with opening snap
Mitral regurgitation (chronic)—holosystolic blowing murmur radiating to axilla
Mitral valve prolapse—mid-systolic click
Hypertrophic cardiomyopathy (HCM)—systolic, brisk upstroke, parasternal lift
Patent ductus arteriosus (PDA)—continuous, machinery murmur
Atrial septal defect (ASD)—fixed, split S_2
Ventricular septal defect (VSD)—systolic, radiates to right
Aortic regurgitation—water-hammer pulse, decrescendo mid-diastolic
Aortic stenosis—harsh, systolic murmur that radiates to carotids, "parvus et tardus"

Signs and Symptoms

- Peripheral edema
- JVD
- Hepatomegaly, ascites, jaundice

Patient with a DVT has a stroke. He has fixed S_2 split. *Think: Atrial septal defect, right-to-left embolization.*

Diagnosis

- Murmur is diastolic, rumbling, low pitched
- Murmur accentuated with inspiration
- Best heard over left sternal border between 4th to 5th interspace
- Echocardiography demonstrates diseased valve.

Treatment

Surgical repair

▶ TRICUSPID REGURGITATION

Right-sided bacterial endocarditis is most frequently associated with nonsterile technique in IV drug abusers.

Etiology

- Increased pulmonary artery pressure (e.g., from left-sided failure or mitral regurgitation/stenosis)
- Right ventricular dilation stretching the outflow tract (e.g., from right heart failure, infarction, or tricuspid regurgitation itself)
- Right papillary muscle rupture from infarction
- Tricuspid valvular lesions (e.g., from rheumatic heart disease or bacterial endocarditis)

Signs and Symptoms

- Signs of right heart failure: Prominent JVD, pulsatile liver

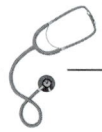

A holosystolic murmur can be due to mitral regurgitation, tricuspid regurgitation, or ventricular septal defect.

Diagnosis

- Holosystolic, blowing, medium-pitched murmur heard best along the left sternal border in the 5th interspace, accentuated with inspiration
- ECG shows right ventricular enlargement.
- Atrial fibrillation is common.
- Echocardiography demonstrates diseased valve.

Treatment

- Treat left heart failure, if applicable.
- Diuresis to reduce volume load
- Surgical repair and endocarditis prophylaxis if valve defective

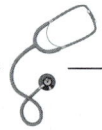

The number one cause of death in patients with CHF is arrhythmia.

DYSRHYTHMIAS

▶ VENTRICULAR FIBRILLATION AND PULSELESS VENTRICULAR TACHYCARDIA

DEFINITION

- Ventricular fibrillation (see Figure 2.1-7) is disorganized electrical activity of the ventricular myocardium. Because the myocardium depolarizes in an irregular, disorganized fashion, regular myocardial contraction does not occur.
- Ventricular tachycardia is organized but inefficient depolarization of the myocardium. It may degenerate into V-fib.

ETIOLOGY

- Ischemic heart disease/myocardial infarction
- Prolonged QT syndrome
- Torsades de pointes
- Wolff–Parkinson–White (WPW) with A-fib and rapid ventricular response
- Administration of antidysrhythmic drugs

SIGNS AND SYMPTOMS

- Ventricular fibrillation is not compatible with life. A patient with V-fib lasting more than 5 to 6 seconds will lose consciousness.

TREATMENT

- Emergent electrical cardioversion (shocking)
- Medications, such as epinephrine, lidocaine, amiodarone

For Prevention

- Cardiac pacemaker
- Implanted cardioverter/defibrillator (ICD)
- Electrophysiologic testing and radiofrequency ablation for accessory bypass tracts, AV nodal reentrant SVT, and others

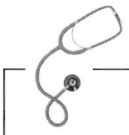

Ventricular fibrillation usually occurs after ventricular tachycardia.

Patient has hyperkalemia and peaked T-waves. First step? Calcium. Why? Stabilizes cardiac membranes

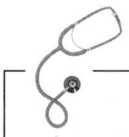

Causes of prolonged QT:
"QT WIDTH"
QT: Prolonged QT syndrome
W: WPW
I: Infarction
D: Drugs
T: Torsades
H: Hypokalemia, hypocalcemia, hypomagnesemia

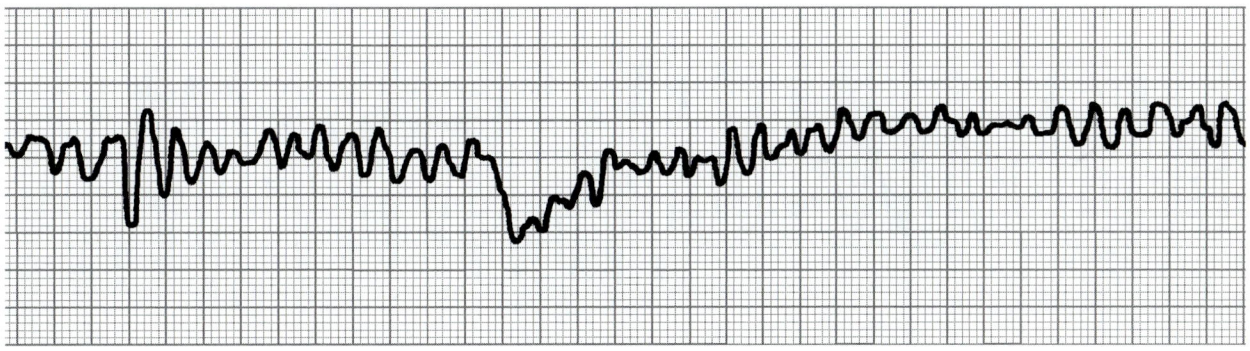

FIGURE 2.1-7. Ventricular fibrillation.

▶ TORSADES DE POINTES

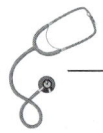

Cause of short QT:
Hypercalcemia

Definition

Arrhythmia with rotating axis and prolonged QT (see Figure 2.1-8)

Etiology

- Hypokalemia
- Hypomagnesemia
- Phenothiazines
- Tricyclic antidepressants
- Intracranial bleed
- Congenital prolonged QT syndrome
- Idiopathic
- Type I antidysrhythmics: Quinidine and procainamide

Treatment

- Magnesium IV
- Overdrive pacing
- Beta blockers for prolonged QT syndrome

Causes of Torsades:
POINTES
Phenothiazines
Other meds (tricyclic antidepressants)
Intracranial bleed
No known cause (idiopathic)
Type I antidysrhythmics
Electrolyte abnormalities
Syndrome of prolonged QT

▶ ATRIAL FIBRILLATION

Definition

- Disorganized electrical activity of the atrial myocardium, causing ineffective atrial contractions

Etiology

Seen often in patients with dilated atria, related to heart failure or valvular disease

Signs and Symptoms

- Sensation of palpitations or skipped beats
- Light-headedness, fatigue
- May develop chest pain

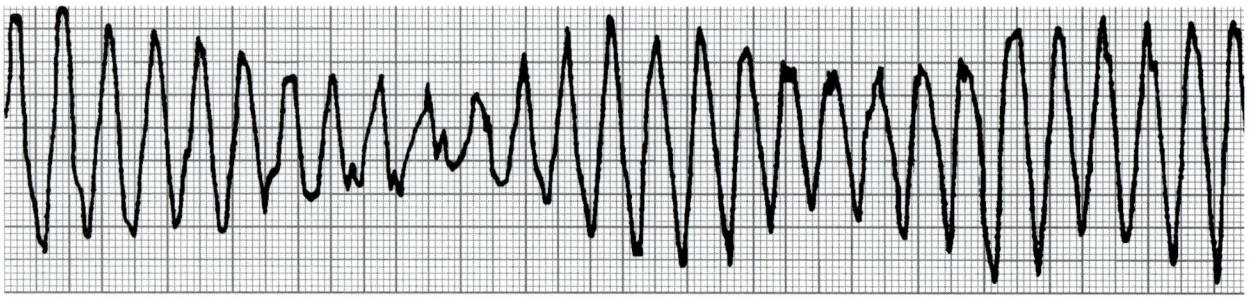

FIGURE 2.1-8. Torsades de pointes. Note bizarre, twisted point of QRS complexes and varying amplitude.

- May develop transient ischemic attack (TIA) or stroke (from embolizing thrombi formed in dyskinetic atrium)

Diagnosis

- Pulse is irregularly irregular.
- ECG: P waves are irregular or difficult to identify; R-R interval is variable (see Figure 2.1-9).
- Echo: May be used to identify presence of clot in the left atrium

Treatment

Rate Control

- Slow rate with calcium channel blocker (diltiazem) or beta blocker.

Rhythm Control

- Goal is to convert back to sinus rhythm.
- If patient has been in A-fib < 48 hours and no evidence of ischemia, synchronized cardioversion can be considered (shocking). Amiodarone and beta blockers can help maintain in sinus rhythm after conversion.
- For all others, anticoagulate with heparin.

For Unstable Patients with Any Rate or Duration of Rhythm

- Immediate synchronized cardioversion (shock)

▶ WOLFF-PARKINSON-WHITE SYNDROME

Definition

- **WPW** is a ventricular preexcitation syndrome: An abnormal bundle of fast-conducting fibers connects the atria and ventricles and allow electrical impulse generated by the sinus node to bypass the normal anatomic conduction pathways.
- Anterograde conduction occurs down the His–Purkinje system and back up the accessory bypass tract (narrow-complex).
- Retrograde conduction occurs down the accessory bypass tract and up the His–Purkinje system (wide-complex).

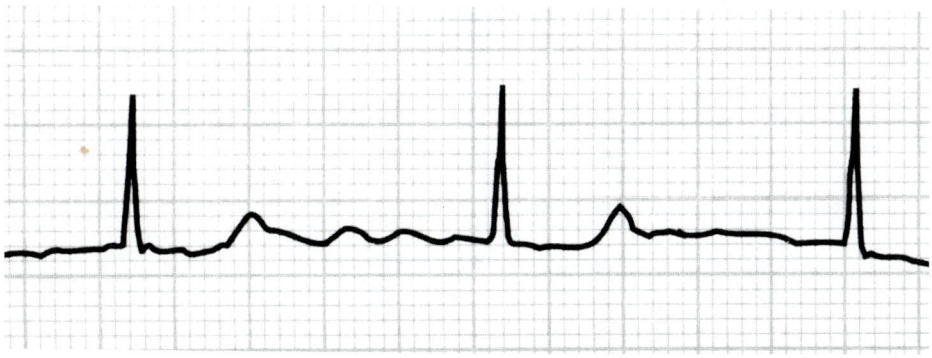

FIGURE 2.1-9. Atrial fibrillation. Note lack of P wave.

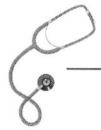

Atrial flutter may be confused with atrial fibrillation at high rates. Atrial flutter is distinguished by regular, distinct P waves in a sawtooth pattern.

Causes of atrial fibrillation:
PIRATES
Pulmonary disease
Ischemia
Rheumatic heart disease
Anemia, atrial myxoma
Thyrotoxicosis
Ethanol
Sepsis

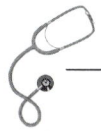

The ineffective atrial contractions of A-fib permit clot formation in the left atrium, which may embolize to the systemic circulation. Unless a patient is unstable, anticoagulate prior to cardioversion.

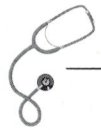

Rapid atrial fibrillation is often difficult to identify. Adenosine can be used to temporarily slow a rapid supraventricular rhythm.

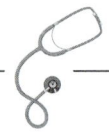

Preexcitation atrial fibrillation may occur in patients who have an accessory bypass tract: Conduction occurs down the bypass tract and up the normal His–Purkinje system. Medications that block conduction at the AV node are contraindicated.

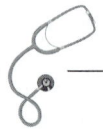

Don't give ABCD (adenosine, beta blockers, calcium channel blocker, or digoxin) to someone with WPW. Procainamide is the classic choice.

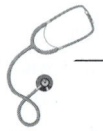

The ECG shows a "delta" wave, a slurred upstroke of the QRS complex (see Figure 2.1-11).

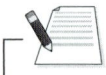

Causes of Mobitz I:
- Inferior wall MI
- Digitalis toxicity
- Increased vagal tone

Causes of Mobitz II:
- Inferior wall or septal MI
- Conduction system disease

Diagnosis

- ECG: Shows a "delta" wave, a slurred upstroke of the QRS complex (see Figure 2.1-10)
- Patients with suspected WPW should have electrophysiologic testing in the cardiac catheterization lab and radiofrequency ablation of the detected bypass tract.

Treatment

- Patients with WPW and rapid atrial fibrillation with rapid ventricular response require emergent synchronized cardioversion.
- Stable patients with WPW and atrial fibrillation or wide-complex SVT are treated with amiodarone, flecanide, procainamide, propafenone, or sotalol.
- Adenosine, beta blockers, calcium channel blockers, and digoxin are *contraindicated* because they preferentially block conduction at the AV node, allowing unopposed conduction down the accessory bypass tract.

▶ HEART BLOCK

First-Degree Heart Block (see Figure 2.1-11)

- Prolonged PR interval (> 0.20 s)
- No treatment required

Second-Degree Heart Block

Mobitz I (Wenckebach) (see Figure 2.1-12)
- Progressive PR prolongation with progressive shortening of the R-R interval until a beat is dropped
- For inadequate perfusion, treat with atropine or temporary pacing.

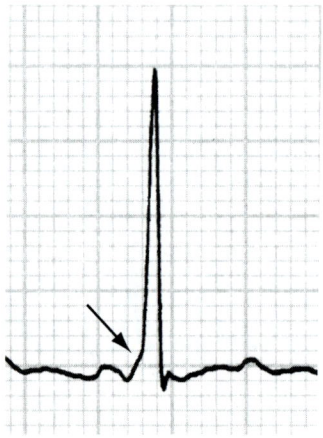

FIGURE 2.1-10. Wolff–Parkinson–White syndrome. Note slurred upstroke of QRS (arrow) known as the "delta" wave.

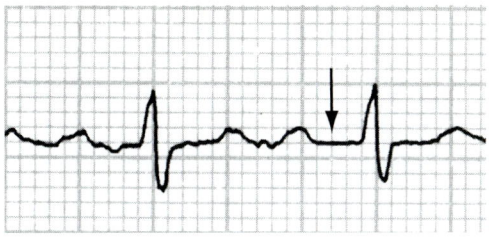

FIGURE 2.1-11. 1st-degree AV block. Note pause (arrow) before QRS complex.

Mobitz II (see Figure 2.1-13)

- Fixed prolonged PR interval followed by a nonconducted beat at a regular interval
- Treat with atropine, temporary pacing, and permanent pacemaker.
- Dangerous! Always place pacemaker!
- Important to treat quickly, as this can rapidly degenerate into complete heart block.

Causes of third-degree heart block:

- Inferior wall MI
- Digitalis toxicity
- Conduction system disease

Third-Degree Heart Block (Complete Heart Block)

- Independent atrial and ventricular activity (see Figure 2.1-14)
- Treat symptomatic patients with atropine and temporary pacing, followed by permanent pacemaker.
- Always needs pacemaker (dangerous rhythm)

Bradycardia:
"One INCH"
If the R-R distance is at least one inch, consider:
O: Overmedication
I: Inferior wall MI
Increased intracranial pressure
N: Normal variant
C: Carotid sinus hypersensitivity
H: Hypothyroidism

▶ SINUS BRADYCARDIA

Definition

- Rate below 60
- Normal P waves, PR intervals

Etiology

- Overmedication
- Inferior wall MI

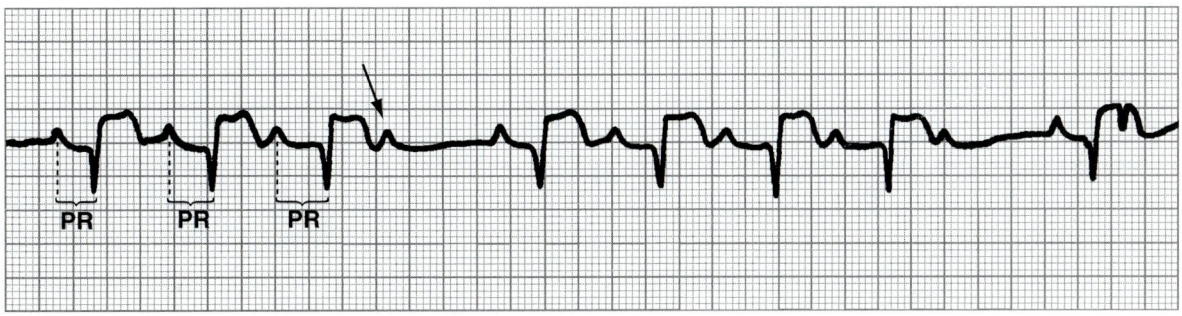

FIGURE 2.1-12. Wenckebach 2nd-degree AV block (Mobitz I). Note progressive lengthening of PR segment until a QRS complex is dropped. Arrow denotes nonconducted P wave.

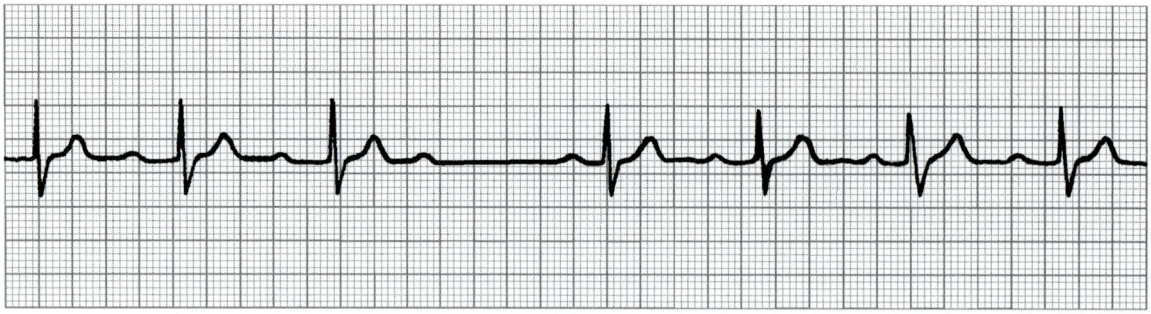

FIGURE 2.1-13. Mobitz II 2nd-degree AV block. Note constant PR interval followed by a nonconducted P at a regular interval.

- Increased intracranial pressure
- Normal variant: Well-trained athletes can have very low resting heart rates.
- Carotid sinus hypersensitivity
- Hypothyroidism

Signs and Symptoms

Often asymptomatic; light-headedness and/or syncope can occur.

Treatment

- Asymptomatic patients do not require immediate treatment: Look for underlying cause.
- Symptomatic patients: Atropine, pacing, pressors for hypotension

Hypertension

▶ OVERVIEW

Definition

Defined as an sBP > 140 or dBP > 90 on two separate occasions (see Table 2.1-3)

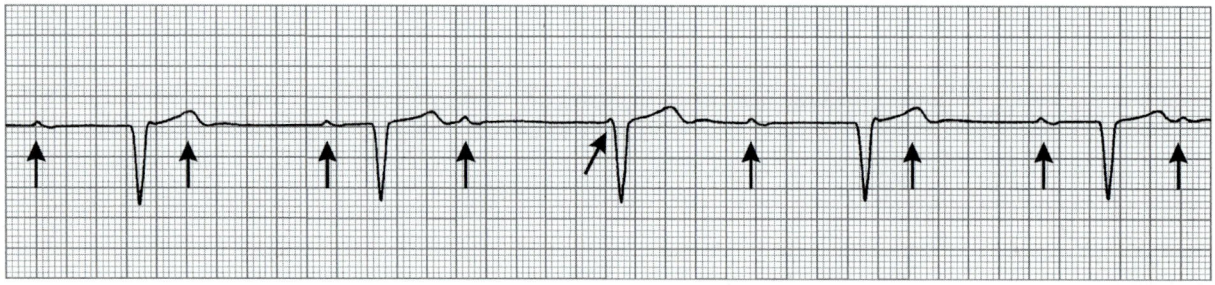

FIGURE 2.1-14. Complete (3rd-degree) AV block. Note dissociation between atrial and ventricular rhythms. Arrows denote P waves.

TABLE 2.1-3. Definition of Hypertension (JNC-7)

Hypertension	Systolic Blood Pressure	Diastolic Blood Pressure
Normal	< 120	< 80
Prehypertension	120–139	80–89
Stage 1	140–159 or	90–99
Stage 2	> 160 or	> 100

If patients do not fit into a discrete category, use the highest (worst) one.

Epidemiology

- 25 to 35% of adults have hypertension

Etiology

- Essential hypertension (primary, idiopathic)
- Secondary causes:
  - Renal parenchymal disease (chronic pyelonephritis)
  - Renal artery stenosis
  - Primary hyperaldosteronism (Cushing's and Conn's syndromes)
  - Pheochromocytoma
  - Eclampsia and preeclampsia
  - Coarctation of the aorta (congenital)

Pathophysiology

Usual mechanism is a normal cardiac output with increased peripheral vascular resistance.

Risk Factors

- Diabetes
- High-sodium diet
- Obesity
- Tobacco use
- Family history of hypertension
- Black race
- Male gender

Signs and Symptoms

Most patients with hypertension have no symptoms. Patients with severe hypertension may present with:

- Light-headedness
- Morning occipital headaches
- Epistaxis
- Hematuria
- Blurred vision
- Angina
- Congestive heart failure

Over 90% of hypertension is essential, or idiopathic.

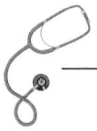

Hypertension due to **pheochromocytoma** is characterized by ectopic production of epinephrine and norepinephrine, causing wide swings in blood pressure.

A 24-year-old woman with preeclampsia treated with IV drip of magnesium complains of difficulty breathing and has diminished reflexes. Next step? Stop magnesium and give IV calcium.

Diagnosis/Evaluation

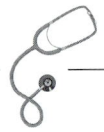

An active urinary sediment contains blood, protein, and red and white cell casts.

- Blood pressure in both arms, repeated if abnormal
- Funduscopic examination to look for AV nicking, hemorrhage, papilledema
- Auscultation for renal artery bruits
- ECG may show LVH or left ventricular strain.
- Urinalysis to look for active sediment, hematuria
- Blood urea nitrogen (BUN)/creatinine, serum potassium (evidence of renal insufficiency)

Treatment

For repeated elevated blood pressure measurements:

- Dietary changes: High fruits, vegetables, and low-fat dairy products, low total and saturated fats, low salt
- Weight loss, physical exercise
- Low-dose thiazide diuretics are first choice for stage 1 hypertension.
- Low-dose ACE inhibitor, calcium channel blockers, or beta blockers are also effective.
- Two- or three-drug therapy for patients not initially controlled (see table on pages 57–59 for commonly used cardiac medications)

Complications of Hypertension

Increases risk of:

- Stroke
- MI
- Atrial fibrillation
- Heart failure
- Peripheral vascular disease
- Renal disease

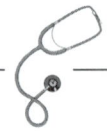

Use parenteral blood pressure–lowering agents only if end-organ damage is found, due to the risk of rapid reduction in coronary and cerebral perfusion.

▶ HYPERTENSIVE EMERGENCY

Definition

Malignant hypertension is characterized by severely elevated blood pressure accompanied by end-organ damage. New-onset neurologic signs, papilledema, chest pain or heart failure, and renal failure should alert the physician to the need for rapid blood pressure reduction.

The **mean arterial pressure** is:
(2dBP + sBP)/3

Diagnosis

- Presence of end-organ damage (ECG changes, new-onset renal failure, active urinary sediment, intracranial bleed, etc.)

Treatment

Reduce the mean arterial pressure by no more than 20%. Common intravenous agents include:

- Labetalol
- Nitroprusside
- Phentolamine for pheochromocytoma
- Hydralazine or magnesium for preeclampsia-related hypertension

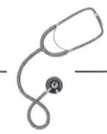

Nitroprusside can cause cyanide toxicity.

▶ AORTIC DISSECTION

Definition

- Usually associated with a transverse tear through the intima and internal media of the aortic wall
- Can lead to death by extension of the intimal tear to a full-thickness tear with hemorrhage into the extravascular space, dissection into the pericardium with tamponade, or extension into the branch arteries, including coronary arteries, carotids, mesenteric, renal, and iliac arteries

Type A involves the ascending aorta and can extend to descending aorta. **Type B** involves only the descending aorta.

Classification

DeBakey Classification
Type I: Ascending plus part of distal aorta (most common)
Type II: Ascending aorta only
Type III: Distal aorta only

Stanford Classification
Type A: Ascending aorta or both ascending and descending
Type B: Descending aorta

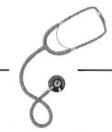

Aortic dissection due to syphilis occurs because the treponema infect the vasa vasorum of the aorta.

Etiology

- Hypertension
- Congenital heart disease
- Connective tissue disease (Marfan's and Ehlers–Danlos syndromes)
- Trauma
- Pregnancy (3rd trimester)
- Aortic coarctation (Turner's syndrome, idiopathic)
- Cocaine use

Causes of aortic dissection:
PATC³H
Pregnancy
Aortic coarctation
Trauma
Cocaine, **C**ongenital, **C**onnective tissue
Hypertension

Signs and Symptoms

- Severe "tearing" chest pain, may radiate to back
- Hypertension
- Unequal pulses distally for descending aortic dissection
- Aortic regurgitation murmur transmitted down right sternal border with ascending aortic dissection

Diagnosis

- CXR: Can be normal but often shows widened mediastinum, apical pleural capping, and loss of the aortic knob
- Helical CT with IV contrast *or* transesophageal echocardiography: May show dissection with extravasation of blood, intimal flap
- If aortic dissection is strongly suspected despite negative studies, the gold standard is angiogram.

Treatment

- Beta blocker + nitroprusside to keep sBP below 120, as long as the patient can maintain organ perfusion. Blood pressure control is crucial!
- Immediate surgical repair for type A dissection (ascending aorta)
- Medical stabilization for type B dissection (descending aorta)

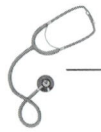

Always get a chest film when you suspect MI: Some of these patients will have aortic dissection, and thrombolysis may kill them.

Complications

- Myocardial infarction (dissection or obstruction of coronary arteries)
- Stroke (dissection or obstruction of carotids)
- Aortic regurgitation (dissection through aortic root)
- Cardiac tamponade (dissection into pericardium)

Infection-Related Cardiac Conditions

▶ BACTERIAL ENDOCARDITIS

Endocarditis prophylaxis is given to patients with VHD and those with previous history of endocarditis 30 minutes prior to:
- Dental procedures
- GI procedures
- Urologic procedures

Bacterial endocarditis is a localized infection of the endocardium characterized by vegetations involving the valve leaflets or walls. It is best categorized by the infecting organism, which determines the course of the disease. It can also be classified as acute (ABE) or subacute (SBE).

ABE
- Infection of **healthy valves** by high-virulence organisms
- Produces metastatic foci
- Usually fatal if not treated within 6 weeks
- Most common organism is *S. aureus*

SBE
- Seeding of **previously damaged valves** (rheumatic heart disease, congenital valve defects: mitral valve prolapse) by low-virulence organisms
- Does not produce metastatic foci
- Most common organism is *Streptococcus viridans*
- Mitral valve is most often affected

There is a strong association between *Streptococcus bovis* endocarditis and colonic neoplasms.

Etiology

- Acute: *S. aureus*, gram negative
- Subacute: *Streptococcus viridans*, other oral flora, group A beta-hemolytic strep, enterococci, *Staphylococcus epidermidis*
- IV drug users: *S. aureus*, streptococci, enterococci, *Candida*
- Prosthetic valves (10 to 20% of cases): *S. aureus*, *Streptococcus viridans*, gram negative bacilli, fungi
- Nosocomial infections: Indwelling venous catheters, hemodialysis, CT surgery

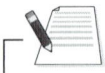

IV drug users: Right-sided ABE most often affects the tricuspid valve, septic pulmonary emboli are common.

Signs and Symptoms

ABE
- Acute onset of fever, chills, rigors
- New cardiac murmur
- Metastatic infections—meningitis, pneumonia

SBE
- Gradual onset of fever, sweats, weakness, arthralgia, anorexia, weight loss, and cutaneous lesions

- New cardiac murmur
- Splenomegaly
- Petechiae: Multiple nonblanching red macules on upper chest and mucous membranes
- **Osler's nodes:** Tender violaceous subcutaneous nodules on fingers and toes (see Figure 2.1-15)
- **Splinter hemorrhages:** Fine linear hemorrhages in middle of nailbed (see Figure 2.1-16)
- **Janeway lesions:** Multiple hemorrhagic nontender macules or nodules on palms and soles (see Figure 2.1-17)
- **Roth's spots:** Retinal hemorrhages seen on funduscopy
- Conjunctival hemorrhages

Diagnosis

Duke's criteria (patient must have 2 major, 1 major + 3 minor, or 5 minor criteria for diagnosis):

Major Criteria

- Two positive blood cultures taken at least 12 hours apart, or 3+ positive cultures taken at least 1 hour apart
- Echocardiography—vegetations are pathognomonic but their absence does not rule out endocarditis; transesophageal echo is more sensitive.

Minor Criteria

- Predisposing lesion on valve or intravenous drug use
- Fever > 38°C
- Arterial emboli (Janeway lesions)
- Osler's nodes, Roth's spots
- Positive blood cultures not meeting major criteria
- Echocardiogram suspicious for endocarditis but not meeting major criteria

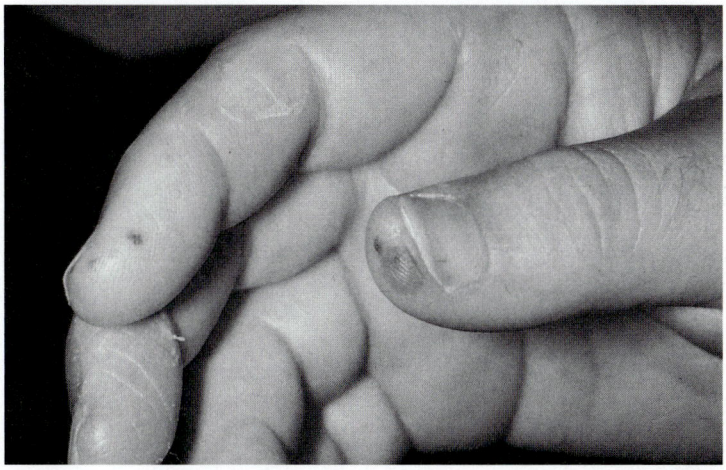

FIGURE 2.1-15. Osler's node.

(Courtesy of the Armed Forces Institute of Pathology, Bethesda, Maryland.)

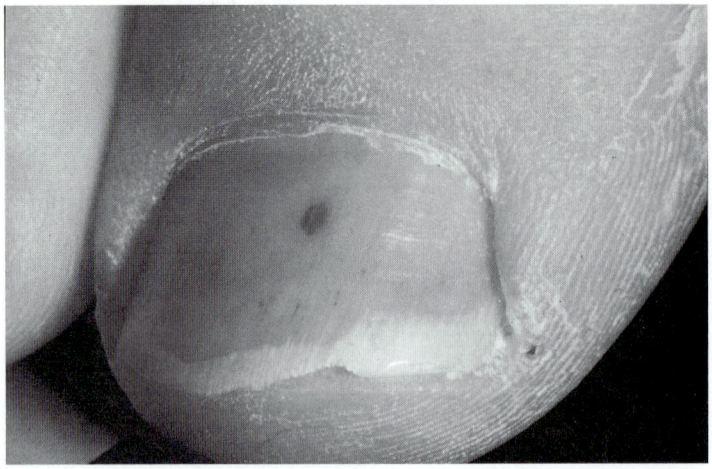

FIGURE 2.1-16. Splinter hemorrhage.

(Courtesy of the Armed Forces Institute of Pathology, Bethesda, Maryland.)

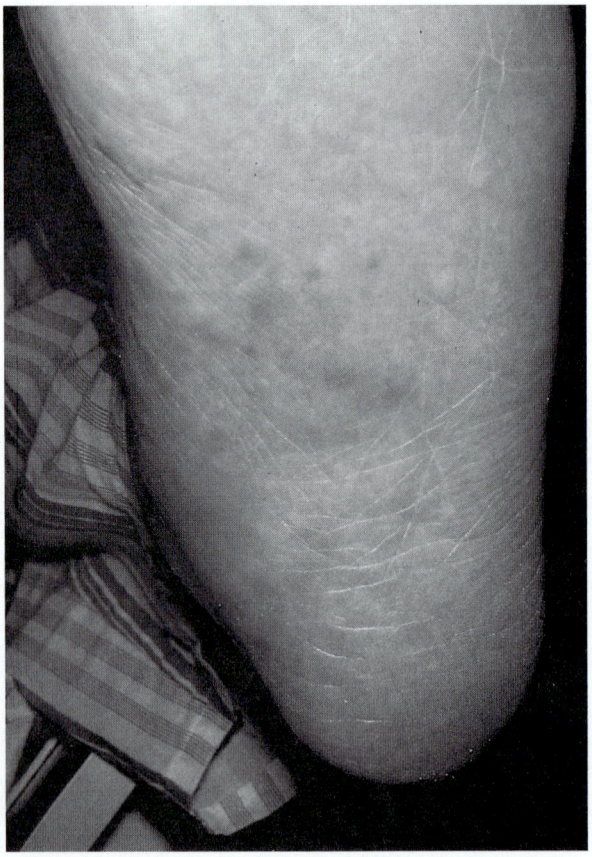

FIGURE 2.1-17. Janeway lesion.

(Courtesy of the Department of Dermatology, Wilford Hall USAF Medical Center and Brooke Army Medical Center, San Antonio, Texas.)

Treatment

- Streptococci: Penicillin G or ceftriaxone × 4 weeks
- Staphylococci: Nafcillin or oxacillin × 4 weeks
- MRSA: Vancomycin × 4 weeks

► RHEUMATIC FEVER

Definition

- Rheumatic fever (RF) is a systemic immune process that usually occurs secondary to pharyngeal streptococcal infection.
- Rheumatic heart disease (RHD) is the occurrence of valvular abnormalities due to immune complex deposition in valve leaflets generated by rheumatic fever.

Etiology

Recent streptococcal infection of pharynx

Diagnosis

Laboratory Findings

- Positive ASLO (antistreptolysin-O) antibody titers
- Elevated erythrocyte sedimentation rate (ESR)

Diagnosis of rheumatic fever requires presence of two major criteria or one major and two minor criteria.

Major Criteria

- Arthritis (migratory, multiple joints)
- Carditis (endo-, myo-, peri-)
- Erythema marginatum rash
- Subcutaneous nodules
- Sydenham's chorea

Minor Criteria

- Fever
- Arthralgias
- Elevated ESR
- Prolonged PR interval
- Recent streptococcal pharyngitis

Treatment

Acute

- Course of penicillin to eradicate throat carriage of group A streptococci
- ASA for arthritis
- Steroids for carditis

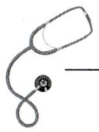

Most common valve affected by RHD is mitral, followed by aortic, then tricuspid.

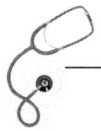

The reason for treating strep throat is to prevent the complication of rheumatic fever, not due to worry of the pharyngitis itself, which would resolve without antibiotics.

Jones Criteria ("JONES")
Joints—arthritis
♡—carditis
Nodules (SO)
Erythema marginatum
Sydenham's chorea

Chronic

- Monthly doses of benzathine penicillin to prevent recurrences
- Follow-up with cardiologist in severe cases

DYSLIPIDEMIA

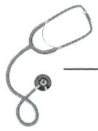

A level of HDL > 60 is cardioprotective.

- About half of all cases of coronary artery disease are associated with disorders of lipid metabolism.

Major Lipoproteins

- Chylomicrons: Transport cholesterol from the gut in the bloodstream
- Chylomicron remnants: Left over after lipoprotein lipase liberates free fatty acids from chylomicrons for use in tissues
- Very low-density lipoprotein (VLDL): Secreted from the liver; carries cholesterol in the bloodstream
- Intermediate-density lipoprotein (IDL): Metabolized from VLDL
- LDL: Metabolized from IDL, it carries cholesterol in the bloodstream to tissues
- HDL: Uptakes free cholesterol secreted by tissues and transports it to the liver

All isolated hypercholesterolemia is type IIa.

Isolated Hypercholesterolemia

- Familial hypercholesterolemia: Elevated LDL (type IIa)
- Familial defective apo B100: Elevated LDL (type IIa)
- Polygenic hypercholesterolemia: Elevated LDL (type IIa)

Isolated Hypertriglyceridemia

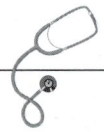

Patients with very high triglyceride levels (> 1,000) are at risk of developing pancreatitis.

- Familial hypertriglyceridemia: Elevated VLDL (type IV)
- Familial lipoprotein lipase deficiency: Elevated chylomicrons (type I, V)
- Familial apo CII deficiency: Elevated chylomicrons (type I, V)

Combined Hypertriglyceridemia and Hypercholesterolemia

- Combined hyperlipidemia: Elevated VLDL, LDL (type IIb)
- Dysbetalipoproteinemia: Elevated VLDL, IDL (type III)

SIGNS AND SYMPTOMS

Certain physical findings are associated with hypercholesterolemia:

- Xanthelasma: Painless, nonpruritic raised yellow plaques that occur on eyelids near inner canthi
- Xanthoma: Reddish brown papules on scalp, face, trunk, and flexor surfaces of limbs

Diagnosis

Serum lipoprotein analysis is done after a 12-hour fast. One-time sample cholesterol levels may not represent true levels in the following circumstances:

- Weight loss
- Pregnancy
- Major surgery
- Severe illness

Note: In patients who have MI, lipoprotein levels obtained within the first 24 hours will more closely approximate true pre-MI levels than later levels, which may not return to baseline for several weeks.

For cholesterol levels, see Table 2.1-4.

Formulae for calculating lipid levels:
LDL = TC – HDL – VLDL
VLDL = Trig/5
Total cholesterol (TC):
Normal: < 200
Borderline: 200–240
High: > 240
Normal HDL: 30–100

Treatment of Hypercholesterolemia

Goals of treatment:

- For a patient with 0–1 risk factors (low risk), keep LDL ≤ 160.
- For a patient with 1–2 risk factors (moderate risk), keep LDL ≤ 130.
- For a patient with known atherosclerotic heart disease (high risk), keep LDL ≤ 100.

For treatment strategies, see Table 2.1-5.

TABLE 2.1-4. Cholesterol Levels Associated with Familial Disease

	Type	Total Cholesterol Level (mg/dL)	LDL Level	VLDL	Chylomicrons
Familial hypercholesterolemia	IIa	275–500	High	Normal	Normal
Familial defective apo B100	IIa	275–500	High	Normal	Normal
Polygenic hypercholesterolemia	IIa	240–350	High	Normal	Normal
Familial hypertriglyceridemia	IV	250–750	Normal/High	High	Normal/High
Familial lipoprotein lipase deficiency	I, (I,V)	> 750	Normal/High	Normal/High	High
Familial apoprotein CII deficiency	I, (I,V)	> 750	Normal/High	Normal/High	High
Familial combined hyperlipidemia	IIb	250–500	High	High	Normal/High
Dysbetalipoproteinemia	III	250–500	Normal	High	Normal/High

TABLE 2.1-5. Treatment of Hypercholesterolemia

Treatment	Mechanism	Results
Diet therapy	Therapeutic Lifestyle Changes (TLC) diet ■ Total fat 25–30% total calories ■ Polyunsaturated fat < 10% ■ Monounsaturated fat < 20% ■ Carbohydrate 50–60% ■ Fiber 20–30 g/day ■ Protein 15% total calories ■ Saturated fat < 10% ■ Dietary cholesterol < 300 mg/day	Step 2 diet reduces total cholesterol by 10–12%. Exercise variably raises HDL. If diet therapy and exercise fail by 6 weeks, progress to medications.
Statins	Statins are HMG-CoA reductase inhibitors and act to reduce LDL and increase HDL.	Can lower LDL cholesterol by 35% and raise HDL by ~8%
Bile acid sequestrants	Cholestyramine and colestipol bind bile acids in the gut.	Reduces LDL cholesterol by 15–20%
Nicotinic acid	Reduces lipolysis in adipose tissue, inhibits hepatic synthesis of cholesterol	Can reduce LDL cholesterol by ~20% over 6 months. Side effects include cutaneous flushing, abdominal pain, nausea.
Fibrinates	Best for reducing triglycerides (in VLDL and chylomicrons)	Increases HDL by 5–30%

Common Cardiac Medications

	Medication	Main Clinical Uses	Adverse Effects
Class I: Sodium channel blockers	Lidocaine	Suppresses ventricular dysrhythmias	Mild: drowsiness, confusion, ataxia Severe: psychosis, seizures, AV block, respiratory depression
	Quinidine	Suppresses ventricular dysrhythmias, atrial premature beats, A-fib	Cinchonism: tinnitus, hearing loss, visual changes, delirium, psychosis. Also causes GI upset, promotes torsades de pointes (prodysrhythmic). Potentates many other medications.
	Procainamide	Suppresses ventricular dysrhythmias and A-fib, A-flutter, WPW	Myocardial depression, prolonged QT and QRS, torsades de pointes, V-fib
Class II: Beta blockers	Propranolol	SVT, thyrotoxicosis, acute MI, HTN	All beta blockers can cause bronchoconstriction; use with caution in asthmatics. Hypotension, light-headedness, fatigue, depression, and elevation of triglycerides can occur.
	Metoprolol	SVT, acute MI, HTN	
	Esmolol	SVT, thyrotoxicosis	
	Labetalol	Hypertension	
Class III: Prolongs action potentials	Amiodarone	VT, VF, A-fib, WPW	Bradycardia, AV block, peripheral neuropathy, pulmonary fibrosis, corneal deposits, skin discoloration, hepato toxicity Due to high iodine content, can cause hypo- or hyperthyroidism
	Bretylium	Ventricular dysrhythmias	Transient hypertension, hypotension
	Sotalol	AV reentry SVT, WPW	Bradycardia, CHF, peripheral edema
Class IV: Calcium channel blockers	Verapamil	Mild to moderate HTN	Calcium channel blockers reduce inotropy and are contraindicated in patients with heart failure, 2nd- or 3rd-degree heart block.
	Diltiazem	Mild to moderate HTN	
	Amlodipine, nifedipine	Mild to moderate HTN	

	Medication	Main Clinical Uses	Adverse Effects
Other antidysrhythmic agents	Adenosine	Supraventricular tachycardia	Transient asystole, hypotension, flushing
	Digoxin	Rate control of atrial tachydysrhythmia, increased inotropy for CHF	Toxicity can occur in therapeutic range. Vomiting, anorexia, confusion, visual changes, AV block, PVCs, VT, VF. Hyperkalemia is seen with acute poisoning. Hypokalemia lowers threshold for toxicity (remember many drugs used for CHF can cause hypokalemia). Chronic therapy can cause gynecomastia.
	Magnesium	Torsades de pointes, HTN due to preeclampsia,	Hypotension, flushing, CNS changes, decreased reflexes, respiratory collapse
	Epinephrine	Asystole, anaphylaxis, pressor	May cause ischemia
Inotropic agents	Dopamine	Increases inotropy, chronotropic, pressor	Increases peripheral vasoconstriction at doses greater than 5–10 μg/kg/min
	Dobutamine	Increases inotropy	Associated with reflex arterial vasodilatation and tachycardia
Chronotropic agents	Atropine	Asystole, symptomatic bradycardia	Anticholinergic
Venous/coronary dilators	Nitroglycerin	Venous and coronary artery dilator, can be used for malignant hypertension	Hypotension, headache
Antihypertensive agents	Nitroprusside	Malignant hypertension	Can cause hypotension, cyanide toxicity, methemoglobinemia
	Minoxidil	Severe hypertension	Can cause hypotension, tachycardia, hair growth
	Hydralazine	Moderate to severe HTN, particularly in the setting of preeclampsia and eclampsia. Hydralazine is a direct vasodilator.	Can cause tachycardia, angina, lupuslike syndrome with a malar rash that disappears after discontinuing the drug
	Clonidine	Central-acting agent for HTN	Hypotension, rebound hypertension after halting medication

	Medication	Main Clinical Uses	Adverse Effects
	Phentolamine	Parenteral alpha blocker used for HTN due to pheochromocytoma, cocaine	Hypotension, tachycardia, light-headedness
	Prazosin	PO alpha-blocker used for mild to moderate HTN	
	ACE inhibitors	Hypertension (decrease preload and afterload), nephroprotective CHF. Decrease cardiovascular events and mortality in high-risk patients > 55 years old.	All ACE inhibitors are variably associated with cough and angioedema and can cause acute renal failure in patients with bilateral renal artery stenosis. Hyperkalemia.
	Angiotensin receptor blockers	Antihypertensive useful as ? protective in patients with proteinuria. Side effects similar to ACE inhibitors but less cough.	
Antiplatelet agents	Aspirin	Used to prevent MI in patients with risk factors, can improve mortality from MI by about 25%	Associated with GI bleed. Some patients can have hypersensitivity reaction to aspirin.
	2b,3a inhibitors	Intravenous adjunct to heparin and thrombolysis in setting of acute MI; best use still being investigated	Can be associated with excessive bleeding
Antithrombotic agents	Warfarins	Long-term prevention of clots in deep vein thrombosis (DVT), A-fib, stroke, and others	Warfarins have an initial *procoagulant* effect. When anticoagulating as an inpatient, use heparin coverage initially. For outpatients, start at very low doses and raise gradually.
	Heparins	Myocardial infarction, pulmonary embolism, deep venous thrombosis	Both low-molecular-weight and unfractionated heparins can be associated with excessive bleeding.
Thrombolytic agents	Streptokinase	Myocardial infarction, pulmonary embolism, embolic cerebrovascular accident (CVA)	Relatively low cost. Cannot be used more than once within a 6-month period. Associated with hemorrhage at various sites.
	Tissue plasminogen activator	Myocardial infarction, pulmonary embolism, embolic CVA	High cost. Associated with hemorrhage at various sites.

NOTES

HIGH-YIELD FACTS IN

Endocrinology

Diabetes Mellitus (DM) 63

- Type 1 DM 63
- Type 2 DM 65
- Diabetic Ketoacidosis 67
- Nonketotic Hyperosmolar Coma (NKHC) 68
- Hypoglycemia 69
- Counterregulatory Hormones 70
- Metabolic Syndrome 71

Pituitary Tumors 72

- Acromegaly 74
- Hypopituitarism 75

Antidiuretic Hormone (ADH) Disorders 76

- Diabetes Insipidus (DI) 76
- Syndrome of Inappropriate Antidiuretic Hormone Secretion (SIADH) 77

Thyroid Disorders 78

- Hyperthyroidism 78
- Thyroid Storm 79
- Graves' Disease 80
- Hypothyroidism 81
- Subclinical Hypothyroidism 83
- Myxedema Coma 84
- Thyroiditis 85
- Evaluation of the Thyroid Nodule 86
- Thyroid Cancer 87

Parathyroid Disorders 87

- Hyperparathyroidism 87
- Hypoparathyroidism 88

Adrenal Disorders 89

- Adrenal Insufficiency 89
- Adrenal Excess: Cushing's Syndrome 92

Hyperaldosteronism 93
Pheochromocytoma 94
Bone Disorders 95
Osteomalacia 95
Osteoporosis 96
Paget's Disease of Bone 97

Diabetes Mellitus (DM)

▶ TYPE 1 DM

Definition

Hyperglycemia resulting from autoimmune destruction of the insulin-producing beta cells of the pancreas

Epidemiology

- Most commonly develops in younger patients. Usually diagnosed before age 30.
- Accounts for < 10% of all DM cases

Etiology

- Eighty percent of type 1 DM patients have HLA phenotypes associated with anticytoplasmic antibodies directed toward pancreatic beta cells (islet cell antibodies) and to glutamic acid decarboxylase (GAD antibodies).
- Glucagon-secreting alpha cells are not involved
- Antibodies detected during the initial stages of the disease usually become undetectable after a few years.
- Environmental factors may also play a role in pathogenesis:
  - Viral infection (congenital rubella, mumps, coxsackie B viruses)
  - Exposure to cow's milk instead of human milk during infancy

Signs and Symptoms

- Usually presents with symptomatic hyperglycemia or diabetic ketoacidosis (discussed later)
- Polyuria
- Polydipsia
- Weight loss
- Dehydration
- Blurred vision
- Fatigue
- Foot ulcers
- Can get restrictive cardiomyopathy without coronary artery disease

Diagnosis

- Confirmed with a fasting serum glucose of > 126 mg/dL
- Glycosuria (causes an osmotic diuresis that leads to the dehydration)
- HbA_{1c} is a measure of glucose control over the past 3 months. Most complications can be prevented if the HbA_{1c} level is kept below 7%.

Treatment

Mainstay of therapy is insulin (see Table 2.2-1 for types).

Initiating Therapy

- Patients are usually hospitalized at the time of initial diagnosis and are treated with regular insulin.

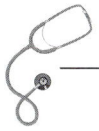

HbA_{1c} and corresponding blood glucose levels:

HbA_{1c}	Blood glucose
6	120
7	150
8	180
9	210

(Increments of 30)

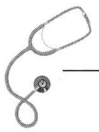

Type 1 DM is also called:
- Juvenile-onset DM
- Insulin-dependent DM

HLA-DR3 and DR4 are the most common HLA genotypes in type 1 DM.

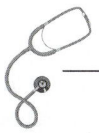

Typical scenario:
A woman presents with a recurrent vaginal candidiasis that is refractory to treatment. *Think: Diabetes mellitus.* Get a blood glucose.

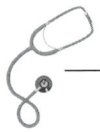

It is important for diabetics to have their feet frequently inspected to look for small cuts that may develop into ulcers. Due to neuropathy, diabetics can often have significant foot pathology and not feel anything.

TABLE 2.2-1. Insulin Preparations

Preparation	Onset of Action	Peak Action	Duration
Regular insulin	30–60 min	2–4 hr	6–8 hr
Rapid-acting (lispro)	15 min	30–90 min	2–4 hr
Intermediate-acting (NPH and Lente)	1–3 hr	6–12 hr	18–26 hr
Long-acting (Ultralente and PZI)	4–8 hr	14–24 hr	28–36 hr
Long-acting (insulin glargine)	1 hr	No peak	24 hr

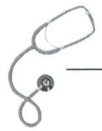

Diabetics have increased susceptibility to infections due to decreased efficacy of granulocytes despite normal number:
- *Pseudomonas*
- Mucormycoses
- Actinomycoses
- Aspergillosis (eosinophilic pneumonia with asthma; treat with steroids)
- Renal abscesses (with urinary tract infections)

- The average total daily dose of regular insulin is used as the initial dose of outpatient insulin therapy (be conservative so as not to induce hypoglycemic episodes).
- Divide the total daily dose to give two thirds before breakfast and one third before dinner if using NPH or 70/30 preparations.
- Initially, the patient should monitor finger-stick glucose levels five times a day and keep a record of the levels:
  - Tighter blood glucose control can be obtained with diet and increase in insulin dose.
  - Some patients may be candidates for rapid-acting insulin analogs (lispro) given right before meals or for continuous subcutaneous insulin infusion (CSII)
  - Choose the regimen that is easiest for the patient to follow while maintaining good blood glucose control.
- Patients must always take insulin to avoid ketosis, even if fasting (may decrease dose).

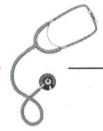

Type 1 DM patients must use insulin. They cannot use oral hypoglycemics because they have no functioning pancreatic beta cells.

Complications of All Diabetes (Types 1 and 2)

- Hypoglycemia (iatrogenic)
- Diabetic ketoacidosis (DKA)
- Nonketotic hyperosmolar coma (usually type 2)
- Retinopathy
- Stroke, MI
- Renal insufficiency
- Neuropathy
- Infections

Dawn Phenomenon

An exaggeration of the normal tendency of the plasma glucose to rise in the early morning hours before breakfast, probably secondary to an increase in growth hormone secretion

Somogyi Effect

- Characterized by nighttime hypoglycemia followed by a dramatic increase in fasting glucose levels and increased plasma ketones
- If Somogyi phenomenon is suspected, patients should check their blood glucose around 3 A.M. Hypoglycemia at this time confirms diagnosis.
- The morning hyperglycemia is a rebound effect.
- Replacement of intermediate-acting insulin with long-acting insulin at bed time can prevent this effect (want to try to avoid peaking of insulin effect in the middle of the night).

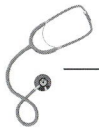

Measure finger-stick glucose levels 5x/day:
- **Morning fasting**
- **Breakfast postprandial**
- **Lunch postprandial**
- **Dinner postprandial**
- **Before bed**

Postprandial is 2 hours after the meal.

▶ TYPE 2 DM

Definition

Hyperglycemia due to insulin resistance

Epidemiology

- Accounts for > 90% of diabetes cases in the United States
- Usually diagnosed in patients > 30 years old, but increasingly seen in adolescents and children due to rising incidence of obesity and sedentary lifestyle.
- Concordance rate for type 2 DM in monozygotic twins is > 90% (< 50% in type 1)
- Commonly associated with obesity, and often presents after period of weight gain

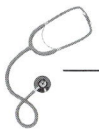

Typical scenario:
A patient presents with persistent morning hyperglycemia, despite steadily increasing his nighttime NPH insulin dose. He also complains of frequent nightmares. His wife brings him now because she witnessed him having a seizure in the middle of the night.
Think: Somogyi effect.

Etiology

- Hyperglycemia is caused by:
  - Impaired secretion of insulin
  - Decreased insulin effectiveness at glucose uptake
  - Impaired inhibition of hepatic gluconeogenesis
- The syndrome of insulin resistance involves hyperglycemia leading to obesity, hypertension, hyperlipidemia, and coronary artery disease.
- Glucose toxicity: Hyperglycemia may cause further glucose intolerance because hyperglycemia decreases insulin sensitivity and increases hepatic glucose production.

Signs and Symptoms

- Patients may be asymptomatic
- Presenting compliant is often a complication of their diabetes, such as a soft tissue infection. Can also present with signs of hyperglycemia.
- Increased susceptibility to fungal infections (cell-mediated immunity is impaired by acute hyperglycemia).
- Patients with type 2 DM will suffer from DKA only in rare instances.
- The nonketotic hyperglycemic–hyperosmolar coma (NKHC) is also a rare presenting situation.

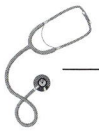

DKA is a complication mostly associated with type 1 DM, while nonketotic hyperglycemic hyperosmolar coma (NKHC) is associated with type 2 DM. However, either can occur with either type of DM.

Diagnosis

- Random glucose > 200 mg/dL
- Asymptomatic patients require a fasting glucose of > 126 mg/dL on two separate occasions.

If a patient has hypoglycemic finger-sticks in A.M., decrease the bedtime NPH, even if the bedtime finger sticks are high.

- If patients have fasting glucose levels of > 110 mg/dL and < 126 mg/dL, an oral glucose tolerance test is indicated.
- Positive oral glucose tolerance test is a plasma glucose > 200 mg/dL at two hours (or at any time up to two hours) after ingesting 75 g of glucose in solution.

Treatment

- Initial management should consist of education, diet, and exercise to achieve weight control.
- Patient education increases compliance with diet, exercise, and medication therapy. Discussions should involve when to seek medical attention, side effects of medications, proper foot care, ophthalmology visits, and symptoms of hyper- and hypoglycemia.
- If glycemic control cannot be obtained with diet and exercise, start oral hypoglycemic.
  - Combination of low-dose insulin secretogogues (Glyburide) plus low-dose insulin sensitizers (metformin) may improve HbA_{1c} with few side effects.
  - Patients not controlled with oral hypoglycemics alone may require insulin.
- Glucose-lowering drugs: See Table 2.2-2.

Table 2.2-2. Glucose-Lowering Drugs

Sulfonylureas	▪ Examples: Chlorpropamide, tolbutamide, glyburide, glipizide ▪ Mechanism: Increase postprandial insulin secretion from beta cells. ▪ Major side effects: Hypoglycemia is the major side effect. First-generation drugs are bound to plasma protein and may displace other meds. Second-generation are not plasma protein bound and are preferred. Second-generation are also excreted by both the kidney and metabolized by the liver so they are safer in patients with renal insufficiency.
Biguanides	▪ Example: Metformin ▪ Mechanism: Sensitize skeletal muscle to insulin which promotes glucose uptake. Inhibits hepatic gluconeogenesis. These meds do not cause hypoglycemia. ▪ Major side effects: Lactic acidosis. GI side effects. Renally excreted so should not be used in patients with compromised renal function (creatinine > 1.5) (increased risk of lactic acidosis). Cannot be given within 24–48 hours of injection of radiographic contrast material.
Thiazolidinediones	▪ Examples: Troglitazone, rosiglitazone, pioglitazone ▪ Mechanism: Reduces insulin resistance. Useful addition to insulin therapy in type 2 DM patients who need > 30 units of insulin/day, as monotherapy or in combination with a sulfonylurea. ▪ Major side effects: Hepatotoxicity
Alpha-glucosidase inhibitors	▪ Example: Acarbose ▪ Mechanism: Competitively inhibits monosaccharide and oligosaccharide hydrolysis in the small intestine, thereby decreasing carbohydrate absorption. ▪ Major side effects: Transient diarrhea and nausea; abdominal pain

▶ DIABETIC KETOACIDOSIS

Definition

Metabolic acidosis due to ketoacid accumulation due to severely depressed insulin levels

Epidemiology

- Common presenting syndrome in IDDM
- Mostly occurs in IDDM, but can also occur in NIDDM (especially in blacks)

Etiology

- Severe insulin deficiency causes the body to switch from metabolizing carbohydrates to metabolizing and oxidizing lipids.
- Usually precipitated by lapse in insulin treatment, acute infection, or major trauma.

Pathophysiology

- Insulin deficiency causes hyperglycemia, which induces an osmotic diuresis.
- Profound dehydration, sodium loss, and potassium loss occurs.
- Ketosis occurs because of the loss of inhibition of free-fatty acid oxidation in the liver.
- Metabolic acidosis ketosis results in respiratory compensation.
- Acetone is produced from spontaneous decarboxylation of acetoacetic acid. The acetone is disposed of by respiration and its odor is present on the patient's breath (fruity odor).
- Plasma ratio of beta-hydroxybutyric acid to acetoacetic acid is usually around 3:1 in DKA but can reach levels of 8:1.

Signs and Symptoms

- Polyuria, nausea, vomiting
- Lethargy and fatigue are later components.
- May progress to coma
- Signs of dehydration are present and patients may be hypotensive and tachycardic.
- Kussmaul respirations (rapid deep breaths) may be present.
- Acetone (fruity) odor may be present on the patient's breath.

Diagnosis

- Anion gap metabolic acidosis (ketones are unmeasured ions)
- Hyperglycemia
- Hyperketonemia
- Usually, the diagnosis can be presumed at the bedside if patient's urine is strongly positive for ketones and the finger-stick glucose is high.
- Glucose is usually between 400 and 800 mg/dL.
- Initially, potassium is high due to acidosis, but drops with treatment (insulin drives K^+ into cells).

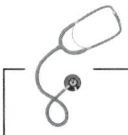

DKA is a life-threatening condition and must be recognized early and treated correctly.

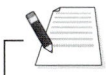

Beta-hydroxybutyric acid and acetoacetic acid are the ketones that are produced.

Treatment

- Goals of treatment are to remove ketones and correct the acidosis.
- Aggressive fluid resuscitation to correct volume deficit
- Correct hyperglycemia with insulin drip.
- Prevent hypokalemia during treatment with judicious potassium administration.
- Correct underlying causes (e.g., infection).
- Bicarbonate may be used to correct severe acidosis (rarely necessary).
- When serum glucose is reduced to 250 to 300 mg/dL, add 5% glucose to the IV fluids to reduce the risk of hypoglycemia.
- Insulin is required in DKA even after blood glucose returns to normal range. Continue to give insulin and glucose-containing IV fluids.
- Admission to intensive care unit (ICU)

Prognosis

Mortality rate is approximately 10%:

- Hypotension or coma present at admission are negative prognostic indicators.
- Major causes of death are circulatory failure, hypokalemia, and infection.

▶ NONKETOTIC HYPEROSMOLAR COMA (NKHC)

Definition

A complication of NIDDM characterized by hyperglycemia and altered mental status. Carries a 50% mortality.

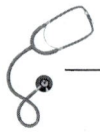

NKHC most commonly occurs in patients unable to affect their own environment, e.g., nursing home residents.

Pathophysiology

- Patients usually have a period of symptomatic hyperglycemia before the syndrome develops.
- When fluid intake becomes insufficient, extreme dehydration ensues because of the hyperglycemia-induced osmotic diuresis.

Etiology

- Sepsis
- Dehydration
- Diuretics
- Glucocorticoids

Signs and Symptoms

- Altered mental status
- Signs of profound dehydration
- Seizures and transient neurologic deficits may occur.

Diagnosis

- Serum glucose levels are usually > 1,000 mg/dL (much higher than in DKA).
- Serum osmolarity is usually around 385 mOsm/kg.
- Blood urea nitrogen (BUN)/creatinine levels are markedly increased from prerenal azotemia.

Treatment

Goal of treatment is to expand the intravascular volume to stabilize vital signs and improve circulation and urine output:

- Infuse 2 to 3 L of normal saline over 1 to 2 hours.
- Once vital signs have stabilized change fluid to D_5 ½ NS and monitor vital signs, urine output, serum electrolytes, and BUN/creatinine carefully.
- Begin potassium replacement with the initial infusion of D_5 ½ NS.
- Withhold insulin therapy for 30 to 60 minutes, because it drives glucose into the cells, exacerbating volume depletion.
- Monitor patient for signs and symptoms of cerebral edema, which may occur if the osmolarity is corrected too quickly.

If insulin is deemed necessary in the initial resuscitation, 5% glucose should be added to the infusion to prevent hypoglycemia when the serum glucose reaches 250 mg/dL.

▶ HYPOGLYCEMIA

Definition

Abnormally low serum glucose level that causes altered mental status and sympathetic stimulation.

Etiology

- Drug-induced (most common cause): Insulin, alcohol, sulfonylureas
- Islet cell carcinoma/adenoma
- Adrenal insufficiency
- Insulin receptor antibodies
- Severe liver or renal disease
- Endotoxic shock
- Hypopituitarism with deficiency of both growth hormone and cortisol

Pathophysiology

- Glucose transport across the blood–brain barrier is regulated by adrenergic nervous system activity (resulting in increased growth hormone and cortisol secretion and decreased insulin secretion.)
- Glucagon is secreted by the pancreatic alpha cells and increases plasma glucose levels and stimulates gluconeogenesis in the liver.
- The adrenergic outflow causes the typical sympathetic stimulatory symptoms of hypoglycemia and the lack of glucose to the brain results in altered mental status.

Signs and Symptoms

- History of insulin or sulfonylurea treatment
- Adrenergic symptoms: Diaphoresis, anxiety, tremor, faintness, palpitations, and hunger
- CNS manifestations: Confusion, inappropriate behavior (sometimes mistaken for alcohol intoxication), visual problems, stupor, and coma.

Whipple's triad of hypoglycemia:

1. Plasma glucose < 60 mg/dL
2. Symptoms of hypoglycemia
3. Improvement of the symptoms with administration of glucose

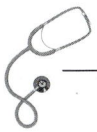

Hypoglycemia is the most common cause of altered mental status in most health care environments.

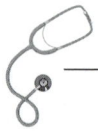

Hypoglycemia due to oral hypoglycemic agents lasts about 24 hours. Patients with sulfonylurea overdose should be admitted to the hospital for 24 hours, for monitoring and continuous glucose administration.

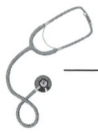

For alcoholics and people with malnutrition, always give thiamine prior to glucose to prevent Wernicke's encephalopathy.

Diagnosis

- Abnormally low serum glucose is < 50 mg/dL.
- Send C-peptide level to distinguish between endogenous (high C-peptide) and exogenous (low C-peptide) insulin because synthetic insulin has no C-peptide.

Treatment

- Once hypoglycemia is confirmed or if serum glucose level is not immediately available, obtain IV access and administer one ampule of 50% dextrose.
- Whenever dextrose is administered for hypoglycemia, and alcoholism or nutritional deficiency is suspected, administer thiamine prior to glucose to prevent Wernicke's encephalopathy.
- If there is not rapid improvement in mental status, repeat D_{50} administration.
- Once mental status has improved, infuse 10% dextrose solution and titrate to maintain a serum glucose level of > 100 mg/dL.
- Finger-stick glucose levels should be obtained every 30 minutes for 2 hours to detect possible rebound hypoglycemia.
- If hypoglycemia is refractory to glucose administration and is associated with signs of adrenal insufficiency, administer hydrocortisone 100 to 200 mg IV.

▶ COUNTERREGULATORY HORMONES

Counterregulatory hormones are hormones that counteract insulin action. Therefore, they can cause insulin resistance and diabetes if there is too much of them, or they can rise in response to hypoglycemia (too much insulin): High-yield facts and potential questions include:

Glucagon:

1. Glucagon is the most important and fastest to act. It acts on the liver to increase gluconeogenesis and glycogenolysis.
2. Glucagon (1 mg IM) is used to resuscitate hypoglycemic coma if you cannot get an IV access. (Never give anything by mouth, including glucose gel.)
3. Glucagon will not work in a patient who is alcoholic with liver failure. Alcohol will suppress gluconeogenesis, and glycogen stores are impaired in severe liver disease.
4. Loss of glucagon's response to hypoglycemia occurs after a long period of diabetes, especially type 1, leading to hypoglycemia unawareness.
5. Too much glucagon (glucagonoma) will present with new-onset diabetes, weight loss and characteristic rash (necrolytic migratory erythema).

Catecholamine:

1. Too much insulin leads to hypoglycemia; catecholamines rise, giving the signs and symptoms of hypoglycemia such as tachycardia, sweating, and anxiety.
2. Pheochromocytoma patients (too much catecholamine) have an increased risk of hyperglycemia and diabetes.

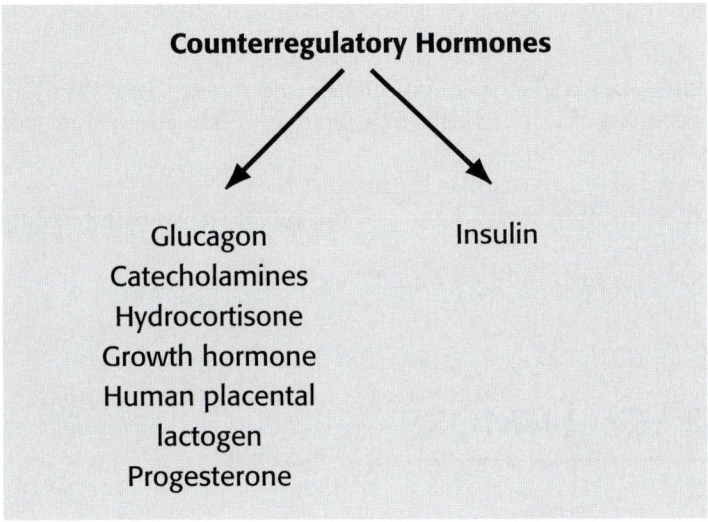

Cortisol:

1. Too much cortisol, as in Cushing's syndrome or in treatment of various diseases such as asthma, leads to hyperglycemia and diabetes.
2. Too little cortisol, as in Addison's disease, leads to hypoglycemia.

Growth hormone:

1. A high level of growth hormone in the early morning leads to hyperglycemia (dawn phenomenon).
2. A high level of growth hormone in acromegaly is associated with hyperglycemia and diabetes in nearly half of cases.
3. In addition to measuring IGF_1, screen for acromegaly by conducting an oral glucose tolerance test to see if the growth hormone will be suppressed in response to insulin release by the glucose given. If there is no suppression, the test is positive for acromegaly.
4. Neonatal hypoglycemia is a cardinal sign of growth hormone deficiency.

Placental secretion hormones, including growth hormone, corticotropin-releasing hormone, progesterone, and human placental lactogen, could lead to gestational diabetes in susceptible individuals, which is why diabetes screening during pregnancy is conducted when these hormone levels are at their peak—around the 24th week of gestation.

▶ METABOLIC SYNDROME

The metabolic syndrome is a constellation of findings that lead to increased risk of cardiovascular disease such as myocardial infarction, stroke, and death. With the growing epidemic of obesity, the prevalence of the metabolic syndrome is rapidly increasing even among adolescents and children.

The definition of metabolic syndrome in adults includes at least three of the following:

1. Fasting plasma glucose ≥ 110 mg/dL (6.1 mmol/L)
2. Abdominal obesity: waist girth in men > 102 cm and in women > 88 cm
3. Serum TG > 150 mg/dL (1.7 mmol/L)
4. HDL-C in men < 40 mg/dL (1 mmol/L); in women < 50 mg/dL (1.3 mmol/L)
5. Blood pressure > 130/85 mm Hg or on medications

Pituitary Tumors

- Anterior pituitary (adenohypophysis): Derivative of Rathke's pouch
- Posterior pituitary (neurohypophysis): Composed of hypothalamic neuronal axon terminals, storage and release site for hormones produced by these neurons
- For specific hormones, see Table 2.2-3.

Pathology

- Constitute ~10% of intracranial tumors
- Most are benign, slow growing
- Anterior pituitary: Craniopharyngiomas, adenomas
- Posterior pituitary: No primary tumors
- Metastases and meningiomas are occasionally seen
- Pathology arises from:
  - Excess hormone production
  - Compression of suprasellar structures
  - Destruction of normal pituitary parenchyma
  - Compression of pituitary stalk

Pituitary Adenomas

Pituitary adenomas are part of MEN type I (pituitary, pancreas, parathyroid).

- **Prolactinoma** is the most common pituitary tumor. It can present with galactorrhea or amenorrhea. Women usually present earlier than men. Prolactin levels correlate with tumor size. Treat with dopamine agonists (bromocriptine).
- **Nonfunctioning tumors** are the second most common pituitary tumors. Symptoms include visual changes or slightly high prolactin levels due to mass effect. Treat with surgery.
- Less common pituitary adenomas include **somatotrophs** (growth hormone; see Acromegaly), **corticotrophs** (ACTH), and thyrotrophs (TSH).
- **Pituitary microadenomas** (< 10 mm) are found in ~15% of asymptomatic women by MRI; in the absence of progression (assessed by follow-up MRI), they are clinically insignificant.

Table 2.2-3. Pituitary Hormones and Their Functions

Anterior Lobe	Main Stimulatory Actions	Hypothalamic Stimulus
Adrenocorticotropic hormone (ACTH, corticotropin)	▪ Growth and secretion of adrenal cortex to make cortisol and sex hormones	CRH
Growth hormone (GH, somatotropin)	▪ Secretion of somatomedin C (insulin-like growth factor) ▪ Body growth	GRH
Thyroid-stimulating hormone (TSH, thyrotropin)	▪ Growth of thyroid gland ▪ Production of T_3 and T_4	TRH
Follicle-stimulating hormone (FSH)	▪ Spermatogenesis in the male ▪ Ovarian follicle growth in the female	GnRH
Luteinizing hormone (LH)	▪ Testosterone secretion in the male ▪ Ovulation in the female	GnRH
Prolactin	▪ Milk production ▪ Maternal behavior	PRH (stimulates) Dopamine (inhibits)
Melanocyte-stimulating hormone (MSH)	▪ Skin pigmentation	
Posterior Lobe		**Releasing Stimulus**
Antidiuretic hormone (ADH, vasopressin, AVP)	▪ Retains sodium and water, producing concentrated urine	Osmoreceptors
Oxytocin	▪ Milk letdown ▪ Contractions of labor	Touch receptors in uterus, genitalia, and breast

Craniopharyngiomas

- Arise from embryologic remnants of Rathke's pouch
- Most common tumors of suprasellar region in children
- Solid or cystic
- Usually calcified

Neurologic Symptoms

- Headache
- Compression of optic chiasm:
  - Superior bitemporal quadrantanopia: Early visual defect, since compression begins on inferior surface of chiasm
  - Bitemporal hemianopia ("tunnel vision"): Classic finding, occurs when tumor has reached significant size

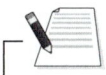

Patients rarely complain of "tunnel vision" or any deficit when the defect is confined to the temporal visual fields. They may report increased clumsiness or bumping into things.

- Signs of increased intracranial pressure (ICP) are rare as tumors are usually diagnosed before they reach the requisite dimensions

Diagnosis

- X-ray: May show enlargement of sella; craniopharyngiomas may show calcifications in suprasellar regions
- Computed tomography (CT): More sensitive than x-ray
- MRI: More sensitive than CT, can detect microadenomas; use with gadolinium contrast
- Hormone studies: Detect excesses or deficiencies, give information about type of tumor; useful when tumor cannot be detected radiographically

Treatment

- Dopamine agonists for prolactinomas (dopamine inhibits prolactin)
- Surgery: Indicated whenever there are neurologic symptoms
- Radiotherapy: Can reduce size of tumor without surgery, sometimes used as surgical adjunct
- Hormone replacement for hypopituitarism

▶ ACROMEGALY

Definition

Disorder marked by progressive enlargement of peripheral body parts resulting from excess pituitary GH production.

Etiology

Pituitary somatotroph adenoma

Signs and Symptoms

- Progressive enlargement of peripheral body parts, particularly head, hands, and feet
- Decreased glucose tolerance due to the anti-insulin actions of GH
- Hyperphosphatemia due to GH's influence on tubular resorption of phosphate
- Gigantism in children due to excess linear growth

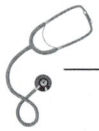

Acromegaly: The changes in a patient's appearance occur over many years, and may not be apparent to the patient or his family. Old photos may suggest the diagnosis.

Diagnosis

- Serum GH levels: Should be measured in the morning while still in bed as GH levels are raised by stress and exercise; may still be normal.
- Lack of GH suppression by glucose load.
- Serum IGF-I levels: Insulin-like growth factor-I is made by the liver under stimulation by GH, elevated in acromegalics

Treatment

- Surgery (transsphenoidal or transfrontal adenectomy, depending on the size and location of the tumor)
- Radiation therapy (takes 6 to 10 years to work)

- Dopamine agonist such as bromocriptine (preferred because of lower cost) or somatostatin analog such as octreotide
- GH receptor blocker such as pegvisomant (Somavert)

► HYPOPITUITARISM

Etiology

- Tumors causing dysfunction either by invasion, replacement, or compression affecting:
  - Normal pituitary parenchyma
  - Pituitary stalk
  - Hypothalamic parenchyma
- Surgical destruction of pituitary or hypothalamus: Either therapeutic or as a casualty of an unrelated neurosurgical procedure
- Sheehan's syndrome: Pituitary gland enlarges during pregnancy due to hyperplasia of lactotrophs without commensurate increase in blood supply; if hypotension occurs during childbirth, pituitary infarction can result
- Systemic (rare): Hemochromatosis, sarcoid
- Infectious (rare): Tuberculosis (TB), neurosyphilis

Typical scenario:
A 29-year-old woman presents with inability to lactate after childbirth. Delivery was complicated by blood loss and hypotension. *Think: Sheehan's syndrome.*

Signs and Symptoms

- ACTH deficiency: See section on adrenal insufficiency
- GH deficiency: Growth retardation in children
- Prolactin:
  - Deficiency: Failure to lactate after childbirth
  - Excess: Amenorrhea and galactorrhea in women, decreased libido and gynecomastia in men
- TSH deficiency: See section on hypothyroidism
- LH and FSH deficiency: Amenorrhea and genital atrophy in women, decreased libido in men
- In slow-growing tumors, GH, FSH, and LH levels are affected early; ACTH and prolactin levels decline only with advanced disease.
- Antidiuretic hormone (ADH) deficiency known as diabetes insipidus (discussed in separate section below).

Typical scenario:
A 36-year-old woman complains of amenorrhea for 1 year, increasingly bad headaches, clumsiness, and sporadic nipple discharge; beta-hCG levels are normal. *Think: Prolactinoma.*

Drugs that inhibit dopamine activity also cause hyperprolactinemia: TCAs, prochlorperazine, haloperidol, methyldopa, metoclopramide, cimetidine.

Diagnosis

- Pituitary hormone levels must be considered with other factors:
  - ACTH levels must be taken with serum cortisol levels, if cortisol is normal or high ACTH is probably low due to feedback inhibition. Insulin-induced hypoglycemia stimulates ACTH secretion and is an effective test of the entire hypothalamic–pituitary–adrenal axis. Test is administered similarly to GH provocation described below.
  - Prolactin levels are normally elevated in the third trimester and in breast-feeding mothers.
  - GH levels cycle daily, peaking in the evening, and decline to minimal levels by age 30. Evaluation requires stimulation testing: Insulin or levodopa stimulate a burst in serum GH, serum levels are drawn at 30, 60, and 90 minutes post-stimulus and compared to normal values.
  - TSH must be taken with serum T_3 and T_4; if they are normal or high, TSH is probably low due to feedback inhibition.

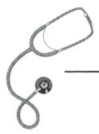

Unlike other pituitary hormones, prolactin secretion is controlled by **inhibitory** hypothalamic input. Destruction of the pituitary stalk or hypothalamus results in release from dopaminergic inhibition causing lactotroph hyperplasia. This results in hyperprolactinemia in the setting of hypopituitarism.

- In women, LH and FSH levels vary with the menstrual cycle so the timing of the levels is important; postmenopausal women have high LH and FSH levels normally.
- ADH levels normally vary according to plasma osmolality; testing is discussed in section on diabetes insipidus.
- Evaluation of target organ function is usually required: Tests include imaging studies, hormone levels, and response to exogenous pituitary hormones

Treatment

- Address underlying cause: Tumor, infection, systemic disease
- Hormone replacement:
  - Cortisol for ACTH deficiency
  - Prolactin:
    - No treatment for deficiency
    - Bromocriptine (dopamine agonist), surgery, or radiation for excess
- GH for GH deficiency in children
- Thyroxine for TSH deficiency
- FSH and LH deficiency can be treated with estrogen/progesterone replacements in women (fertility is usually not restored) and testosterone replacements in men.
- DDAVP for ADH deficiency

Antidiuretic Hormone (ADH) Disorders

▶ DIABETES INSIPIDUS (DI)

Psychogenic polydipsia: Psychiatric disorder of compulsive water drinking most common in young to middle-aged women. Presents with polyuria and dilute urine, distinguished from DI by low plasma osmolality.

Definitions

- Central DI: Inadequate pituitary secretion of ADH
- Nephrogenic DI: Lack of renal response to ADH

Etiology

Central DI

- Idiopathic: Accounts for 50% of cases
- Posterior pituitary or hypothalamic damage (tumor, trauma, neurosurgery)
- Systemic: Sarcoidosis, neurosyphilis, encephalitis

Nephrogenic DI

- Familial
- Chronic renal disease
- Sickle cell anemia (renal papillary necrosis)
- Hypokalemia
- Hypercalcemia
- Drugs: Lithium, demeclocycline, methoxyflurane

Signs and Symptoms

- Polyuria (3 to 15 L/day)
- Thirst
- Dilute urine (specific gravity < 1.005)

Diagnosis

- High plasma osmolality (280 to 310) due to incomplete compensation for the inability to resorb free water
- Water deprivation followed by exogenous ADH:
- Central DI: Low urine osm → high urine osm
- Nephrogenic DI: Low urine osm → low urine osm
- Normal: High urine osm → high urine osm
- Infusion of hypertonic saline normally results in a sharp decrease in urine output; patients with DI do respond.

Treatment

- Desmopressin (DDAVP): Analog of ADH, useful in central DI
- Thiazide diuretics: Paradoxically decrease urine output in patients with DI by increasing sodium and water resorption in the proximal tubule. They are the only therapy useful in nephrogenic DI.
- Chlorpropamide: Oral hypoglycemic with side effect of potentiating secretion and action of endogenous ADH. Partial function must exist for this therapy to be of use.

▶ SYNDROME OF INAPPROPRIATE ANTIDIURETIC HORMONE SECRETION (SIADH)

Definition

Excess production of ADH

Etiology

- Idiopathic overproduction via the hypothalamic-posterior pituitary axis: often associated with disorders of the CNS (encephalitis, stroke, head trauma) and pulmonary disease (TB, pneumonia)
- Ectopic production by malignant tumors, particularly small cell lung cancer and pancreatic carcinoma
- Pharmacologic stimulation of the hypothalamic–pituitary axis: Carbamazepine, chlorpropamide, clofibrate, vincristine

Other causes of excess ADH secretion:
- **Adrenal failure**
- **Renal failure**
- **Edema**
- **Fluid loss**

Signs and Symptoms

Attributable to hyponatremia—see chapter on fluid and electrolytes

Diagnosis

- Hyponatremia
- Low serum osmolality
- High urinary sodium
- Osmolality of urine > serum

Treatment

- Fluid restriction
- Hypertonic saline in severe hyponatremia
- Demeclocycline: Has side effect of decreasing collecting duct response to ADH

Thyroid Disorders

▶ HYPERTHYROIDISM

Causes of large tongue (macroglossia):
- **Acromegaly**
- **Myxedema**
- **Amyloidosis**

Definition

Increased synthesis and secretion of free thyroid hormones resulting in hypermetabolism

Epidemiology

- Ten times more common in women than in men
- Annual incidence is 1 in 1,000 women.

Etiology

- Graves' disease (most common cause, 80% of cases in the United States)
- Toxic multinodular goiter
- Toxic adenoma (Plummer's disease)
- Iatrogenic (lithium therapy), inadvertent toxic ingestion, or factitious (thyrotoxicosis factitia)
- Transient hyperthyroidism (subacute thyroiditis)

Pathophysiology

High levels of free thyroid hormones increase levels of cellular metabolism and cause multiple effects, resulting in a general state of hypermetabolism.

Signs and Symptoms

- Heat intolerance, sweating
- Palpitations (hyperthyroidism is a common cause of atrial fibrillation)
- Weight loss
- Tremor
- Nervousness and anxiety
- Weakness and fatigue
- Hyperdefecation

Diagnosis

Measure TSH, free T_4, and free T_3 (if the T_4 level is normal) (see Table 2.2-4)

Treatment

Depends on underlying disorder

TABLE 2.2-4. Laboratory Evaluation of Thyroid Function

Thyroid State	T_4	FT_{4I}	T_3	FT_{3I}	TSH	TRH
Hypothyroidism						
1°	↓	↓	↓	↓	↑	↑
2°	↓	↓	↓	↓	↓/N	↓
3°	↓	↓	↓	↓	↓/N	N
Peripheral unresponsiveness	↑/N	↑/N	↑/N	↑	↓/N	↑/N
Hyperthyroidism						
Pituitary tumor (secretes TSH)	↑	↑	↑	↑	↑	↓
Graves' disease	↑	↑	↑	↑	↓	↓
T_3 thyrotoxicosis	N	N	↑	↑	↓	↓
T_4 thyrotoxicosis	↑	↑	N	N	↓	↓
Toxic nodular goiter	↑	↑	↑	↑	↓	↓

► THYROID STORM

Definition

Exaggerated manifestation of hyperthyroidism

Epidemiology

Mortality is high (20 to 50%) even with the correct treatment.

Etiology

- Infection
- Trauma and major surgical procedures
- DKA
- MI, cerebrovascular accident (CVA), pulmonary embolism (PE)
- Withdrawal of antihyperthyroid medications, iodine administration, thyroid hormone ingestion
- Idiopathic

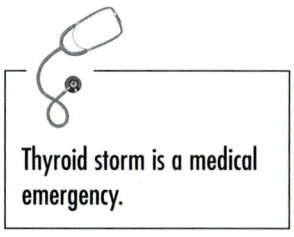

Thyroid storm is a medical emergency.

Signs and Symptoms

Overactivated sympathetic nervous system causes most of the signs and symptoms of this syndrome:

- Fever > 101°
- Tachycardia (out of proportion to fever)
- High-output congestive heart failure (CHF) and volume depletion
- Exhaustion
- GI manifestations: Diarrhea, abdominal pain

- Continuum of CNS alterations (from agitation to confusion when moderate, to stupor or coma with or without seizures when most severe)
- Jaundice is a late and ominous manifestation.

Diagnosis

- This is a clinical diagnosis, and since most patients present in need of emergent stabilization, treatment is initiated empirically.
- Patients may have improperly treated hyperthyroidism.
- May also occur in the setting of unintentional or intentional toxic ingestion of synthetic thyroid hormone in the hypothyroid patient.

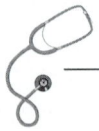

In initial stabilization of thyroid storm, cooling blankets can be applied to treat hyperpyrexia, if present.

Treatment

- Primary stabilization:
  - Airway protection
  - Oxygenation
  - Assess circulation (pulse/BP) and continuous cardiac monitoring
  - IV hydration
- Beta-blocker therapy (e.g., propranolol) to block adrenergic effects
- Treat fever with acetaminophen (not aspirin, which displaces T_4 from thyroid binding protein).
- Propylthiouracil (PTU) or methimazole to block synthesis of new thyroid hormone
- Iodine to decrease release of preformed thyroid hormone. Do not give iodine until the PTU has taken effect (1.5 hours) because more thyroid hormone will be produced.
- Treat any possible precipitating factors that may be present.

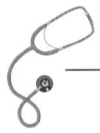

Never send any thyroid storm patient for a procedure involving iodine contrast before giving PTU.

▶ GRAVES' DISEASE

Definition

Autoimmune disease causing hyperthyroidism due to antibody, which stimulates TSH receptor

Pathophysiology

- Antibody is produced that interacts with the receptor for TSH resulting in continuous excess secretion.
- Cause of the exophthalmos (infiltrative opthalmopathy) in Graves' is unknown, but is thought to be due to immunoglobulins that interact with self-antigens in the extraocular muscles and on orbital fibroblasts. These antibodies are not the same antibodies as those interacting with the TSH receptor.

Graves' disease is the most common cause of hyperthyroidism.

Signs and Symptoms

- Diffusely enlarged thyroid
- Exophthalmos
- Pretibial myxedema
- Tachycardia, palpitations
- In elderly patients the presentation is less classic. Apathy can be present without the common hyperactivity signs (apathetic hyperthyroidism). Cardiovascular features may be prominent and hyperthyroidism may not be suspected initially.

Diagnosis

- High radioactive iodine uptake on a radionuclide scan. (If uptake is present but low, then diagnosis is thyroiditis or factitious hyperthyroidism.)
- Elevated free thyroid hormones (T_3, T_4)
- Undetectable TSH levels
- High thyroglobulin level

Graves' (and Hashimoto's thyroiditis) are sometimes associated with other autoimmune diseases (type I diabetes mellitus, vitiligo, myasthenia, pernicious anemia, collagen diseases).

Treatment

Long-Term Antithyroid Therapy

- Usually accomplished with propylthiouracil (PTU)
- Methimazole is as effective as PTU when administered at one tenth of the PTU dosage.
- PTU has the advantage of inhibiting the peripheral conversion of T_4 to T_3, thus there is usually a more rapid symptomatic improvement.
- Twelve- to 24-month course is usually used and one third to one half of patients remain well indefinitely.
- *Complications:* Leukopenia (check CBC before initiating therapy). Stop medication if absolute PMN drops below 1,500 cells/μL. If patient develops fever or sore throat, he or she should be instructed to return.

Radioactive Iodine Ablation Therapy (Preferred Treatment)

- Can produce the same effects as surgery without the surgical complications
- Tends to produce hypothyroidism over time. Forty to 70% for patients will develop hypothyroidism within 10 years of therapy.
- Some prefer to reserve radioactive iodine ablation therapy for patients over 30 years of age because of a higher incidence of hypothyroidism in younger patients.
- **Complications:** Radiation thyroiditis commonly appears within 7 to 10 days after therapy and is associated with accelerated release of thyroid hormone into the blood. Rarely, this results in thyrotoxic crisis.

Adrenergic Antagonists

- Propranolol is the agent of choice.
- Should be used only as adjunctive therapy because it does not treat the underlying problem.

Subtotal Thyroidectomy

- Still used for younger patients or when ablation therapy is unsuccessful
- Prior to surgery, patients should be euthyroid (pre-treated with PTU); then give iodine to cause involution of thyroid gland.
- Immediate complications include hemorrhage, which can result in airway compromise.
- Delayed complications include hypoparathyroidism (can be life threatening) and hypothyroidism.

▶ HYPOTHYROIDISM

Definition

- TSH levels greater than twice the upper limit of normal in primary hypothyroidism

- Can be clinically evident hypothyroidism with classic physical findings or subclinical hypothyroidism detectable only upon laboratory analysis

Epidemiology

- Clinically evident hypothyroidism occurs in 1.5 to 2% of women and in 0.2% of men.
- The incidence increases with age, usually between 40 and 60.
- In people over age 60, 6% of women and 2.5% of men have TSH levels greater than twice the upper limit of normal.

Etiology

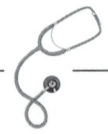

Hashimoto's thyroiditis (chronic lymphocytic thyroiditis) is the most common cause of hypothyroidism in patients older than 8 years of age.

Primary Hypothyroidism (Thyroid Gland Dysfunction)
- Hashimoto's thyroiditis
- Previous treatment for hyperthyroidism
- Subacute thyroiditis
- Radiation therapy to the neck (for other malignancy)
- Iodine deficiency or excess
- Medications (lithium is the most common)
- Prolonged treatment with iodine-containing substances

Secondary Hypothyroidism (Pituitary Dysfunction)
- Postpartum necrosis (Sheehan's syndrome)
- Space-occupying pituitary neoplasm
- Infiltrating disease (TB) causing TSH deficiency

Tertiary Hypothyroidism (Deficiency in TRH [Thyroid-Releasing Hormone] Secretion) (Hypothalamic Dysfunction)
- Granuloma
- Neoplasm
- Hypothalamic radiation

Signs and Symptoms

Muscle weakness and cramps occur in both hyper- and hypothyroidism. In hyperthyroidism, CPK will be normal. In hypothyroidism, it will be elevated.

- Fatigue, lethargy, weakness
- Constipation, weight gain (usually > 15 pounds)
- Muscle weakness, cramps, arthralgias
- Cold intolerance
- Slow speech with hoarse voice (from myxedematous changes in vocal cords)
- Slow thinking with poor memory
- Skin: Dry, coarse, thick, and cool; nonpitting edema of the skin and eyelids
- Hair: Brittle and coarse; loss of outer one-third of eyebrows
- Thyroid gland: May or may not be palpable (depending on the etiology of the hypothyroidism)
- Heart: Distant heart sounds may be present if pericardial effusion is present. Bradycardia may occur.
- Neurologic: **Delayed relaxation phase of deep tendon reflexes** (very specific). Cerebellar ataxia can be present. Peripheral neuropathies with paresthesias; carpal tunnel syndrome.
- Musculoskeletal: Muscular stiffness and weakness

Diagnosis

- See Table 2.2-4 for results of thyroid tests.
- Serum cholesterol, triglycerides may be elevated.
- LDH, AST, ALT, and the MM fraction of CPK may be elevated.
- Hematocrit and hemoglobin may be decreased.
- Hyponatremia may be present.
- Hashimoto's thyroiditis: May show increased antithyroglobulin and antimicrosomal antibody titers.

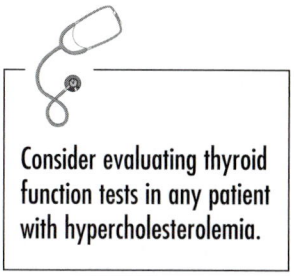

The TRH stimulation test is useful in distinguishing secondary from tertiary hypothyroidism.

Treatment

Therapy

- Start therapy with low-dose levothyroxine and increase dose every 6 to 8 weeks, depending on the patient's response (start low, go slow).
- Elderly patients and patients with coronary artery disease should be started on a low dose of levothyroxine because high doses may precipitate angina pectoris.

Monitoring Therapy

- In 1° hypothyroidism, it is adequate to measure the TSH level, which should fall well within the normal range.
- In 2° hypothyroidism, measure the T_4 level, which should fall well within the normal range.

▶ SUBCLINICAL HYPOTHYROIDISM

Definition

Elevated TSH level with normal thyroid hormone levels in the absence of overt clinical symptoms

Clinical Course

This is not usually a precursor to 1° hypothyroidism. There are usually two distinct patterns:

- Patients who will eventually develop 1° hypothyroidism: Women who have both elevated TSH and detectable antithyroid antibodies have a 5% annual incidence of overt hypothyroidism. Patients over age 65 with this combination will usually develop clinical hypothyroidism within 4 years.
- Euthyroidism with reset thyrostat: Permanent state without definitive progression to 1° hypothyroidism. Probably due to subtle damage to the thyroid gland from another cause.

Treatment

Replacement therapy:

- All patients with TSH > 10
- Patients with TSH > 5 and goiter or antithyroid Ab
- All patients with a history of iodine therapy

▶ MYXEDEMA COMA

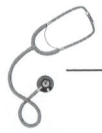

Hypothermia is often missed by tympanic thermometers. Use a rectal probe if hypothermia is suspected.

Definition

Life-threatening complication of hypothyroidism with profound lethargy or coma usually accompanied by hypothermia. Mortality is 20 to 50% even if treated early.

Etiology

- Sepsis
- Prolonged exposure to cold weather
- CNS depressants (sedatives, narcotics)
- Trauma or surgery

Differential diagnosis of myxedema coma:
- Severe depression or primary psychosis
- Drug overdose or toxic exposure
- CVA
- Liver failure
- Hypoglycemia
- CO_2 narcosis
- CNS infection

Signs and Symptoms

- Profound lethargy or coma is obvious.
- Hypothermia: Rectal T < 35°C (95°F)
- Bradycardia or circulatory collapse
- Delayed relaxation phase of DTRs, areflexia if severe (this can be a very important clue).

Diagnosis

Lab tests for the patient presenting with profound altered mental status:

- CBC with differential
- Blood and urine cultures
- Serum electrolytes
- BUN and creatinine
- Blood glucose
- Urine toxicology screen
- Serum transaminases and LDH
- Arterial blood gas (ABG) to rule out hypoxemia and CO_2 retention
- Cortisol level
- Carboxyhemoglobin
- Chest radiograph
- Brain CT

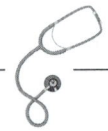

Corticosteroids are given empirically in myxedema coma before thyroxine is given due to concern that associated Addison's disease exists. Giving only thyroxine could precipitate an addisonian crisis.

Treatment

- Airway management with mechanical ventilation if necessary.
- Prevent further heat loss.
- Monitor patient in intensive care unit.
- Pharmacologic therapy:
  - Intravenous levothyroxine
  - Glucocorticoids (until coexisting adrenal insufficiency is excluded)
  - IV hydration (D_5 ½ NS)
  - Rule out and treat any precipitating causes (antibiotics for suspected infection).

▶ THYROIDITIS

Definition

- Inflammation of the thyroid
- Can be divided into three common types (Hashimoto's, subacute, and silent), and two rarer forms (suppurative and Riedel's)

Etiology

- Hashimoto's thyroiditis: Autoimmune disorder that involves CD_4 lymphocyte-mediated destruction of the thyroid. The lymphocytes are specific for thyroid antigens. Cause for activation of these cells is unknown.
- Subacute thyroiditis: Possibly a postviral condition because it usually follows a viral URI. Not considered an autoimmune reaction.
- Silent thyroiditis: Usually occurs postpartum and is thought to be autoimmune mediated
- Suppurative thyroiditis: Usually, a bacterial infection, but fungi and parasites have also been implicated in some cases. Commonly seen in HIV^+ patients with PCP.
- Riedel's thyroiditis: Also called fibrous thyroiditis, fibrous infiltration of the thyroid of unknown etiology.

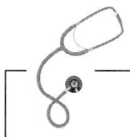

The thyroid in Hashimoto's is nontender, which distinguishes it from other forms of thyroiditis.

Signs and Symptoms

- Hashimoto's: There may be signs of hyper- or hypothyroidism depending on the stage. Usually, there is diffuse, firm enlargement of the gland, but it may be of normal size if the disease has progressed.
- Subacute: Tender, enlarged gland. Fever, and signs of hyperthyroidism are initially present. Hypothyroidism may develop.
- Silent: Similar to subacute except there is no tenderness of the gland (painless thyroiditis).
- Suppurative: Fever with severe neck pain. Focal tenderness of involved portion of the gland.
- Riedel's: Slowly enlarging rock-hard mass in the anterior neck. Tight, stiff neck. Must differentiate from thyroid CA. Hypothyroidism may occur if advanced. Fibrosis may involve mediastinum.

Typical scenario:
A 35-year-old female with a history of hyperthyroidism and a recent flu presents with neck pain and an elevated ESR. *Think: Subacute thyroiditis.*

Diagnosis

History

- Presentation following viral URI is suggestive of subacute thyroiditis.
- Presentation after penetrating injury to the neck is suggestive of suppurative processes.
- Postpartum presentation is suggestive of silent thyroiditis.

Laboratory Examination

- TSH and free T_4 may be normal or indicative of hypo- or hyperthyroidism.
- WBC with differential should be obtained to look for leukocytosis and left shift (subacute and suppurative).
- Antimicrosomal antibodies are present in > 90% with Hashimoto's and 50 to 80% with silent thyroiditis.
- Serum thyroglobulin levels are elevated in subacute and silent thyroiditis (test is very nonspecific).

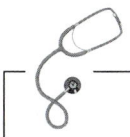

Differential diagnosis of thyroiditis:
- The hyperthyroid stage of Hashimoto's, subacute, or silent, may mimic Graves' disease.
- Riedel's must be differentiated from thyroid CA.
- Subacute can be mistaken for oropharyngeal or tracheal infections or for suppurative thyroiditis.

Imaging Studies

- Radioactive iodine uptake (RAIU) can be useful to distinguish Graves' disease (increased RAIU) from Hashimoto's thyroiditis (decreased RAIU).

Treatment

- Treat hypothyroidism, if present, with levothyroxine for 6 to 8 weeks. Reevaluate the TSH level.
- Control symptoms of hyperthyroidism, if present, with propranolol.
- Pain management in patients with subacute thyroiditis should be accomplished with NSAIDs. If ineffective, begin steroids.
- IV antibiotics and abscess drainage, if present, should be performed in suppurative thyroiditis.
- Do not give PTU or methimazole in thyroiditis.

Prognosis

- Hashimoto's: Most patients do not completely recover their total thyroid function.
- Subacute: Hypothyroidism persists in 10%.
- Silent: Hypothyroidism persists in 6%.
- Suppurative: Full recovery is common.
- Riedel's thyroiditis: Hypothyroidism occurs when the entire gland undergoes fibrosis.

▶ EVALUATION OF THE THYROID NODULE

Epidemiology

- Common (0.8% of men and 5.0% of women)
- Incidence increases after age 45
- History of neck irradiation (increased CA risk)
- Family history of pheochromocytoma, thyroid CA, or hyperparathyroidism (MEN II)

Signs and Symptoms

- Dysphagia, hoarseness
- Physical exam: Likelihood of malignancy increases with nodule > 2 cm, regional lymphadenopathy, fixation to tissues, age < 40, male sex.

Diagnosis

- Fine-needle aspiration is the best initial study. Accuracy can be > 90%.
- Thyroid ultrasound is performed to evaluate the size and number of thyroid nodules. It also evaluates whether the nodules are cystic or solid.
- Thyroid scan with technetium 99m classifies nodules as hyperfunctioning (hot nodules, less likely to be malignant) or hypofunctioning (cold nodules, more likely to be malignant).

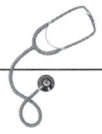

If thyroidectomy is planned, obtain a thyroglobulin level. A return to normal following thyroidectomy suggests the absence of metastatic thyroid tissue.

▶ THYROID CANCER

Epidemiology

- Incidence ~ 9/100,000
- 2:1 female predominance
- Increases with age and plateaus after age 50
- Worse prognosis if < 20 years old or > 65 years old

Risk Factors

- History of childhood head or neck irradiation
- Large nodule (> 4 cm)
- Enlarging neck mass
- Family history

Classification

Two types—follicular (epithelial) and parafollicular:

- **Epithelial** (three histologic types):
  - Papillary: Most common, has best prognosis
  - Follicular: Early metastasis
  - Anaplastic: Rare, worst prognosis
- **Parafollicular** (also called medullary thyroid cancer):
  - Calcitonin is increased from parafollicular C-cells
  - Seen in MEN II and III

Treatment

- Thyroidectomy
- Oral thyroxine supplement after surgery
- Careful monitoring of TSH and thyroglobulin levels (a rise indicates recurrence of the cancer)

Parathyroid Disorders

▶ HYPERPARATHYROIDISM

Definitions

- Primary: Hypersecretion of PTH by the parathyroid glands; *the rest of the section refers to 1° only.*
- Secondary: Glandular hyperplasia and elevated PTH in an appropriate response to hypocalcemia (due to renal failure, GI disturbances, etc.)
- Tertiary: Continued elevation of PTH after the disturbance causing 2° hyperparathyroidism has been corrected

Epidemiology

- Most common in middle-aged and elderly women
- Common: Present in 0.1% of the population

Etiology

- Parathyroid adenoma: 85%, 1 gland involved
- Parathyroid hyperplasia: 14%, all four glands involved
- Parathyroid carcinoma: 1%, 1 gland involved
- Associated with MEN II and III
- Neck irradiation increases risk.

Other causes of hypercalcemia:
- **Bone metastases**
- **Sarcoidosis**
- **Hyperthyroidism**
- **Thiazide diuretics**
- **Immobilization**
- **Paget's disease (only if patient is immobilized)**

Pathophysiology

- Parathyroid hormone (PTH) increases serum Ca^{2+} levels:
  - Stimulates renal hydroxylation of vitamin D (necessary for GI absorption of Ca^{2+})
  - Increases renal resorption of Ca^{2+}
  - Decreases renal resorption of PO_4^-
  - Increases resorption of bone (increases osteoclastic activity)
- PTH secretion is stimulated by decreased serum levels of Ca^{2+} and inhibited by high levels, except in adenomas and carcinomas in which feedback inhibition is lost.

Signs and Symptoms

Attributable to hypercalcemia (see chapter on nephrology and acid–base disorders)

Diagnosis

- Elevated serum Ca^{2+}, low serum PO_4^-
- High serum PTH
- Hypercalciuria

Treatment

- Older asymptomatic patients with serum $Ca^{2+} < 12$ should just be followed for progression.
- Surgery:
  - Adenomas should be completely excised.
  - In hyperplasia, all four glands are removed and a small portion is reinserted in an easily accessible place such as the sternocleidomastoid so that it can function, but if hyperplasia recurs, subsequent surgical intervention is simplified.
- Emergency measures:
  - Hydration with furosemide diuresis
  - Bisphosphonates to block bone resorption
  - Calcitonin acts rapidly but loses its efficacy after several days

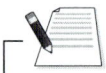

Mg deficiency is seen in alcoholism, SIADH, and pancreatitis.

▶ HYPOPARATHYROIDISM

Definition

Condition characterized by PTH deficiency

Etiology

- Idiopathic
- DiGeorge syndrome (see chapter on infectious disease)
- Postsurgical

- Infiltrative carcinoma
- Irradiation
- Hypomagnesemia (magnesium is necessary for parathyroid gland to secrete PTH)

Epidemiology

Equal incidence in men and women

Signs and Symptoms

Signs and symptoms of hypocalcemia (see chapter on nephrology and acid–base disorders):

- Seizures
- Perioral paresthesia
- Fasciculations, tetany, and muscle weakness
- CNS depression, irritability, confusion
- Chvostek's and Trousseau's signs
- Faint heart sounds
- Bronchospasm
- Anxiety, psychosis

Diagnosis

- QT prolongation on ECG
- Low serum calcium
- High serum phosphorus
- Normal or low PTH
- Normal 25-OH vit D
- Low 1,25-$(OH)_2$ vit D

Treatment

- Treat severe, life-threatening hypocalcemia with intravenous calcium.
- Maintenance therapy with calcitriol and oral calcium supplementation

Typical scenario:
A 30-year-old woman presents with perioral paresthesias and a long QT interval on ECG. She recently had surgery for a thyroid goiter. *Think: Hypoparathyroidism* (due to neck surgery with probable accidental resection of the parathyroids).

Vitamin D acts on the intestines to increase absorption of calcium and phosphate. It enters the skin via sunlight as a previtamin and is converted to an inactive intermediate (25-OH vit D) in the liver before being converted to its active form 1,25-$(OH)_2$ vit D (calcitriol) in the kidney.

Adrenal Disorders

ADRENAL INSUFFICIENCY

Definition

- Primary insufficiency is due to a problem with the adrenal gland itself, in which it does not produce hormones.
- In secondary insufficiency, the adrenal gland is intact, but the pituitary does not produce ACTH, so that there is no stimulus for the adrenal gland to secrete its hormones.
- Tertiary insufficiency is due to hypothalamic failure

Epidemiology

More common in women (2:1)

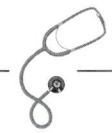

Pseudohypoparathyroidism presents the same as hypoparathyroidism, except that the pathophysiology in pseudohypoparathyroidism is tissue resistance to PTH, so that PTH is high (distinguishing feature). Pseudohypoparathyroidism is associated with Albright's hereditary osteodystrophy.

Primary adrenal insufficiency is known as Addison's disease.

Addisonian or adrenal crisis is an acute complication of adrenal insufficiency characterized by shock, dehydration, confusion, vomiting, hyperkalemia, and hypoglycemia. It is precipitated by sepsis, hemorrhage, trauma, and other stressors.

Primary insufficiency results in increased levels of ACTH. Melanocyte-stimulating hormone (MSH) and ACTH are cleaved from the same propeptide, so elevated ACTH results in increased skin pigmentation.

Etiology

Primary Insufficiency (Addison's Disease)

- Autoimmune (80%)
- Tuberculosis (15%)
- Neoplastic disease
- Sarcoidosis
- Amyloidosis
- Blastomycosis
- Hemochromatosis
- AIDS
- Adrenal hemorrhage due to trauma, anticoagulants, or coagulopathies
- Congenital adrenal hyperplasia
- Waterhouse–Friderichsen syndrome (fulminant septicemia in newborns)
- Adrenalectomy

Secondary Insufficiency

- Suppression of hypothalamic–pituitary–adrenal axis by exogenous steroids (most common)
- Sheehan's syndrome (postpartum pituitary necrosis)
- Pituitary infarct
- Autoimmune destruction of pituitary

Anatomy

The adrenal cortex consists of three zones:

- Zona glomerulosa—produces aldosterone.
- Zona fasciculata and zona reticularis—produce cortisol and androgens (sex hormones)

The adrenal medulla produces catecholamines.

Pathophysiology

Aldosterone

- Produced when angiotensin II acts on the zona glomerulosa to convert corticosterone to aldosterone

Addison's Disease	Cushing's Disease
Cortisol deficiency	Cortisol excess
Patient is thin	Patient is obese
Hyponatremia	Hypernatremia
Hyperkalemia	Hypokalemia
Metabolic acidosis	Metabolic alkalosis
Hypotension	Hypertension
Hypoglycemia	Hyperglycemia (or diabetes)
Lymphocytosis	Lymphopenia
Eosinophilia	No eosinophilia

- Principal function is to increase renal sodium reabsorption in the distal tubule and collecting ducts, causing secretion of potassium and hydrogen ions
- Deficiency results in hyperkalemia and hyponatremia.

Cortisol

- Stimulates gluconeogenesis by increasing protein and fat catabolism and decreasing utilization of glucose and tissue sensitivity to insulin
- Promotes anti-inflammatory state via inhibition of arachidonic acid, inhibition of interleukin-2 production, and inhibiting release of histamine from mast cells
- Has widespread effects on carbohydrate and protein metabolism
- Acts to counteract the effects of insulin and maintain blood glucose levels
- Governs body water distribution
- Enhances the pressor effects of catecholamine on heart muscle
- Inhibits inflammatory and allergic reactions
- Deficiency results in impairment of body's ability to handle stress

Typical scenario:
An 18-year-old man with hemophilia A who was recently mugged (receiving multiple blows to the back and abdomen) is now complaining of dizziness, abdominal pain, dark patches on his elbows and knees, and uncontrollable cravings for pizza and french fries. *Think: 1° adrenal insufficiency.*

Signs and Symptoms

- Hyperpigmentation of mucosa, areolae, hand creases, knees, elbows, and knuckles (1° only)
- Salt craving (1° only)
- Orthostatic hypotension (1° only)
- Weakness
- Amenorrhea, loss of axillary hair (due to absence of androgens)
- Anorexia
- Weight loss
- Abdominal pain

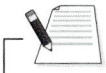

Secondary adrenal insufficiency can be distinguished from Addison's disease by:

- Absence of hyperpigmentation
- Normal aldosterone secretion
- Other signs of hypopituitarism such as hypothyroidism and hypogonadism

Diagnosis

ACTH (Cortrosyn) Test

- Give test dose of ACTH and measure serum cortisol levels at 0 and 30 minutes. A level < 18 μg/dL at 30 minutes suggests adrenal insufficiency.
- Measuring the plasma ACTH after test will tell you whether it is primary (high ACTH) or secondary (low or normal ACTH).
- Hyperkalemia, hyponatremia, extracellular fluid (ECF) volume contraction and metabolic acidosis due to aldosterone deficiency (1° only)
- Hypoglycemia
- Anemia
- Elevated BUN and creatinine
- Elevated ACTH, low serum cortisol

Treatment

- Glucocorticoid replacement for all patients
- Instruct patients to increase their glucocorticoid dose in times of stress and infection.
- Patients with Addison's disease should also receive mineralocorticoid replacement therapy.

▶ ADRENAL EXCESS: CUSHING'S SYNDROME

Definition

- Cushing's syndrome: Symptoms caused by excess cortisol production
- Cushing's disease: Cushing's syndrome caused by excess ACTH secretion by pituitary

Small (oat) cell lung carcinoma is frequently associated with ectopic ACTH production.

Epidemiology

More common in females

Etiology

- Exogenous corticosteroid therapy
- Adrenal neoplasm
- Ectopic ACTH production
- Cushing's disease

Patients with ectopic ACTH production often do not have all the mentioned symptoms; they usually have only weight gain and weakness because the ACTH they secrete is usually an inactive form.

Signs and Symptoms

- Hypertension
- Facial plethora
- Hair loss
- Central obesity (apple-shaped habitus, moon facies, thin extremities)
- Hump on back of neck (Buffalo's hump)
- Fragile, easily bruised skin
- Abdominal purplish striae
- Proximal muscle weakness
- Hirsutism
- Emotional lability
- Osteoporosis

Cushing's disease can be distinguished from Cushing's syndrome by the presence of hyperpigmentation.

Diagnosis

Overnight Dexamethasone Suppression Test

- 1 mg dexamethasone is given at night, plasma cortisol measured in the A.M.
- If < 5 μg/100 mL, excludes Cushing's as a diagnosis

High-Dose Dexamethasone Suppression Test

- Give 8 mg dexamethasone, then measure ACTH.
- If ACTH is undetectable or decreased and there is no suppression, likely adrenal etiology
- If ACTH normal or increased and there is no suppression, likely ectopic ACTH etiology
- If ACTH high with partial suppression, likely pituitary etiology

Other Findings

- Increased 24-hour urinary free cortisol (> 100 μg/24 hr)
- Hypokalemia, hypochloremia, metabolic alkalosis
- Hyperglycemia, hypercholesterolemia
- CT of adrenals to look for mass
- MRI of pituitary to look for mass
- Malignancy workup if ectopic ACTH production is suspected

Typical scenario:
A 42-year-old woman on long-term steroids for asthma has excess adipose tissue in her neck and upper trunk, a wide "moon face," and very fine hair. *Think: Cushing's syndrome* (due to exogenous steroids).

Treatment

Pituitary Adenomas (see Figure 2.2-1)
- Transsphenoidal surgery
- Radiation for children and cases refractory to surgery

Adrenal Adenoma
- Unilateral resection, followed by 3 to 12 months of glucocorticoid replacement (normal adrenal needs time to come out of suppression)

Bilateral Adrenal Hyperplasia
- Bilateral resection with lifelong replacement of glucocorticoids and mineralocorticoids

Ectopic ACTH Production
- Remove source of neoplasm if possible

▶ HYPERALDOSTERONISM

Definition

- Isolated excess production of aldosterone
- Also called Conn's syndrome

Epidemiology

- One to 2% of all patients with hypertension
- Most frequent in ages 30 to 60
- Adrenal tumor more common in women

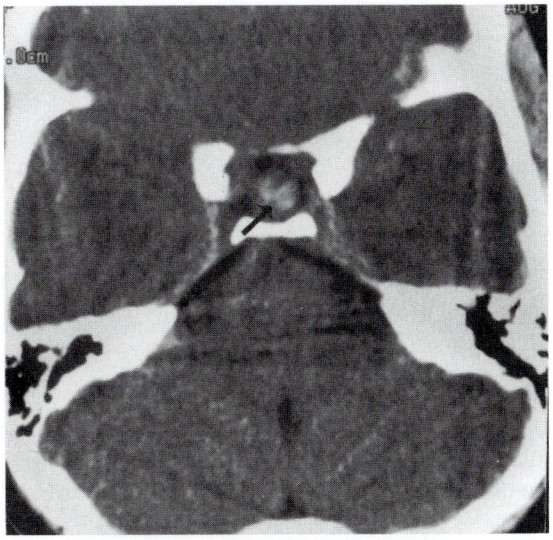

FIGURE 2.2-1. Pituitary adenoma (arrow).

(Reproduced, with permission, from Lee SH, Rao K, Zimmerman RA. *Cranial MRI and CT*, 4th ed. New York: McGraw-Hill, 1999:653.)

Etiology

- Unilateral aldosterone producing adenoma (most common cause)
- Bilateral hyperplasia of zona glomerulosa (idiopathic)

Signs and Symptoms

- Usually asymptomatic
- Hypertension
- May see signs of hypokalemia (muscle cramps, palpitations)
- May see signs of glucose intolerance (polyuria, polydipsia)

Diagnosis

Typical scenario:
A 44-year-old woman has hypertension, muscle cramps, and excessive thirst. *Think: Hyperaldosteronism.*

Measure plasma aldosterone to plasma renin activity ratio; a ratio > 20 suggests hyperaldosteronism.

Other Findings

- Hypokalemia, hypernatremia, and metabolic alkalosis
- High serum aldosterone, low renin levels
- Glucose intolerance
- 24-hour urine high in potassium and aldosterone
- Evidence of adrenal mass on abdominal CT
- Aldosterone escape: After initial edema and weight gain, patients usually diurese and shed the edema.

Treatment

- Adrenalectomy for tumor
- Medical management for hyperplasia:
  - Spironolactone (potassium sparing) or ACE inhibitors to control blood pressure
  - Low-sodium diet
  - Maintenance of ideal body weight, regular exercise, smoking cessation

▶ PHEOCHROMOCYTOMA

Definition

Tumor of the adrenal medulla resulting in catecholamine excess

Epidemiology

Pheochromocytoma:
Rule of 10s:
10% are extra-adrenal
10% are bilateral
10% are malignant
10% are familial
10% are pediatric
10% calcify
10% recur after resection

Equal incidence in men and women. Tumors in women are three times as likely to be malignant.

Etiology

- Multiple endocrine neoplasia types II and III
- MEN II: Pheochromocytoma, parathyroid tumor, and medullary thyroid tumor
- MEN III: Pheochromocytoma, parathyroid tumor, and mucosal neuromas
- Neurofibromatosis

- Von Hippel–Lindau disease: Pheochromocytoma, retinal angiomas, CNS hemangioblastomas, renal cell carcinoma, pancreatic pseudocysts, ependymal cystadenoma

Signs and Symptoms

Patients experience "paroxysmal attacks" of high blood pressure. Physical exam usually normal outside of an attack. Symptoms of catecholamine (sympathetic) excess will predominate during an attack.

5H's
- Headache
- Hypertension
- Hot (diaphoretic)
- Heart (palpitations)
- Hyperhidrosis

Other Symptoms
- Tremor
- Anxiety
- Weight loss

Typical scenario:
A 38-year-old woman on labetalol presents with poorly controlled hypertension, frequent headaches, and palpitations. *Think: Pheochomocytoma.*

Diagnosis

- Elevated urine vanillylmandelic acid (urine catecholamines)
- Hypercalcemia
- Hyperglycemia
- CT to look for adrenal mass

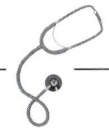

Patients with pheochromocytoma may carry an incorrect diagnosis of anxiety disorder.

Treatment

- Surgical resection
- Alpha-adrenergic blockade (may also add beta blocker)

Bone Disorders

▶ OSTEOMALACIA

Definition

- Disease of impaired bone mineralization
- Termed *rickets* in the pediatric population

Etiology

- Decreased Ca^{2+} absorption
- Dietary calcium deficiency: Rare, avoidance of dairy products:
  - GI disorders: Malabsorption syndromes, gastrectomy, dumping syndrome
- Vitamin D deficiency:
  - Hepatobiliary and pancreatic disease: Loss of bile acids or pancreatic lipase reduce absorption of fat soluble vitamins

- Extremely low-fat diets
  - Renal osteodystrophy: Decreased renal hydroxylation of vitamin D
- Decreased serum PO_4^-:
- More common cause than calcium deficiency in United States
  - Renal tubular acidosis, Fanconi's syndrome, hypophosphatasia

Signs and Symptoms

- Bone pain
- Weakness
- Difficulty walking: Broad-based waddling gait with short strides
- Thoracic kyphosis

Diagnosis

Radiographs

- Show diffuse, nonspecific osteopenia
- Vertebrae may be biconcave from compression by intervertebral disks
- Pseudofractures (radiolucent lines perpendicular to bone cortex)

Labs

- Ca^{2+} and PO_4^- low to normal
- High alkaline phosphatase
- PTH may be elevated in response to low Ca^{2+}

Treatment

- Address underlying disorder
- Calcium, vitamin D supplements

▶ OSTEOPOROSIS

Definition

Systemic disorder resulting in a reduction of bone mass that leads to increased risk of fracture.

Epidemiology

Risk factors for osteoporosis include:

- Female and elderly
- Postmenopause
- Family history of osteoporosis
- Cigarette smoking
- Thin body habitus
- Sedentary lifestyle

Pathophysiology

- Reduction in bone mass occurs due to an imbalance between bone acquisition and bone reabsorption.
- There is no change in the ratio of mineral to organic bone.
- Histology: Decreased cortical thickness and decreased number and size of cancellous bone trabeculae (especially horizontal).

Clinical Findings

- Osteoporosis is asymptomatic until fracture occurs (see Figure 2.8-1).
- Vertebral body fractures:
  - Pain in the lumbar region
  - Acute in onset
  - Radiating to the flank
  - Usually occur after sudden bending or lifting
  - Radiation of the pain down one leg is common
  - Spinal cord compression is rare
- Hip fractures:
  - Most serious complication
  - Most resulting from a fall from a standing position
  - Incidence of fracture increases with age in both men and women

Laboratory Findings

- Serum calcium and phosphorus usually *normal*
- Alkaline phosphatase is increased after fractures but is usually normal if fractures aren't present.
- Bone-specific alkaline phosphatase assays are useful for monitoring response to therapy.
- Twenty percent of postmenopausal women have hypercalciuria.

Bone Mineral Density Scoring
T score ≤ 2.5 = osteoporosis
T score −2.5 to −1 = osteopenia

Diagnosis

- Since bone loss is a universal process of aging, secondary osteoporosis should be diagnosed definitively and other causes should be ruled out.
- Biconcavity of vertebral bodies with pathologic fractures is highly suggestive of osteoporosis.
- Bone densitometry establishes the diagnosis.
- Measure bone mineral density using dual x-ray absorptiometry (DEXA) scan (not a bone scan).

Differential in osteoporosis:
- Malignancy: Multiple myeloma, lymphoma, leukemia, and metastatic carcinoma
- Hyperparathyroidism
- Osteomalacia
- Paget's disease of bone

Prevention and Therapy

- Prevention of low bone mass by adequate dietary calcium and weight-bearing exercise. These measures increase peak bone mass earlier in life and prevent accelerated bone loss later in life.
- Estrogen replacement therapy prevents rapid bone loss and subsequently decreases rate of fractures.
- Calcitonin decreases bone reabsorption.
- Bisphosphonates (alendronate) increase density of spinal bone and decreases incidence of fractures when used in conjunction with vitamin D and calcium supplementation.

▶ PAGET'S DISEASE OF BONE

Definition

Chronic disease of adult bone in which localized areas of bone become hyperactive, and the normal bone matrix is replaced by softened and enlarged bone.

Etiology

Cause is unknown, but it is suspected that a viral infection plays a role.

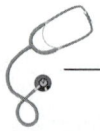

When alkaline phosphatase is elevated, send GGT to determine if hepatic or bone (elevated in liver but not bone).

Alkaline phosphatase of bony origin is heat labile, whereas the hepatic variant is not.

Typical scenario:
A patient is found to have an elevated alkaline phosphatase during a routine blood test. No other abnormalities were found. Further workup revealed the enzyme to be heat labile. *Think: Paget's disease.*

Epidemiology

- 3% of people > 40 years
- 3:2 male predominance

Pathophysiology

- Hyperactive bone turnover
- Increased bone formation
- Pelvis, femur, skull, tibiae, and vertebrae all affected
- Enlarged multinucleated osteoclasts

Clinical Findings

- Most patients asymptomatic, diagnosis made at autopsy
- Incidental radiographic findings: Area of hyperlucency surrounded by a hyperdense border
- Elevated alkaline phosphatase
- Symptomatic patients:
  - Increasing hat size due to skull involvement
  - Swelling or lengthening of a long bone causing gait disturbance
  - Dull aching pain, usually in the back, may radiate to the buttocks or lower extremities.
  - Rarely hearing loss due to involvement of the ossicles or auditory canal impinging on CN VIII
- Complications:
  - Pathologic fractures
  - Rarely "high-output" cardiac failure due to high vascularity of lesions
  - Urinary stones due to high calcium excretion
  - Sarcoma occurs in 1% of patients, poor prognosis

Treatment

- Most patients require no treatment.
- Indications for therapy are excessive pain, neural compression, profound alteration in posture or gait, high-output heart failure, hypercalcemia, and excessive calciuria, with or without renal calculi.
- Indomethacin is usually satisfactory for pain relief.
- Osteotomy is useful in selected cases of anatomic deformity or impingement.
- Bisphosphonates decrease bone reabsorption and are usually well tolerated.
- Calcitonin may be instituted in cases with cardiac failure or neurologic deficits. Calcitonin also has an analgesic effect.

HIGH-YIELD FACTS IN

Gastroenterology

Abdominal Pain 101

Vascular Problems of the Abdomen 103
- Abdominal Aortic Aneurysm (AAA) 103
- Mesenteric Ischemia 104

Disorders of the Esophagus 104
- Infectious Esophagitis 104
- Esophageal Perforation or Rupture 105
- Zenker's Diverticulum 106
- Esophageal Spasm and Achalasia 106
- GI Webs and Rings 107
- Gastroesophageal Reflux Disease (GERD) 109

Disorders of the Stomach 110
- Peptic Ulcer Disease (PUD) 110
- Duodenal Ulcer (DU) 111
- Gastric Ulcer (GU) 113
- Gastritis 114

Disorders of the Pancreas 114
- Acute Pancreatitis 114
- Chronic Pancreatitis 116

Disorders of the Biliary Tree 117
- Bile Storage and Release 117
- Cholelithiasis 117
- Cholecystitis 118
- Acalculous Cholecystitis 119
- Ascending Cholangitis 119
- Primary Sclerosing Cholangitis 120

Disorders of the Liver 120
- Normal Function of the Liver 120
- Cirrhosis 121
- Alcoholic Cirrhosis 121
- Primary Biliary Cirrhosis 122
- Portal Hypertension 122
- Esophageal Variceal Bleeding 123
- Hepatic Encephalopathy 123
- Spontaneous Bacterial Peritonitis 124
- Hepatorenal Syndrome 124

Hepatitis 124
Liver Transplantation 127

Disorders of the Colon 128
Carcinoid Tumor 128
Diverticulosis 129
Diverticulitis 129
Pseudomembranous Colitis 131
Irritable Bowel Syndrome 131
Inflammatory Bowel Disease 132
Colorectal Cancer 134
Hereditary Colon Cancer Syndromes 136

Gastrointestinal Bleeds 136
General Approach to GI Bleeding 136
Upper GI Bleeds 137
Lower GI Bleeds 138

Diarrhea 139
Acute Diarrhea 139
Chronic Diarrhea 140

Major Types of Malabsorption 142
Celiac Sprue 142
Tropical Sprue 142
Lactase Deficiency 143
Whipple's Disease 144
Protein-Losing Enteropathy 145
Ménétrier's Disease 145
Constipation 146

Abdominal Pain

Types of Pain

Visceral Pain

- Vague, dull, and poorly localized pain
- Midline location due to bilateral innervation of organs based on their embryological origin
- Associated with stretching, inflammation, or ischemia, involving bowel walls or organ capsules

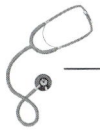

Visceral pain is **V**ague. **Example:** Early appendicitis; initially dull, periumbilical pain.

Parietal Pain

- Sharp, well-localized pain; peritonitis associated with rebound and involuntary guarding
- Pain location correlates with associated dermatomes.
- Occurs commonly with inflammation, frank pus, blood, or bile in or adjacent to the peritoneum

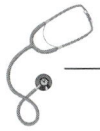

Parietal pain is **P**inpoint. **Example:** Late appendicitis; local inflammation leads to tenderness in the right lower quadrant.

Peritonitis is associated with rebound tenderness and involuntary guarding.

Referred Pain

- Pain stimuli generated at an afflicted location are perceived as originating from a site in which there is no current pathology.
- These sites are usually related by a common embryological origin.
- The pain can sometimes be perceived in both locations.

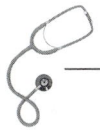

Example of referred pain: Ureteral obstruction can produce pain in the ipsilateral testicle.

Causes of Abdominal Pain

There are no hard-and-fast rules for localizing different types of abdominal pain. The following are classic examples for the exam:

Epigastric, Upper Abdominal Pain

- Gastroduodenal: Gastritis, peptic ulcer/perforation
- Pancreatic: Acute/chronic pancreatitis
- Aorta: Ruptured abdominal aortic aneurysm, dissecting abdominal aortic aneurysm
- Cardiac: Angina, myocardial infarction pericarditis

Typical scenario: A 45-year-old obese woman complains of fever, RUQ pain, and nausea that is worse when she eats fatty foods. *Think: Cholecystitis.*

Right Upper Quadrant

- Hepatobiliary: Cholelithiasis, cholecystitis, cholangitis, hepatitis
- Peptic ulcer

Left Upper Quadrant

- Spleen: Trauma, infarction, abscess, rupture (mononucleosis)
- Gastric ulcer

Right Lower Quadrant

- Appendicitis
- Small bowel obstruction
- Crohn's disease

Left Lower Quadrant

- Diverticulitis
- Inflammatory bowel disease

Typical scenario:
A 26-year-old woman complains of severe left lower quadrant pain, vaginal bleeding, and light-headedness. Last menstrual period was 6 weeks ago.
Think: Ectopic pregnancy.

Typical scenario:
A 28-year-old woman presents with diffuse abdominal pain, nausea, and confusion. She is not pregnant. She currently takes a stained-glass class.
Think: Lead poisoning.

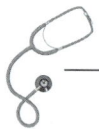

In elderly patients with abdominal pain, always consider vascular causes, including:
- AAA
- Mesenteric ischemia
- Myocardial infarction

Flank Pain
- Nephrolithiasis
- Pyelonephritis
- Testicular torsion
- Prostatitis
- Epididymitis

Adnexal (Lower Abdominal Pain)
- Ectopic pregnancy
- Tubo-ovarian abscess
- Pelvic inflammatory disease
- Ovarian torsion
- Salpingitis
- Cystitis

Anywhere
- Strangulated hernia
- Large bowel obstruction
- Sigmoid volvulus
- Mesenteric ischemia

Note: All premenopausal women with abdominal pain must have a pregnancy test, even if they say they are not sexually active.

Other Causes of Abdominal Pain

Abdominal Wall
- Hernia
- Rectus sheath hematoma

Metabolic
- Diabetic ketoacidosis
- Acute intermittent porphyria
- Hypercalcemia

Infectious
- Herpes zoster
- Mononucleosis
- HIV

Drugs/Toxins
- Heavy metal poisoning
- Black widow spider envenomation

Other
- Sickle cell anemia
- Mesenteric ischemia

Abdominal Pain in the Elderly

Elderly patients who present with abdominal pain must be treated with particular caution. Common problems include:
- Difficulty communicating
- Comorbid disease

- Inability to tolerate intravascular volume loss
- Unusual presentation of common disease
- May not mount a white blood cell count or a fever
- Complaint often incommensurate with severity of disease

Note: Up to 2% of elderly patients with an MI will present with abdominal pain.

Vascular Problems of the Abdomen

▶ ABDOMINAL AORTIC ANEURYSM (AAA)

Definition

Dilation of the abdominal aorta, usually below the renal arteries. Abdominal aortic aneurysms are associated with atherosclerosis. Acute expansion or leak of an AAA causes pain and may precede rupture, a life-threatening emergency.

Risk Factors

- Atherosclerosis
- Aneurysms > 5 cm associated with 20 to 40% 5-year risk of rupture

Typical scenario:
A 63-year-old obese man complains of pain in his "kidney" for 3 days. He has a history of MI × 2. He has no back tenderness. *Think: Abdominal aortic aneurysm.*

Signs and Symptoms

- Abdominal or back pain
- Pulsatile mass in abdomen
- Hypotension (or symptoms of)
- History of vascular disease or atherosclerosis

Diagnosis

MRI or CT scan with IV contrast: Can demonstrate size of aneurysm and location of leak or rupture. May replace angiogram as gold standard.
Angiogram: Can demonstrate size of aneurysm and location of leak or rupture. Can underestimate size of aneurysm with mural thrombus. Gold standard.

Treatment

All patients should have good IV access and a type and cross. Patients with a suspected rupture in progress require emergent surgical repair.

▶ MESENTERIC ISCHEMIA

Typical scenario:
A 72-year-old man with history of A-fib, on digoxin, complains of severe abdominal pain out of proportion to the exam. *Think: Acute mesenteric ischemia.*

Definition

Ischemia of the small bowel due to compromised mesenteric blood supply. This can be chronic, caused by atherosclerotic disease, or acute, caused by an embolus.

Causes

- Atherosclerosis causing obstruction of SMA, IMA, or celiac artery (chronic)
- Atrial fibrillation: Embolus (acute)
- Low-flow state: Hypotension, poor cardiac output
- Hypercoagulability (acute)

Signs and Symptoms

- Severe abdominal pain out of proportion to exam
- History of gnawing abdominal pain after eating
- History of sudden onset of abdominal pain and history of atrial fibrillation or hypercoagulable state
- Labs may show increased lactate, metabolic acidosis

Typical scenario:
A 75-year-old woman with a history of myocardial infarction complains of gnawing abdominal pain after eating. She has lost 15 pounds in the past month. *Think: Chronic mesenteric ischemia.*

Diagnosis

- Gold standard is angiography.
- Spiral CT scan with PO and IV contrast is often useful.
- MRA

Treatment

- Maintain tissue perfusion with fluids.
- Surgery (bypass)

Disorders of the Esophagus

INFECTIOUS ESOPHAGITIS

Etiology

Viral Esophagitis
- Herpes simplex virus
- Varicella-zoster virus
- Cytomegalovirus

Bacterial Esophagitis
- *Lactobacillus*
- *Streptococcus*
- *Cryptosporidium*
- *Pneumocystis carinii*
- *Mycobacterium tuberculosis*

Other Causes
- *Candida*
- Radiation exposure or therapy
- Corrosive exposure

Signs and Symptoms

- Odynophagia
- Dysphagia
- Esophageal bleeding
- Nausea/vomiting
- Chest pain
- May be asymptomatic

Diagnosis

Candida: Nodular filling defects on barium esophagogram
HSV, VZV: Vesicles and discrete erosions on endoscopy
CMV: Intranuclear inclusions on biopsy via endoscopy

Treatment

Candida: Fluconazole PO
HSV: Acyclovir IV
CMV: Ganciclovir IV

Differential: A patient with HIV and odynophagia (pain on swallowing) has esophagitis most likely due to:
- ***Candida***
- **CMV**
- **Herpes**

▶ ESOPHAGEAL PERFORATION OR RUPTURE

Definition

Iatrogenic or pathologic trauma to the esophagus, which may result in leakage of air and esophageal contents into the mediastinum. Carries a 50% mortality.

Etiology

Iatrogenic: This often occurs in an already diseased esophagus. Comprises 50 to 75% of cases of esophageal rupture:
- Endoscopy
- Dilation
- Blakemore tubes
- Intubation of the esophagus
- Nasogastric tube placement

Boerhaave's syndrome: A *full-thickness* tear. Generally occurs in the relatively weak left posterolateral wall of distal esophagus. Due to:
- Forceful vomiting
- Cough
- Trauma

Mallory–Weiss syndrome: A *partial-thickness* tear. Usually occurs in the right posterolateral wall of the distal esophagus and results in bleeding that generally resolves spontaneously. Due to:
- Forceful vomiting

Foreign body ingestion: Objects usually lodge near anatomic narrowings:
- Distal to the upper esophageal sphincter
- Near the aortic arch
- At lower esophageal sphincter

Typical scenario:
An alcoholic man presents after severe retching, complaining of retrosternal and upper abdominal pain. ***Think: Boerhaave's syndrome (full thickness) or Mallory–Weiss syndrome (partial thickness).***

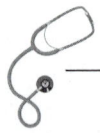

Subcutaneous and mediastinal emphysema are due to a full-thickness tear.

Signs and Symptoms

- Severe, constant pain in chest, abdomen, and back
- Dysphagia
- Dyspnea
- Subcutaneous emphysema
- Mediastinal emphysema heard as a "crunching sound" with heartbeat (Hammon's crunch)

Diagnosis

- **Chest x-ray:** Left-sided pleural effusion, mediastinal or subcutaneous emphysema
- **Esophagogram with *water-soluble* contrast:** Shows extravasation of contrast
- **Other studies:** Endoscopy, CT, and pleurocentesis (check fluid for low pH and high amylase)

Treatment

Surgical repair of full-thickness tears. Partial-thickness tears may resolve spontaneously.

▶ ZENKER'S DIVERTICULUM

Definition

Pharyngeal or esophageal pouch due to a defect in the muscular wall of the posterior hypopharynx

Signs and Symptoms

- Halitosis
- Regurgitation of food days after eating it
- Frequent aspiration
- Esophageal obstruction

Diagnosis

- Barium swallow
- Endoscopy

Treatment

Surgical removal or cricopharyngeal myotomy

Typical scenario:
A 56-year-old man complains of food feeling "stuck" on its way down and vomiting food he ate days ago. *Think: Zenker's diverticulum.*

▶ ESOPHAGEAL SPASM AND ACHALASIA

Definition

- **Achalasia:** A neurogenic disorder of esophageal motility with absence of normal peristalsis and impaired relaxation of lower esophageal sphincter
- **Diffuse esophageal spasm (DES):** Motility disorder with frequent nonperistaltic contractions

See Table 2.3-1.

TABLE 2.3-1. Comparison of Achalasia and Diffuse Esophageal Spasm

	Achalasia	Diffuse Esophageal Spasm
Signs and symptoms	Weight loss, cough, diffuse chest pain	Dysphagia, diffuse chest pain
Pattern of contraction	Failure of LES to relax on swallowing Classic: Simultaneous small wave Vigorous: Simultaneous large wave	Swallow-induced large wave
Relieved by	Nitroglycerin	Nitroglycerin
X-ray findings	"Bird's beak" narrowing of terminal esophagus	Corkscrew appearance
Treatment	Nitroglycerin, local botulinum toxin, balloon dilatation, sphincter myotomy	Nitroglycerin, anticholinergics

Etiology

- Achalasia is thought to arise from scarring in Auerbach's plexus.
- DES shows no physical abnormality in Auerbach's plexus but is thought to arise from hypoactive inhibitory interneurons within it.

Epidemiology

Achalasia has equal incidence in males and females. Ratio not known for diffuse esophageal spasm (DES).

Diagnosis

- Barium swallow (see Figures 2.3-1 and 2.3-2)
- Manometry: Achalasia will show normal to increased pressure at LES with no relaxation upon swallowing; DES will show high-amplitude contractions, possibly including proximal esophagus.

Dysphagia to solids **and** liquids often indicates a motility problem (i.e., achalasia and esophageal spasm). Dysphagia to **only** solids indicates mechanical obstruction (i.e., tumor or Schatzki's ring).

Barium swallow:
- Bird's beak or steeple sign: Achalasia
- Corkscrew-shaped: DES

▶ GI WEBS AND RINGS

The following conditions are anatomical obstructions, usually presenting with dysphagia to solids.

Plummer–Vinson Syndrome

Hypopharyngeal webs (thin mucosal structures protruding into lumen) associated with iron deficiency anemia

Schatzki's Ring

A narrow lower esophageal ringlike outgrowth associated with dysphagia (see Figure 2.3-3)

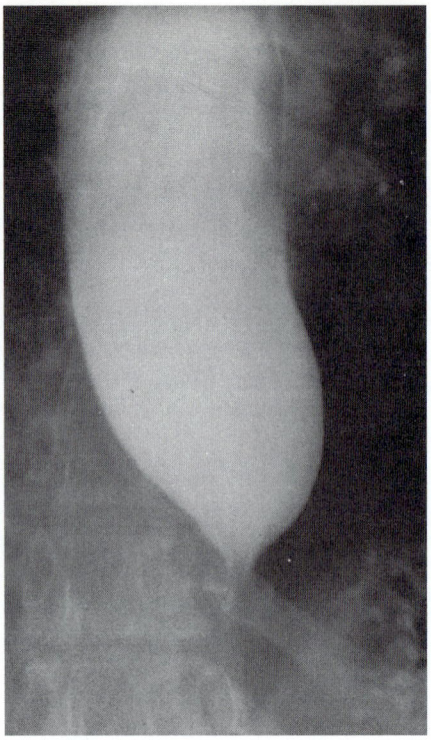

FIGURE 2.3-1. Achalasia.

Barium esophagogram in a patient with achalasia demonstrates a dilated esophagus with a sharply tapered "bird's beak" narrowing. (Reproduced, with permission, from Waters PF, DeMeester TR. Foregut motor disorders and their surgical management. *Med Clin North Am* 65:1244, 1981.)

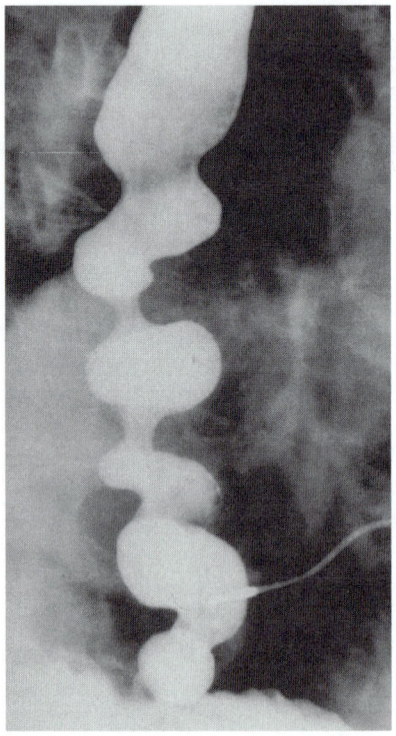

FIGURE 2.3-2. Diffuse esophageal spasm.

Barium esophagogram in a patient with diffuse esophageal spasm demonstrates the characteristic "corkscrew" pattern. (Reproduced, with permission, from *Schwartz's Principles of Surgery*, 7th ed. New York: McGraw-Hill, 2000:1129.)

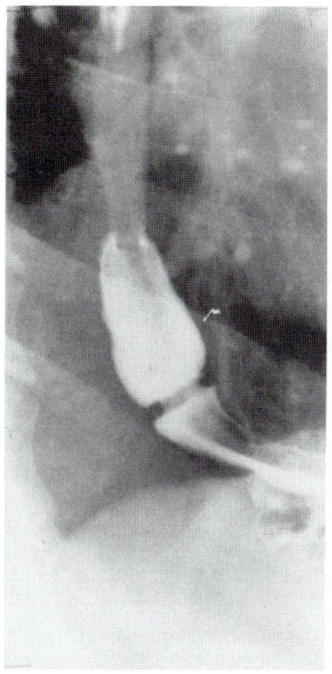

FIGURE 2.3-3. Schatzki's ring.

Barium esophagogram in a patient with Schatzki's ring demonstrates a distal esophageal ring at the gastroesophageal junction. (Reproduced, with permission, from *Schwartz's Principles of Surgery*, 7th ed. New York: McGraw-Hill, 2000:1168.)

▶ GASTROESOPHAGEAL REFLUX DISEASE (GERD)

Definition

Reflux of acidic gastric contents into the esophagus

Causes of GERD

- Relaxed or incompetent lower esophageal sphincter (LES)
- Hiatal hernia
- Delayed gastric emptying
- Decreased esophageal motility

Causes of Lowered LES Tone

- Foods: Coffee, chocolate
- Alcohol
- Cigarettes
- Drugs: Nitrates, calcium channel blockers
- Hormones: Estrogen, progesterone

Signs and Symptoms

- Substernal burning pain
- Dysphagia (secondary to stricture formation)

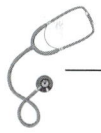

Causes of delayed gastric emptying:
- Diabetes mellitus
- Gastroparesis
- Gastric outlet obstruction
- Anticholinergic use
- Fatty foods

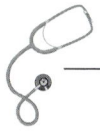

Differential of chronic cough:
- Asthma
- GERD
- Postnasal drip

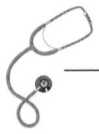

A majority of patients with asthma have associated GERD.

- Hypersalivation (water brash)
- Cough (particularly nocturnal)
- Wheezing

Diagnosis

Often, a trial of proton pump inhibitor will be given to relieve symptoms without further workup. However, if "alarm signals" (weight loss, advanced age, nausea, guaiac +), an endoscopy to rule out cancer is required.

Treatment

Lifestyle Modification
- Elevate head of bed.
- Discontinue foods that decrease LES tone; avoid food < 3 hours before bed

Pharmacologic
- H_2 blocker
- Proton pump inhibitor (continued indefinitely if severe)

Surgical
- Surgical correction such as fundoplication if all else fails

Complications of GERD

Barrett's esophagus carries a 2 to 5% risk of development of esophageal adenocarcinoma, which carries a < 5% chance of 5-year survival.

- **Esophagitis:** Esophageal damage, bleeding, and friability due to prolonged exposure to gastric contents
- **Peptic stricture:** Occurs in about 10% of patients with GERD
- **Barrett's esophagus:** Transformation of normal squamous epithelium to columnar epithelium, sometimes accompanied by an ulcer or stricture. This carries a significant risk of cancerous transformation. High-grade Barrett's requires resection. Other grades of Barrett's require surveillance endoscopy regularly for **life;** Barrett's does **not** regress, even if GERD is successfully treated.
- **Esophageal cancer:** Upper ⅔ squamous, lower ⅓ adenocarcinoma

Disorders of the Stomach

▶ PEPTIC ULCER DISEASE (PUD)

PUD consists of duodenal ulcers (DU) and gastric ulcers (GU).

Epidemiology

- Two times more common in men
- Incidence increases with age.
- Smoking increases risk.

Pathophysiology

Key Concepts

- Parietal cells secrete HCl into the gastric lumen and bicarbonate into the gastric venous circulation (alkaline tide) and into the protective gastric mucous gel.
- A proton pump exchanges potassium in the gastric lumen for protons.
- The parietal cells are stimulated by gastrin and the vagus nerve.
- Gastrin release is stimulated by gastrin-releasing peptide and is inhibited by somatostatin.
- Histamine receptors on parietal cells also stimulate HCl secretion.
- Gastric bicarbonate secretion into the mucous gel is inhibited by nonsteroidal anti-inflammatory drugs (NSAIDs), acetazolamide, alpha blockers, and alcohol.
- Gel thickness is increased by prostaglandin E (PGE) and reduced by steroids and NSAIDs.

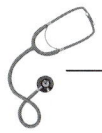

Typical scenario:
A patient with known PUD presents with sudden onset of severe epigastric pain. Physical exam reveals guarding and rebound tenderness.
Think: Perforation.

Complications

- **Bleeding:** 20% incidence
- **Perforation:**
  - 7% incidence
  - Posterior perforation of a duodenal ulcer will cause pain that radiates to the back and can cause pancreatitis. A chest or abdominal film will not show free air because the posterior duodenum is retroperitoneal.
  - Anterior perforation will show free air under the diaphragm in 70% of cases (see Figure 2.3-4).
- **Gastric outlet obstruction,** due to scarring and edema (can also be a complication of neoplasm)

Typical scenario:
A 52-year-old woman presents due to 3 months of early satiety, weight loss, and vomiting.
Think: Gastric outlet obstruction.

► DUODENAL ULCER (DU)

Pathophysiology

Increased acid production

Etiology

H. pylori

- A bacterium that produces urease, which decreases gastric mucosal defenses. Ten to 20% of persons with *H. pylori* develop PUD.

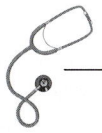

Over 90% of patients with ZE have peptic ulcer disease.

NSAIDs/Steroids

- Inhibit production of PGE thereby inhibiting mucosal barrier production

Zollinger–Ellison Syndrome (ZE)

- A gastrin-secreting tumor in or near the pancreas. ZE can be part of multiple endocrine neoplasia type I (MEN I). Diarrhea is common.
- ZE has a triad of PUD, gastric acid hypersecretion, and an elevated gastrin level.

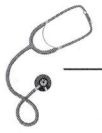

H. pylori may colonize 90% of the population—infection does not necessitate disease.

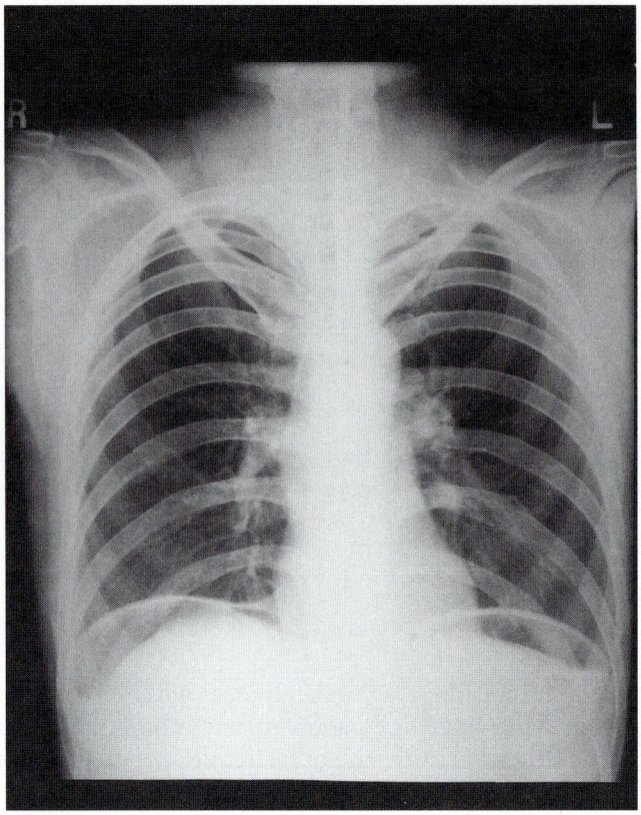

FIGURE 2.3-4. Free air.

Upright chest film in a patient with perforated duodenal ulcer demonstrates free air underneath both right and left hemidiaphragms (Reproduced, with permission, from *Schwartz's Principles of Surgery*, 7th ed. New York: McGraw-Hill, 2000:1195.)

Typical scenario:
A 33-year-old female smoker presents with burning epigastric pain that is improved after eating a meal. *Think: Duodenal ulcer.*

Clinical Features

- Burning gnawing epigastric pain that occurs with an empty stomach: Pain is relieved within 30 minutes by food.
- Nighttime awakening (when stomach empties)
- Nausea, vomiting
- Associated with blood type O
- When bleeding, melena or hematochezia is present.

Diagnosis

Duodenal Ulcer (DU)

- Via endoscopy; however, most symptomatic cases of DU are easily diagnosed clinically. If patient responds to DU therapy, there is no need to do the biopsy.

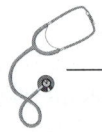

Gastric ulcer pain is typically exacerbated by food. Duodenal ulcer pain is typically relieved by food.

H. pylori

- Endoscopy with biopsy—allows culture and sensitivity for *H. pylori* (organism is notoriously hard to culture—multiple specimens required during biopsy)
- Serology: Anti–*H. pylori* IgG indicates current or prior infection.
- *Urease breath test:* $C^{13/14}$ labeled urea is ingested. If gastric urease is present, the carbon isotope can be detected as CO_2 isotopes in the breath.

ZE

- Secretin stimulation test: Secretin, a gastrin inhibitor, is delivered parenterally (usually with Ca^{2+}), and its effect on gastrin secretion is measured. In ZE syndrome, there is a paradoxical astronomic rise in serum gastrin.
- Gastrin level (must be taken when off antacid meds): If elevated, test for hyperacidity with gastric pH monitor.

Treatment

Treatment of PUD mainly depends on the cause.

- Discontinue NSAIDs, steroids, and smoking.
- Triple therapy for *H. pylori* (e.g., proton pump inhibitor, amoxicillin, and clarithromycin)
- H_2 blockers
- Proton pump inhibitors
- If bleeding, endoscopy is done and sucralfate (enhances mucosal barrier) or misoprostol (prostaglandin analog) is used.
- Surgery is indicated when ulcer is refractory to 12 weeks of medical treatment, or if hemorrhage, obstruction, or perforation is present.

Causes of Peptic Ulcer Disease

- NSAIDs and steroids inhibit production of PGE, which helps produce the gastric mucosal barrier.
- *H. pylori* produces urease, which breaks down the gastric mucosal barrier.

▶ GASTRIC ULCER (GU)

Definition

Ulcer located in the stomach

Pathophysiology

Decreased protection against acid: *normal or low acid production*

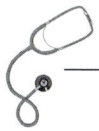

Gastric ulcers can even occur with achlorhydria.

Etiology

- *H. pylori* (less than for duodenal)
- NSAIDs/steroids

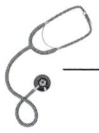

Smoking is a risk factor for gastric ulcer.

Clinical Features

- Burning gnawing epigastric pain that occurs with anything in the stomach: Pain is **worst 30 minutes after food.**
- Anorexia/weight loss
- Vomiting
- Associated with blood type A

Typical scenario:
A 45-year-old Japanese male smoker presents with epigastric pain, exacerbated by eating, and weight loss. *Think: Gastric ulcer.*

Diagnosis

Via endoscopy; 3% of GUs are associated with gastric cancer, so all GUs are biopsied.

Treatment

Same as for DU

▶ GASTRITIS

Definition

- Acute or chronic inflammation of the stomach lining

Etiologies of gastritis: "GNASHING"
- **G**astric reflux (bile or pancreatic secretions)
- **N**icotine
- **A**lcohol
- **S**tress
- ***H**elicobacter pylori* and other infections
- **I**schemia
- **N**SAIDs
- **G**lucocorticoids (long-term use)

Etiology

- Increased acid: Smoking, alcohol, stress
- Decreased mucosal barrier: NSAIDs, steroids, *H. pylori*
- Direct irritant: Pancreatic and biliary reflux, infection
- Autoimmune

Signs and Symptoms

- Burning or gnawing pain
- Pain *usually worsened with food* and relieved by antacids
- Vomiting may relieve the pain after eating.

Diagnosis

Diagnosis is made by endoscopy.

Treatment

- Dicontinue NSAIDs.
- Triple therapy to eradicate *H. pylori* if present (proton pump inhibitor, amoxicillin, clarithromycin)
- Abstain from cigarettes and alcohol.
- H_2 blockers (e.g., cimetidine, ranitidine), sucralfate, or misoprostol
- Over-the-counter antacids

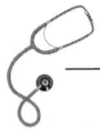

Cimetidine is a p450 inhibitor and, therefore, prolongs the action of drugs cleared in the liver by this system.

Complications

Chronic gastritis leads to:

- Gastric atrophy
- Gastric metaplasia
- Pernicious anemia (decreased production of intrinsic factor from gastric parietal cells due to **idiopathic** atrophy of the gastric mucosa and subsequent malabsorption of vitamin B_{12})
- Gastric carcinoma, gastric lymphoma

Disorders of the Pancreas

▶ ACUTE PANCREATITIS

Definition

- Inflammation of the pancreas due to parenchymal autodigestion by proteolytic enzymes
- In severe cases, it can be associated with a *systemic inflammatory response syndrome* (SIRS), which can progress to multi-organ system failure and ARDS.

Normal Function of the Pancreas

Exocrine: Bicarbonate, amylase, lipase, tyrosine, and other digestive enzymes
Endocrine: Insulin, glucagon, somatostatin

Etiologies

- Gallstones
- EtOH
- Hypertriglycerides
- Endoscopic retrograde cholangiopancreatography (ERCP)
- Drugs (thiazides, furosemide, estrogen, antiretrovirals)
- Structural problems (neoplasm)

Signs and Symptoms

- Severe, constant midepigastric or LUQ pain, *radiates to the back*
- Pain sometimes improved when patient sits up and leans forward
- Nausea, vomiting
- Low-grade fever
- Tachypnea
- Abdomen is usually tender with guarding, but no rebound.

Diagnostic Markers

Amylase

- Secreted by the pancreas to break down carbohydrates
- Also found in salivary glands, small bowel, ovaries, testes, skeletal muscle
- May be persistently elevated in renal insufficiency
- A level three times the upper limit of normal is 75% specific and 80 to 90% sensitive for pancreatitis.

Lipase

- Secreted by the pancreas to break down triglycerides
- Also found in gastric and intestinal mucosa, and liver
- A level two times the upper limit of normal is 90% specific and 80 to 90% sensitive.

Imaging Pancreatitis

- Abdominal film: May see calcification of pancreas, which is indicative of chronic pancreatitis or the "sentinel loop" of a localized small bowel ileus.
- Ultrasound: May identify gallstones as the cause
- ERCP: Allows direct visualization and sphincterotomy of ampulla of Vater for relief of biliary obstruction
- Contrast-enhanced dynamic CT (CECT): May show degree of pancreatic necrosis

Prognosis

Ranson's criteria (see Table 2.3-2)

A patient with a history of EtOH abuse has abdominal pain and calcifications on abdominal x-ray. *Think: Chronic pancreatitis.*

*Hyper*calcemia can cause pancreatitis, and pancreatitis can cause *hypo*calcemia.

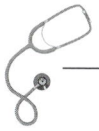

Most common causes of pancreatitis: Gallstones and EtOH

Typical scenario:
A 50-year-old male alcoholic presents with midepigastric pain radiating to the back. He is leaning forward on his stretcher and vomiting. *Think: Pancreatitis.*

Typical scenario:
A 66-year-old female with HTN and seizures for which she is on furosemide and valproic acid, presents with abdominal pain, back pain, and fever. Her nonfasting glucose is noted to be 300. *Think: Pancreatitis.*

TABLE 2.3-2. Ranson's Criteria (Predicts Risk of Mortality in Pancreatitis)

On Admission	After 48 hours
Age > 55	Drop in hematocrit > 10%
Blood sugar > 200	Increase in BUN > 5
WBC > 16,000	Calcium < 8
SGOT > 250	PO_2 < 60 mm Hg
LDH > 700	Base deficit > 4
	Fluid deficit > 6 L

Number of Risk Factors	Mortality
< 3	1%
3 or 4	16%
5 or 6	40%
> 6	Approaches 100%

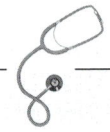

Elevated lipase is more specific than amylase for diagnosing pancreatitis.

Treatment

- IV hydration
- Bowel rest, NG tube for vomiting or associated ileus
- Analgesics and antiemetics as needed
- Antibiotics (e.g., imipenem) if infection is suspected

A sentinel loop is distention and/or air–fluid levels near a site of abdominal distention. In pancreatitis, it is secondary to pancreatitis-associated ileus.

Sequelae

- < 48 hours: Pleural effusion containing high-amylase peripancreatic fluid
- 1 to 4 weeks: Pseudocyst (diagnosed by CT); if it persists it can rupture or create a fistula, so surgical drainage is required.
- 4 to 6 weeks: Abscess; requires surgical drainage

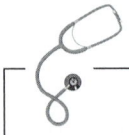

Gastric varices (without esopohageal varices) indicates splenic vein thrombosis, which is a complication of pancreatitis.

▶ CHRONIC PANCREATITIS

Definition

Recurrent episodes of acute pancreatitis, usually from alcohol abuse (70 to 80%), which leads to inflammation, scarring, and duct obstruction

Signs and Symptoms

- Pain similar to acute pancreatitis
- Malabsorption
- Steatorrhea
- Elevated blood sugars
- Polyuria
- Associated with chronic liver disease

Diagnosis

Pancreatic calcifications on x-ray, diabetes, steatorrhea

Workup

Do x-ray, get trypsin level (low indicates poorly functioning pancreas). If these are inconclusive, do CT and/or ERCP (looking for abnormal duct anatomy). Finally, if all is still inconclusive, do secretin test.

Treatment

Same as for acute pancreatitis, with emphasis on pain control and abstinence from alcohol and fatty foods. May need pancreatic enzyme supplements.

A patient with history of EtOH abuse presents with severe abdominal pain exacerbated by food. Imaging shows calcifications of pancreas. *Diagnosis: Chronic pancreatitis.*

Disorders of the Biliary Tree

▶ BILE STORAGE AND RELEASE

Bile is produced in the liver and stored in the gallbladder where it is acidified and concentrated. The presence of fat and amino acids in the proximal duodenum causes release of cholecystokinin, which stimulates gallbladder contraction.

CHOLELITHIASIS

Definition

Gallstones

Mechanisms of Gallstone Formation

- Increased secretion of cholesterol in bile
- Increased formation of solid cholesterol nuclei
- Decreased gallbladder emptying

Signs and Symptoms

- RUQ pain that lasts between 2 and 6 hours. About two thirds of patients will have pain after meals—often worse with fatty foods.
- Nausea and vomiting are common.

Risk factors for cholelithiasis: **(8 Fs)**
Female
Fat
Fertile
Forty
Fibrosis, cystic
Familial
Fasting
F-Hgb (sickle cell disease)
Also:
Diabetes
Oral contraceptives

Gallstone composition:
- **Cholesterol (70%): Radiolucent (seen in rapid weight loss, oral contraception, ileal disease)**
- **Pigment (20%): Radiodense (seen in hemolysis)**
- **Mixed (10%)**

- On exam, the patient will be mildly tender in the RUQ *without* guarding or rebound.

Diagnosis

- AST/ALT to evaluate for hepatitis
- Alkaline phosphatase and bilirubin (direct fraction more elevated than indirect) to evaluate for common duct stones
- Amylase/lipase for concomitant pancreatitis
- RUQ ultrasound to detect gallstones

Treatment

- Chenodeoxycholate to dissolve stones (not very effective)
- Lithotripsy (extracorporeal shock wave treatment; breaks up stones)
- Low-fat diet
- Cholecystectomy is definitive; if asymptomatic, do nothing, as only 20% develop symptoms.

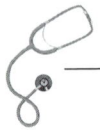

Note: **Meperidine (Demerol) is thought to produce less spasm of the Sphincter of Oddi than morphine, *although clinical evidence is lacking.***

CHOLECYSTITIS

Definition

Gallbladder inflammation, ischemia, or infection usually due to an obstructing stone

Note: Infection *is not necessary* to make the diagnosis of acute cholecystitis but may complicate up to 75% of the cases.

Etiology

- Tumor
- Abscess
- Infection (*E. coli, Klebsiella, Enterococcus, Bacteroides*)

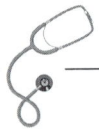

Murphy's sign: The arrest of inspiration while palpating the RUQ. This test is > 95% sensitive for acute cholecystitis, but less sensitive in the elderly.

Signs and Symptoms

- RUQ pain often longer than the 6 hours' duration
- Guarding and rebound may occur
- Fever
- Tachycardia
- Murphy's sign (see box)

Diagnosis

- Elevated white cell count with increased PMNs
- Ultrasound findings: Presence of gallstones, thickened gallbladder wall, pericholecystic fluid (presence of all three has a positive predictive value of > 90%)
- **HIDA** *(the study of choice)*: For this test, technetium 99m-labeled iminodiacetic acid is injected IV and is taken up by hepatocytes. In normals, the gallbladder is outlined within 1 hour; absence of visible gallbladder on HIDA = cholecystitis.

Treatment

- Pain control
- Administration of second- or third-generation cephalosporin
- The definitive treatment is cholecystectomy.

Complications

Fistula, gallstone ileus, perforation, pancreatitis, gangrene

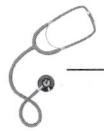

Gold standard test for cholecystitis is HIDA scan.

▶ ACALCULOUS CHOLECYSTITIS

Definition

Cholecystitis without stones

- 5 to 10% of cases of cholecystitis (usually occurs in seriously ill patients [e.g., trauma, burns])
- More rapid downhill clinical course
- Increased morbidity and mortality

Risk factors include increased age, DM, multiple trauma, HIV, extensive burn, major surgery, prolonged labor, systemic vasculitides, gallbladder torsion, and infections of the biliary tract.

▶ ASCENDING CHOLANGITIS

Definition

Complete obstruction of the biliary outflow tract due to a stone obstructing the common bile duct (choledocholelithiasis), a stricture or tumor. The patient becomes septic, and it is life threatening.

Signs and Symptoms

- *Charcot's triad* (see box) occurs in only about 25% of patients and lacks specificity.
- Patients may also develop shock and altered mental status (Reynolds' pentad), which carries a worse prognosis.

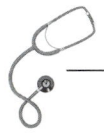

Charcot's triad:
- **RUQ pain**
- **Jaundice**
- **Fever**

Reynolds' pentad:
- **Shock (hypotension)**
- **Altered mental status**

Diagnosis

Ultrasound may show stones in the common bile duct.

Treatment

- ERCP with endoscopic sphincterotomy is crucial (diagnostic and therapeutic).
- Fluid resuscitation, vasopressors as needed
- Antibiotics to cover *E. coli*, *Klebsiella*, *Enterococcus*, and *Bacteroides*

Typical scenario:
A 34-year-old man with a history of ulcerative colitis presents with jaundice and elevated GGT and alkaline phosphatase. *Think: Primary sclerosing cholangitis.*

▶ PRIMARY SCLEROSING CHOLANGITIS

Definition

Chronic progressive disorder of unknown etiology characterized by inflammation, fibrosis, and strictures of the medium- and large-diameter intrahepatic and extrahepatic biliary tree. Many develop cholangiocarcinoma. There is a strong association with ulcerative colitis.

Treatment

Balloon dilatation of obstructed biliary tree. The only cure is a liver transplant.

Disorders of the Liver

▶ NORMAL FUNCTION OF THE LIVER

- Carbohydrate metabolism (glucose homeostasis)
- Plasma protein synthesis
- Bile acid synthesis
- Coagulation factor synthesis
- Lipid synthesis
- Vitamin storage
- Detoxification of many endogenous and exogenous substances
- Hormone metabolism
- Nitrogenous waste processing (urea cycle)

See Table 2.3-3 for explanation of liver function tests.

TABLE 2.3-3. A Comparison of Lab Findings in Obstructive and Parenchymal Liver Disease

Test	Obstructive	Parenchymal
AST/ALT	Slight elevation	Very high
Alkaline phosphatase	Very high	Slight elevation
Albumin	Normal	Decreased
PT	Normal–slight elevation	Very high
Bilirubin: Direct (conjugated)	Normal–very high	Normal–very high
Bilirubin: Indirect (unconjugated)	Normal–slight elevation	Normal–very high
GGT	Very high	Normal–very high

PT and albumin are the only true tests of liver function; they are both synthesized by the liver.

▶ CIRRHOSIS

Definition

Chronic hepatic injury associated with hepatocellular necrosis, fibrosis, and nodular regeneration. There are many causes of cirrhosis (EtOH, hepatitis, etc.) listed below. They all share a similar clinical picture.

Signs and Symptoms

- Loss of appetite, nausea, vomiting
- Jaundice (from high bilirubin)
- Signs of portal hypertension (varices, spider angiomata, ascites, edema)
- Tender hepatomegaly
- Bleeding (from decreased clotting factors made in liver)
- Encephalopathy (from increased NH_4)
- Palmar erythema
- Dupuytren's contractures (contractures of palmar fascia resulting in flexion of 4th digit)
- Gynecomastia and hypogonadism

A patient with alcoholic cirrhosis comes in vomiting blood. He is stabilized with fluid. What is the next step? *Octreotide*

▶ ALCOHOLIC CIRRHOSIS

Most common cause of cirrhosis in North America

Etiology

Caused by chronic alcoholism. *Alcoholic fatty liver,* a mostly asymptomatic, reversible form of liver injury, often precedes cirrhosis. *Alcoholic hepatitis* initiates the necrosis.

Diagnosis

Common Laboratory Abnormalities/Tests

- Liver biopsy
- Anemia
- Elevated bilirubin (direct and indirect)
- AST/ALT ratio > 2
- Elevated GGT
- In severe disease: Prolonged PT and low albumin

Treatment

- Cease alcohol consumption.
- High-protein diet (1 g/kg body weight) and multivitamins
- Avoid hepatotoxins (e.g., acetaminophen, INH).
- Consider glucocorticoids and colchicine to decrease inflammation.
- Spironolactone (potassium-sparing diuretic) for ascites
- Lactulose for hepatic encephalopathy (broken down by colonic bacteria and causes NH_3 to convert to NH_4, which cannot cross the blood–brain barrier)

Nonalcoholic causes of cirrhosis:

- Postviral
- Primary biliary cirrhosis
- Secondary biliary cirrhosis
- Cardiac cirrhosis
- Wilson's disease
- Alpha-1-antitrypsin deficiency
- Hemochromatosis

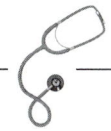

GGT is the most sensitive serum marker for recent alcohol bingeing.

▶ PRIMARY BILIARY CIRRHOSIS

Primary biliary cirrhosis: Women, autoimmune diseases
vs.
Primary sclerosing cholangitis: Men, ulcerative colitis

Definition

Autoimmune disease causing destruction of *intrahepatic* bile ducts

Etiology

Unknown, but *antimitochondrial antibodies* are the serologic hallmark and the pathology results from an autoimmune response to the biliary epithelium.

Epidemiology

More common in middle-aged women, often associated with autoimmune disease (scleroderma, Sjögren's)

Signs and Symptoms

- Pruritus
- Jaundice
- Xanthelasmas, xanthomas (from high cholesterol)
- Presence of an additional (extrahepatic) autoimmune disorder (e.g., RA or Sjögren's)

Diagnosis

Presence of antimitochondrial antibodies (90% sensitive)

Treatment

- Liver transplant is the only cure.
- Ursodiol (ursodeoxycholate [synthetic bile acid]) may slow progression.

▶ PORTAL HYPERTENSION

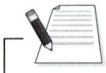

Schistosomiasis is the most common cause of portal hypertension worldwide.

Definition

Increased portal vascular resistance caused by cirrhosis, portal vein obstruction, or hepatic vein thrombosis

Complications

- Esophageal varices
- Splenomegaly
- Ascites
- Hemorrhoids
- Caput medusae (periumbilical collaterals visible on abdomen)

Treatment

- Portosystemic shunt surgery
- TIPS (transjugular intrahepatic portacaval shunt) between hepatic and portal veins

- Propranolol reduces portal pressure and prevents variceal bleeds.
- Liver transplant

ESOPHAGEAL VARICEAL BLEEDING

Definition

Bleeding from esophageal vessels that have increased pressure 2° to portal hypertension. **Variceal bleeding** presents as hematemesis or postural hypotension in a patient with known or suspected portal hypertension.

Treatment

- Maintain perfusion pressure with normal saline and blood as needed.
- Replace clotting factors with FFP.
- Somatostatin (octreotide)
- Beta blockade
- Endoscopic sclerotherapy or banding
- Balloon tamponade

HEPATIC ENCEPHALOPATHY

Definition

Neurobehavioral changes associated with hepatocellular dysfunction

Etiology

- Increased CNS GABA due to high circulating precursor amino acids
- Increased endogenous benzodiazepines
- Cerebral edema
- The direct role of ammonia is questioned.

Signs and Symptoms

- Mental status progression from mild to moderate to marked confusion, to coma
- Asterixis (unless patient is in coma)
- Fetor hepaticus (peculiar breath smell) may be present.

Diagnosis

- Exclude acute alcohol intoxication, delirium tremens, infection, trauma, and metabolic disorders.

Treatment

- Protein restriction
- Lactulose (is metabolized by gut bacteria to small acids. The acidification of the stool favors conversion of ammonia to ammonium ion, which gets trapped in the colonic lumen)
- Neomycin (kills urease-producing bacteria in the gut, so that urea can be excreted, rather than ammonia reabsorbed)
- Look for source of infection and consider empiric antibiotics.

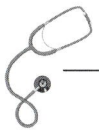

Acute variceal bleeds have a 50% mortality.

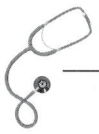

GI functions of somatostatin:
- Inhibit visceral blood flow
- Inhibit gastric acid secretion
- Inhibit gastric motility
- Inhibit gallbladder emptying
- Inhibit pancreatic enzyme and bicarbonate secretion
- Inhibit intestinal absorption of glucose, water, amino acids, and triglycerides

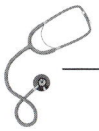

Hepatic encephalopathy precipitated by:
- Gastrointestinal bleed
- Increased dietary protein
- Infection

A patient presents with bleeding esophageal varices. After stabilizing with IV fluid, what is the next step? *Octreotide.*

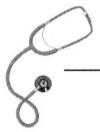

In early liver disease, patients are placed on a high-protein diet because the general state of protein malnutrition puts the body at a disadvantage to fight other stresses such as infection. In end-stage liver disease, the liver cannot break down protein, and the excess accumulation can cause encephalopathy. At this stage, the patient is protein restricted.

Most common organism in SBP: *E. coli*

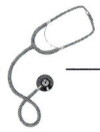

Hepatorenal syndrome can be precipitated by fluid shifts (aggressive diuresis, bleeding paracentesis, contrast dye).

▶ SPONTANEOUS BACTERIAL PERITONITIS

Definition

An acute bacterial peritonitis in patients with ascites

Signs and Symptoms

- Presence of ascites
- Fever, chills
- Generalized abdominal pain with rebound
- May progress to sepsis with change in level of consciousness

Diagnosis

Via Paracentesis (Abdominal Tap)

- > 250 polymorphonuclear cells/μL considered diagnostic
- Gram stain
- Culture and sensitivity

Treatment

- Cover enteric gram negatives (e.g., cefuroxime).
- Monitor electrolytes carefully (hypokalemia and hypernatremia common)

▶ HEPATORENAL SYNDROME

Definition

The development of acute renal failure in patients with advanced hepatic disease, characterized by azotemia, sodium retention, and oliguria

Signs and Symptoms

- Worsening azotemia
- Oliguria
- Hypotension

Diagnosis

- Urine sodium < 10 meq/L
- Hyponatremia

Treatment

- None proven effective
- Restoring plasma volume if low is occasionally successful.

▶ HEPATITIS

Definition

Systemic infection or inflammation of the liver due to viral agents, toxins, or alcohol

Etiology

- Viral hepatitis A, B, C, D ("delta"), E, or G
- Alcohol
- Toxins: Acetaminophen, aflatoxin (found in peanuts)

Signs and Symptoms

- Right upper quadrant pain
- Nausea, vomiting, malaise, fever
- Jaundice

Etiology of viral hepatitis:
- **Vowels from the bowels (A and E, fecal–oral route)**
- **Consonants from "consumance" (B, C, D, G from sex and blood)**

Hepatitis A Virus

Definition

- RNA virus
- Spread by fecal–oral route
- 15- to 50-day incubation
- No chronic carrier or infection state

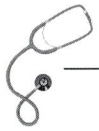

Hepatotoxicity due to acetaminophen (APAP) can be *prevented* by early determination of APAP levels and administration of *N*-acetylcysteine.

Diagnosis

- Anti-HAV IgM = acute infection
- Anti-HAV IgG = immunity from prior infection

Treatment

- Treatment is symptomatic.
- Self-limited, no progression to chronic liver disease
- Prevention:
  - Anti-HAV immunoglobulin is 90% effective if given within 2 weeks of exposure.
  - HAV vaccine is given to all with chronic liver disease (especially hepatitis C), travel to high-risk countries, high-risk behavior, high-risk communities

Hepatitis B Virus

Definition

- DNA virus
- Spread by percutaneous or mucous membrane exposure to blood, semen, and saliva
- 45- to 160-day incubation

HBV is the *only* DNA hepatic virus.

Diagnosis

- HbsAg positive = infection is present
- Anti-HBc IgM = the infection is acute (window period)
- Anti-HBs IgG = past infection or vaccine (indicates immunity)

For explanation of more Hep B markers, see Table 2.3-4.

TABLE 2.3-4. Hepatitis B Markers

Disease State	Marker	Approximate Time from Exposure to Detection in Serum	Explanation
Early infection	HBcAg (hepatitis B core antigen)	Never detectable	Intracellular antigen expressed in infected hepatocytes; not detectable in the serum
Acute infection	Anti-HBc IgM	1.5–6 months	Window period (there can be a several week gap between the disappearance of HBsAg and the appearance of anti-HBs in the serum, during this time infection can be detected with anti-HBc IgM)
Active hepatitis or carrier	HBsAg	1–6 months	Viral protein coat
High infectivity, chronic hepatitis	HBeAg	1–4 months	Indicates ongoing viral replication
Low infectivity	Anti-HBe	4 months–years	Present in acute phase
Immunity (past infection or vaccine)	Anti-HBs IgG	6 months–years	In serum after disappearance of HBsAg
Remote infection	Anti-HBc IgG	6 months–years	Remains detectable longest

Hepatitis B Exposure Scenarios

- Exposed newborn: Give HBIG vaccine.
- Infected blood exposure: Test for hepatitis B and if negative, give HBIG alone.
- Vaccine is okay in pregnancy.

PREVENTION

- Vaccine
- Hepatitis B immune globulin (HBIG) (if < 7 days of exposure)

TREATMENT

Lamivudine

COMPLICATIONS

- 1% will develop fulminant hepatic necrosis.
- 10% of adults (90% neonates) will develop chronic carrier state or chronic hepatitis with an increased hepatocellular cancer risk.

Hepatitis C Virus

Note: Hepatitis G virus is very similar to HCV.

DEFINITION

- RNA virus
- Spread by blood and body fluid contact (common from past blood transfusions and tattoos, IV drugs)

- Incubation 15 to 160 days
- Most common hepatitis in the United States

Diagnosis

- Anti-HCV IgG presents 1 to 6 months after infectivity and indicates chronic or past infection.
- PCR for hepatitis C RNA measures viral load or disease activity.

Treatment

Interferon and ribavirin (reduce risk of hepatoma)

Complications

Seventy to 80% develop chronic hepatitis and 25% of these develop cirrhosis and/or hepatocellular carcinoma.

Hepatitis D Virus or "Delta" Agent

- "Defective" RNA virus; requires HBV for replication and expression
- Spread by blood or body fluid exposure as a *coinfection* (simultaneously with HBV) or a *superinfection* (patient already infected with HBV)
- If coinfection of hepatitis B and D, infection and complications are more severe.
- Diagnosis is anti-HDV IgM.

Hepatitis E Virus

- RNA virus
- Incubation 15 to 60 days
- Fecal–oral transmission
- Occurs in India, Asia, Africa, and Central America
- High rate of fulminant liver failure, especially if pregnant
- No chronic carrier or infection state
- Only supportive treatment

Typical scenario:
A medical resident develops fever, jaundice, and fatigue 2 weeks after returning from a trip to India.
Think: Hepatitis E.

▶ LIVER TRANSPLANTATION

Definition

- Used in selected cases of severe, irreversible liver disease
- Currently has a 5-year survival rate of better than 80%
- Factors to determine eligibility reflect severity of disease: Bilirubin, INR, creatinine

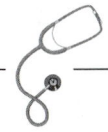

Indications for liver transplant:
- Cirrhosis (biliary, alcoholic.)
- 1° sclerosing cholangitis
- Hepatitis (chronic, fulminant)
- Hepatocellular carcinoma
- Hepatic vein thrombosis

Immunosuppression

- Cyclophosphamide
- Tacrolimus
- OKT3

Acute Rejection

Suspect in transplant recipients with:
- RUQ pain, fever
- Increased serum bilirubin, transaminases
- Treat with steroids, lymphocyte antibodies

Donor Liver

- Needs to be size and ABO matched
- Does not require Rh or HLA matching

Disorders of the Colon

▶ CARCINOID TUMOR

Carcinoid constitutes one third of all primary gut neoplasms.

Types of GI cancer differ based on region:
- Esophagus: Squamous and adenocarcinoma
- Duodenum and jejunum: Adenocarcinoma
- Ileum: Carcinoid, lipoma, and lymphoma

Definition

- Neuroendocrine tumor arising from ectodermal stem cells in the gut
- Generally slow growing
- 90% in ileum—most in appendix
- Secretes neurotransmitters and hormones, commonly:
  - Serotonin (5-HT), bradykinin, histamine
- Metastases (in order of frequency):
  - Regional lymph nodes
  - Liver (graver prognosis)
  - Lung

Etiology

- Most idiopathic
- Part of MEN type I

Signs and Symptoms

- Carcinoid syndrome:
  - Occurs in only 5 to 10% of carcinoid tumors
  - Classic triad:
    1. Flushing, hypotension—bradykinin
    2. Diarrhea—serotonin
    3. Right-sided valvular heart disease—serotonin
  - Wheezing is also common (histamine).
  - Small bowel obstruction, appendicitis

Diagnosis

- > 10 mg/24 hr urine 5-HIAA is 75% sensitive and 100% specific.
- Elevated serum and urinary 5-HT
- Abdominal CT for primary tumors, lymph nodes, and liver metastases

Treatment

- Surgical excision
- Radiation therapy
- Antihormonal therapy as needed

Prognosis

- With carcinoid syndrome, median survival is 3 years.
- Appendiceal primaries have 99% 5-year survival.
- Extra-appendiceal primaries have 50% 5-year survival.

▶ DIVERTICULOSIS

Definition

- An *acquired* condition of the colon in which saclike protrusions of colonic mucosa herniate through a defect in the muscle layer (where nutrient arteries insert) (see Figure 2.3-5)
- Diverticulae are most common in the sigmoid colon, probably because this is the narrowest area of the colon and therefore subject to the highest pressures.

Etiology

- Low-fiber diet, less bulk in the stool
- Frequency increases directly with age—50% affected by age 65 in the United States

Diverticulosis is the most common cause of massive lower GI bleeding in patients over age 60.

Signs and Symptoms

Can cause **painless** rectal **bleeding**

Pathophysiology of Diverticular Bleeding

- An inflamed diverticulum erodes through a colonic artery causing sudden, profuse, painless bleeding, usually from right-sided diverticula.
- Seventy-five to 95% of the cases stop bleeding spontaneously.

Treatment of Diverticular Bleeding

Bleeding scan and embolization; surgery if refractory

▶ DIVERTICULITIS

Definition

Inflammation and or infection of a diverticulum due to impaction of fecal material in the diverticular neck

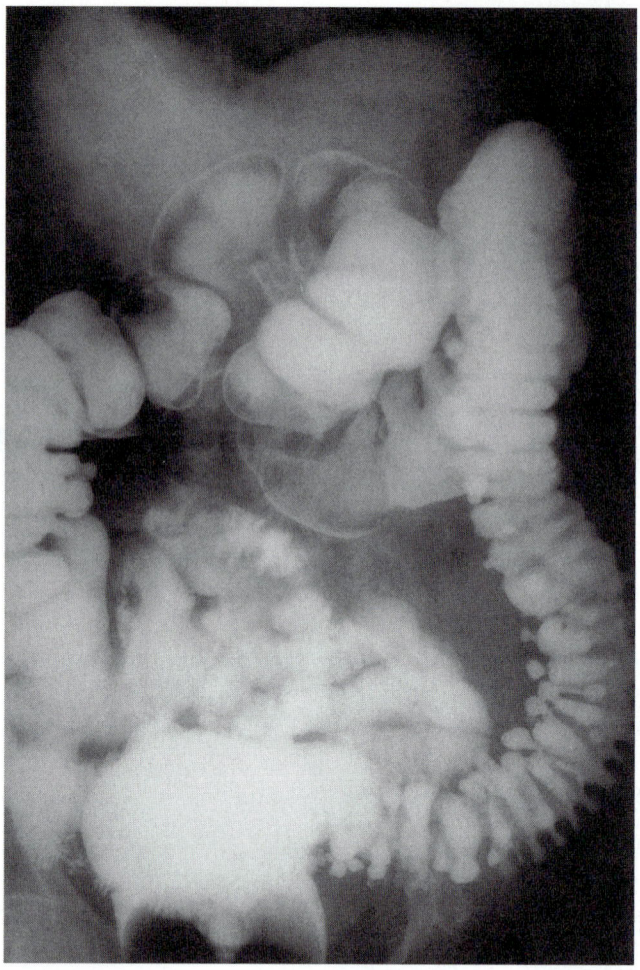

FIGURE 2.3-5. Diverticulosis.

Barium study in a patient with diverticulosis demonstrates many small contrast-filled outpouchings in the sigmoid colon. (Reproduced, with permission, from *Schwartz's Principles of Surgery*, 7th ed. New York: McGraw-Hill, 2000:1277.)

Signs and Symptoms

- LLQ pain
- Fever
- High WBC
- May have sigmoid mass on exam

Diagnosis

- Abdominal CT may help define the extent of disease:
  - CT findings are inflammation of pericolic fat, diverticula, bowel-wall thickening, +/– abscess
- **Never** do colonoscopy (risk of perforation)

Treatment

- NPO, IV fluids, pain control
- Antibiotics to cover gram-negative anaerobes, particularly *E. coli*, *Klebsiella*, *Enterobacter*, *Bacteroides*, and *Enterococcus* (typically ciprofloxacin and metronidazole [Flagyl] or clindamycin and gentamicin)

▶ PSEUDOMEMBRANOUS COLITIS

Definition

Colonic infection caused by *Clostridium difficile*, a spore-forming anaerobe found normally in GI tract. When *C. difficile* overgrows, due to eradication of competing gut flora by antibiotics, it may release a toxin, which damages colon mucosa.

Classically caused by clindamycin, but any antibiotic can do it—even metronidazole and vancomycin, which are used to treat it.

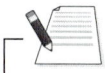

C. difficile is the most common cause of nosocomial enteric infection.

Signs and Symptoms

- Crampy, diffuse abdominal pain
- Fever
- Watery (occasionally bloody) diarrhea

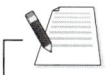

Typical scenario:
A 68-year-old man in the hospital for 3 weeks for pneumonia returns with new-onset diarrhea.
Think: C. difficile.

Diagnosis

- *C. difficile* toxin in stool (insensitive)
- Fecal leukocytes
- Sigmoidoscopy: Yellowish membranous plaques (pseudomembranes) adherent to colonic mucosa are pathognomonic.

Treatment

- Stop the offending antibiotic if possible.
- Metronidazole PO or vancomycin PO

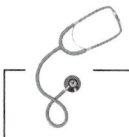

Vancomycin is almost never given PO, except in the case of pseudomembranous colitis. The reason is because it has such poor GI absorption.

Complications

Toxic megacolon can occur when inflammation and infection spread through all layers of the colon wall. Severe diarrhea and toxicity develop. Plain radiography may show a long, colon loop with diameter > 6 cm and "thumbprinting" (bowel-wall edema)—these patients will likely need a colectomy.

▶ IRRITABLE BOWEL SYNDROME

An alteration of intestinal motility that leads to changes in bowel habits. The "resting pressures" in patients with IBS may fluctuate between spasm (constipation) and laxity (diarrhea). It typically presents in young people and is twice as common in females. Diagnosis requires that other causes of diarrhea are ruled out.

There is a strong relationship between symptoms and psychosocial stress in irritable bowel syndrome.

Signs and Symptoms

- Fluctuating constipation and diarrhea
- Increased with stress
- Lack of systemic symptoms

Treatment

- Reassurance
- High-fiber and low-fat diet
- Anxiolytic, antispasmodic, or antidiarrheal may help with more severe cases.

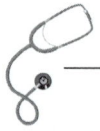

Giardia infection and lactose intolerance may present similarly to IBS, so they must be ruled out.

▶ INFLAMMATORY BOWEL DISEASE

Definition

A chronic, inflammatory disease affecting GI tract. Two major types are Crohn's disease (CD) and ulcerative colitis (UC).

Epidemiology

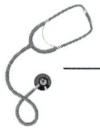

Crohn's: Lower incidence, lower risk of cancer, more common in men than UC.

- More common in people of Caucasian and Jewish background
- Peak incidence in ages 15 to 35
- Occurs with familial clustering
- Incidence: UC = 2–10/100,000; CD = 1–6/100,000
- UC more common in women
- CD more common in men
- Associated risk of colon cancer is 10 to 30 times for UC and 3 times for CD.

Signs and Symptoms

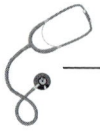

Inflammatory bowel disease symptoms improve with nicotine. Patients can wear dermal patches.

UC
- Bloody diarrhea (more prominent than in CD)
- Rectal pain
- More acute flares

CD
- Tender RLQ mass
- More indolent, chronic

Extraintestinal manifestations affect 20% of patients with IBD (see Table 2.3-5).

Pathology

UC
- Inflammation of the **mucosa only** (exudate of pus, blood, and mucous from the *crypt abscess*)
- Always **starts in rectum** (up to ⅓ don't progress).

CD
- Inflammation involves **all bowel-wall layers,** which is what may lead to fistulas and abscess.
- Rectal sparing in 50%
- Granulomas

TABLE 2.3-5. Extraintestinal Manifestations of Inflammatory Bowel Disease

Eye involvement	▪ Uveitis ▪ Episcleritis	CD > UC Uveitis, erythema nodosum, and colitic arthritis are commonly seen together.
Dermatologic	▪ Erythema nodosum ▪ Pyoderma gangrenosum ▪ Aphthous ulcers	CD, especially in children > UC Parallels disease course (gets better as IBD improves) UC > CD May or may not follow disease course CD
Arthritis	▪ Colitic arthritis ▪ Ankylosing spondylitis	CD > UC Parallels disease course 30 times more common in UC Unrelated to disease course
Hematologic	▪ Anemia ▪ Thromboembolism	
Hepatobiliary	▪ Fatty liver ▪ Hepatitis ▪ Cholelithiasis ▪ Primary sclerosing cholangitis	 UC > CD
Renal	▪ Secondary amyloidosis leading to renal failure	CD Unrelated to disease course

Diagnosis (Colonoscopy Findings)

UC

- **Continuous lesions** (always includes rectum)
- **Apthous ulcers rare**
- **Lead pipe colon** appearance due to chronic scarring and subsequent retraction and loss of haustra

CD

- **Skip lesions:** Interspersed normal and diseased bowel
- **Aphthous ulcers common**
- **Cobblestone** appearance (from submucosal thickening interspersed with mucosal ulceration)

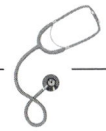

Sulfasalazine is also used to treat rheumatoid arthritis, but in RA, it is the sulfapyridine component that is the active one.

Complications

UC

- Perforation
- Stricture
- Megacolon

CD

- Abscess
- Fistulas
- Perianal disease (abscess, fistula)

Treatment

Sulfasalazine

- Consists of 5-ASA (active component) and sulfapyridine (toxic effects are due to this moiety)

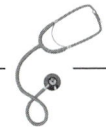

Drugs with only the 5-ASA component are not effective.

- How it works in IBD is unknown (because other NSAIDs do not work). It is activated in the colon by colonic bacteria, so it is ineffective for small bowel.

Mesalamine
- Like sulfasalazine but active in small bowel if taken orally; active in colon if given by enema

Corticosteroids
- May be given as enemas (decreases systemic absorption)or orally
- Work better in UC than CD

Antibiotics (Used for CD)
- Metronidazole and has been used to induce disease remission with some success.

Immunomodulators
- Used in refractory cases, especially in CD on chronic steroids
- Include azathioprine and 6-mercaptopurine (both purine analogs) and methotrexate
- Infliximab (Remicade) (antibody to TNF-α) is used in severe CD.

▶ COLORECTAL CANCER

Definition

Colorectal cancer is the second most common cause of cancer death in the United States. Most cases are thought to arise from adenomatous polyps, usually sessile, villous polyps.

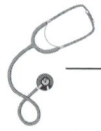

Villous polyps are the villain in colorectal cancer.

Signs and Symptoms

Constitutional Symptoms
- Weight loss
- Anorexia
- Malaise

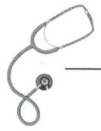

Fifty percent of colorectal cancer is within reach of the examiner's finger on rectal exam.

Right Colon
- Signs of anemia: Pallor, weakness
- Dull abdominal pain may or may not be present.

Left Colon
- Pencil-thin stools
- Rectal bleeding
- Signs of obstruction (constipation, vomiting)
- Mass on rectal exam

Signs Related to Metastases
- Hepatomegaly
- Palpable abdominal masses

Screening/Diagnosis

American Cancer Society recommendations for screening:

- Annual digital rectal exam beginning at age 40
- Annual fecal occult blood test (FOBT) screening beginning at age 50
- Flexible sigmoidoscopy—every 3 to 5 years beginning at age 50, if asymptomatic with no risk factors
- Colonoscopy is recommended for positive FOBT or sigmoidoscopy and for patients with inflammatory bowel disease or hereditary colorectal cancer syndromes. Colonoscopy has been used with increasing frequency over flexible sigmoidoscopy (it views entire colon rather than just sigmoid). Diagnosis requires biopsy (see Figure 2.3-6).

Lab Findings

- Anemia (iron deficiency)
- Elevated CEA (carcinoembryonic antigen)
- Check LFTs (elevations may indicate metastases).

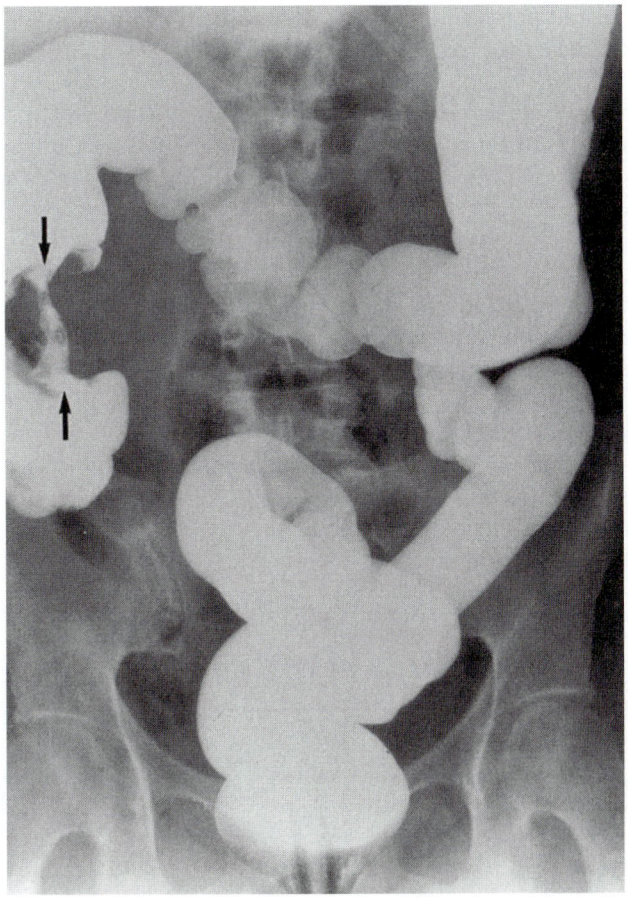

FIGURE 2.3-6. Colon cancer.

Barium study in a patient with colon cancer demonstrates an "apple core"–shaped filling defect at the site of a circumferential neoplasm. (Reproduced, with permission, from *Schwartz's Principles of Surgery*, 7th ed. New York: McGraw-Hill, 2000:1347.)

Typical scenario:
A 70-year-old woman presents with microcytic anemia, weight loss, and a vague abdominal pain that is not related to food or time of day. *Think: Colorectal cancer.*

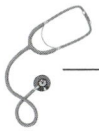

Up to 50% of patients with colorectal cancer can have a negative FOBT.

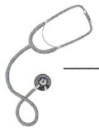

Polyps

- Tubular—benign
- Villous or tubulovillous—have malignant potential
- The larger the polyp, the more malignant potential (> 1 cm)

If a polyp is found on colonoscopy, perform polypectomy/biopsy and repeat colonoscopy in 3 years.

Endocarditis with *Streptococcus bovis* or *Clostridium septicum* is associated with colon cancer.

Duke's Classification for Staging and Prognosis

Staging		5-Year Survival
A	Confined to mucosa and submucosa	> 80%
B	Invasion of muscularis propria	60%
C	Local node involvement	20%
D	Distant metastases	3%

TREATMENT

- Surgical resection: Cures about 50% of cases (stages A and B)
- Chemotherapy: 5-Fluorouracil (FU) and levimasole for stages B at high risk and all C and D. Oxaliplatinum or irinotecan is often added.
- Radiation is used only for rectal involvement.

▶ HEREDITARY COLON CANCER SYNDROMES

Familial polyposis coli (high risk for colorectal cancer):
- Autosomal dominant condition in which thousands of adenomatous polyps appear throughout the colon by age 25
- Most untreated patients develop colon cancer by age 40.
- Do prophylactic total colectomy.

Hereditary nonpolyposis colon cancer (HNPCC) (high risk):
- Autosomal dominant condition in which three or more relatives of a patient, and at least one first-degree relative, develop colon cancer at an early age
- Often multiple other primary cancers in family

Gardner's syndrome (high risk):
- Autosomal dominant disorder characterized by polyposis coli, supernumerary teeth, osteomas, and fibrous dysplasia of the skull

Peutz–Jeghers syndrome (low to moderate risk):
- Multiple polyposis of small intestine with multiple pigmented melanin macules in oral mucosa
- Associated with gynecological cancers

GASTROINTESTINAL BLEEDS

▶ GENERAL APPROACH TO GI BLEEDING

Resuscitation

- Establish IV access with two large-bore IV catheters.
- Evaluate patient for hemodynamic instability:
  - Hypotension
  - Tachycardia
  - Orthostatic hypotension

- Type and cross, CBC, coagulation studies
- IV fluid resuscitation and blood transfusion as needed
- Vasopressors if BP does not respond to aggressive fluid resuscitation
- GI evaluation
- Surgical evaluation in the setting of lower GI bleeds

Determining the Source of Bleed

- Upper GI (UGI) vs. lower GI (LGI) bleed (upper GI bleed anatomically defined as bleeding above the ligament of Treitz)
- Targeted history and physical including presence/absence and localization of abdominal pain or tenderness; significant past medical history including peptic ulcer disease, chronic NSAID use, liver disease, recent vomiting or retching
- UGI bleed may present as:
  - Hematemesis (bloody vomitus)
  - Coffee ground emesis (dark-colored material representing a mixture of blood and gastric acid)
  - Melena
  - Hematochezia (bright red blood per rectum) or maroon-colored stools with severe GI bleeds
- LGI bleeds may present as:
  - Hematochezia
  - Melena (less commonly) with cecal or right colonic bleeds with slow transit
- Rectal examination, looking for:
  - Hemorrhoids
  - Rectal mass
  - Rectal tenderness
  - Stool examination for evidence of frank blood, stool color, melena, guiac test for occult blood
- Nasogastric lavage, looking for:
  - Bright red blood or coffee grounds indicate UGI bleed
  - Clear bilious drainage, indicating acute UGI bleed as an unlikely source

▶ UPPER GI BLEEDS

Etiology

- **M**allory–Weiss tear
- **V**arices
- **G**astritis
- **A**rteriovenous malformation
- **U**lcer (peptic)

Etiology of UGI bleeds: Mallory's Vices Gave (her) An Ulcer.

Signs and Symptoms

- Hematemesis (bright red or coffee grounds)
- Hypotension
- Tachycardia
- Bleeding that produces 60 cc of blood or more will produce black, tarry stool.
- Very brisk upper GI bleeds can be associated with bright red blood per rectum.

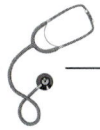

Coffee grounds **is the term used to describe old, brown, digested blood found on gastric lavage. It usually indicates a source of bleeding proximal to the ligament of Treitz.**

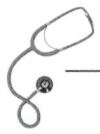

A bleeding scan detects *active* bleeding by infusing a radioactive colloid or radiolabeled autologous RBCs and watching for their collection in the GI tract.

A patient comes in vomiting blood. What do you do?
1. Two large-bore IVs and fluid
2. EGD

Diagnosis

- Gastric lavage with normal saline or free water to assess severity of bleeding (old versus new blood)
- Rectal exam with fecal occult blood testing
- CBC
- Endoscopy
- Bleeding scan
- Arteriography

Treatment

- Depends on etiology and severity
- IV fluids and blood
- Endoscopy with epinephrine injection; cautery or ligation is used with bleeding ulcers and varices
- IV proton pump inhibitor
- Most Mallory–Weiss tears resolve spontaneously.
- For bleeding varices:
  - Somatostatin (inhibits gastric, intestinal, and biliary motility, decreases visceral blood flow)
  - Consider balloon tamponade (rarely used at present).

▶ LOWER GI BLEEDS

Etiology of UGI bleeds: **C**an **U** **C**ure **A**unt **D**i's **H**emorrhoids.

Etiology

- **C**ancer or polyps
- **U**pper GI bleed (need to rule it out)
- **C**olitis (infectious, inflammatory bowel disease, ischemic, etc.)
- **A**ngiodysplasia
- **D**iverticulosis
- **H**emorrhoids

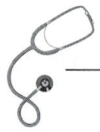

CBC in hemorrhage will not reflect the true severity of the bleed for 4 to 6 hours, as it takes time for the concentration to change.

Signs and Symptoms

- Bright red blood per rectum (hematochezia)
- Melena (black or maroon tarry stool)
- Signs of blood loss (tachycardia, hypotension)
- Diarrhea (as seen with colitis)

Diagnosis

- Gastric lavage to rule out upper GI source
- Rectal exam
- CBC
- Colonoscopy
- Bleeding scan
- Arteriography

Treatment

- Fluids
- Blood (RBCs)
- Embolization or surgery

Diarrhea

Definition

Abnormal passage of fluid or semisolid stool with increased frequency

General Approach

Primary evaluation targeted at differentiating between an infectious versus noninfectious etiology

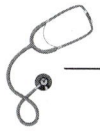

Opiate antidiarrheal agents such as loperamide are *contraindicated* in diarrhea due to infectious agents; they promote longer contact time between bacteria and intestinal mucosa.

History

- Quantity of diarrhea:
  - Small bowel involvement usually large-volume, watery diarrhea
  - Large bowel involvement usually small-volume diarrhea
- Quality of stool: Color, foul odor, blood, mucus, fatty consistency
- Length of symptoms:
  - Acute: < 2 weeks
  - Persistent: > 2 weeks
  - Chronic: > 4 weeks
- Associated symptoms: Fever, chills, abdominal pain, nausea, vomiting, weight loss
- Food intake prior to onset of diarrhea
- Travel history
- Pertinent past medical/surgical history: Predisposing conditions (IBD, small bowel resection, pancreatic disease, immunodeficiency, etc.)
- Medications
- Recent antibiotic use or hospitalization increasing risk for *Clostridium difficile* colitis
- Lactose intolerance
- Sick contacts

Bloody diarrhea: "CASES"
- **C***ampylobacter*
- **A**moeba *(E. histolytica)*
- **S***higella*
- **E.** *coli*
- **S***almonella*

Diagnosis

- General appearance: Does the patient look ill?
- Vital signs: Fever, tachycardia, hypotension, orthostatic hypotension
- Abdominal exam: Tenderness, distention, hepatomegaly, ascites
- Rectal exam: Tenderness, mass, stool appearance, occult blood
- Skin: Turgor, rash

ACUTE DIARRHEA

Less than 2 to 4 weeks in duration; usually due to infectious etiology

Workup

- **Fecal leukocytes** (may be suggestive of infectious or inflammatory causes)
- **Stool culture** for enteric pathogens
- **Stool test for C. *difficile* toxins** (for pseudomembranous colitis)
- **Stool examination for ova and parasites** (insensitive—must do with three different bowel movements over 3 days)

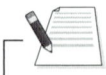

Typical scenario:
A patient vomits within 6 hours of eating something with mayonnaise (e.g., potato salad at a picnic on a hot day. *Think: Staphylococcus.*

Typical scenario:
A patient has vomiting/diarrhea after eating reheated rice from leftover Chinese food. *Think: Bacillus cereus.*

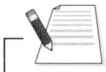

Typical scenario:
A patient has vomiting and severe watery diarrhea after eating spoiled shellfish. *Think: Vibrio cholerae.*

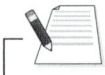

Typical scenario:
A patient has flatulence and foul-smelling diarrhea after a camping trip. *Think: Giardia lamblia.* Treat with metronidazole.

Typical scenario:
A patient has watery diarrhea following a recent course of antibiotics. *Think: Clostridium difficile.* Treat with *oral* metronidazole or vancomycin.

Common Infectious Pathogens

- Bacterial:
  - Noninvasive, all foodborne: *Staphylococcus aureus* (quick onset, mostly vomiting), *Bacillus cereus* (Chinese food), *Clostridium perfringens*, *Vibrio cholerae* (contaminated water in third-world countries), enterotoxigenic *Escherichia coli* (most common cause of traveler's diarrhea)
  - Invasive (bloody): *Campylobacter* (associated with Guillain–Barré syndrome), *Yersinia*, *Shigella*, *Salmonella* (raw eggs), enterohemorrhagic *E. coli*, *C. difficile* (pseudomembranous colitis)
- Viral: Rotavirus, Norwalk virus, cytomegalovirus (CMV) (in the immunocompromised patient)
- Protozoa (can also cause chronic diarrhea): *Giardia lamblia* (after hiking trip), *Entamoeba histolytica*, *Cryptosporidium* (common in AIDS)

Management

- Oral or intravenous rehydration
- Electrolyte replacement
- Antibiotic therapy when infectious etiology is suspected and patient is moderately to severely ill: Empiric treatment with ciprofloxacin or trimethoprim–sulfamethoxazole (TMP-SMX); Flagyl (metronidazole) if *C. difficile* is suspected
- Treat the underlying disorder (e.g., IBD, bacterial overgrowth).
- Antimotility agents in noninfectious diarrhea

CHRONIC DIARRHEA

Classification

- **Osmotic:** Ingestion of nonabsorbable solutes leading to osmotic water loss in the stool
  - Causes/examples: Magnesium-containing antacids, sodium phosphates, carbohydrates (lactose intolerance)
- **Secretory:** Oversecretion of water by the small and large bowel, which may be caused by bacteria, bacterial toxins, medications, gastrointestinal hormones (e.g., VIP), unabsorbed dietary fat.
  - Causes/examples: Enteroinvasive bacteria, laxatives, hyperthyroidism, neuroendocrine tumors (e.g., carcinoid, VIPoma), irritable bowel syndrome, microscopic colitis)
- **Inflammatory**: Gastrointestinal mucosal irritation and inflammation leading to an exudative diarrhea
  - Causes/examples: Inflammatory bowel disease (Crohn's, ulcerative colitis), invasive bacteria and viruses, vasculitides
- **Malabsorption:** A problem with either digestion (i.e., lack of digestive enzymes or bile acids) or transport (i.e., problem with the small bowel mucosa)
  - Causes/examples: Chronic pancreatitis, bile acid malabsorption, celiac sprue, bacterial overgrowth of small bowel, tropical sprue, Whipple's disease, eosinophilic gastroenteritis, MALToma, chronic mesenteric ischemia

- **Decreased transit time:** May lead to diarrhea by an osmotic mechanism.
  - Causes/examples: Dumping syndrome, short gut syndrome, neuroendocrine tumors

Workup

- **As with acute diarrhea (above):** Check stool for fecal leukocytes, stool culture, *C. difficile* toxin, and ova and parasites
- **Fecal electrolytes and calculation of osmotic gap:** Osmotic gap = 290 – 2(Na + K) > 50 mOsm suggestive of an unmeasured solute indicating osmotic component to diarrhea
- **Fecal pH:** < 5.5 suggestive of carbohydrate malabsorption
- **D-xylose test:** Distinguishes digestion problem vs. transport problem. A set amount of D-xylose given PO followed by measuring blood and urine levels to assess for adequate absorption. Xylose requires transport but not digestive enzymes to be absorbed; therefore, adequate amounts in blood/urine demonstrate intact absorption. Low levels of xylose indicate a problem with the small bowel mucosal transport.
- **Small bowel biopsy:** If a transport problem is suspected in the small bowel, a biopsy will diagnose the cause (e.g., Whipple's disease, celiac sprue)
- **72-hour fecal fat analysis:** Steatorrhea (increased fecal fat) may be seen in pancreatic exocrine insufficiency due to malabsorption.
- **Sigmoidoscopy/colonoscopy** in certain cases of colitis will show pseudomembranes or inflammation.

Distinguishing Types of Chronic Diarrhea

Osmotic vs. Secretory Diarrhea

- **Calculation of osmotic gap** with fecal electrolytes (osmotic gap = 290 – 2(Na + K))
  - > 50 mOsm suggestive of an unmeasured solute indicating osmotic component to diarrhea
  - Secretory diarrhea (and other nonosmotic diarrheas) has normal osmotic gap (< 50)
- **24-hour fasting:** Secretory diarrhea does not resolve with fasting; osmotic diarrhea resolves.

Malabsorption: Digestion vs. Transport Problems

- **D-xylose test:** A set amount of D-xylose given PO followed by measuring blood and urine levels to assess for adequate absorption. Xylose requires transport but not digestive enzymes to be absorbed.
  - Adequate amounts in blood/urine demonstrate intact absorption.
  - Low levels of xylose indicate a problem with the small bowel mucosal transport.

Major Types of Malabsorption

▶ CELIAC SPRUE

Definition

A gluten-induced enteropathy in susceptible persons diffusely affecting the entire small bowel (also called celiac disease, nontropical sprue, gluten-induced enteropathy). Glutens are a class of high-molecular-weight proteins found in wheat, rye, and barley.

Epidemiology

- More common in women (3:2)
- Associated with HLA DR3 and HLA DQw2

Signs and Symptoms

- Malabsorption (diarrhea, bloating abdominal pain, steatorrhea, weight loss)
- Signs of vitamin deficiency from malabsorption (↑ PT/INR from vitamin K deficiency, iron deficiency, low calcium)
- Rash (dermatitis herpetiformis)

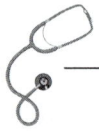

Dermatitis herpetiformis is a pruritic rash associated with celiac sprue, responds to treatment of topical sulfone, resolves with regression of disease.

Pathology (from small bowel biopsy)

- Very flattened intestinal villi
- Infiltration of **lymphocytes**
- Hyperplasia and lengthening of intestinal crypts

Diagnosis

- Small bowel biopsy
- Antibody tests (antigliadal IgG/IgA, antiendomysial antibody)
- Tissue transglutaminase
- Barium swallow shows clumping of barium and loss of mucosal folds (see Figure 2.3-7).

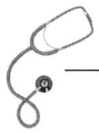

Treatment of celiac sprue: All grains are to be eliminated from diet, except rice and corn.

Treatment

- Avoid gluten-containing foods.
- Consider course of glucocorticoids for severe cases.

▶ TROPICAL SPRUE

Definition

- Malabsorption disease with flattened villi in the jejunum similar to celiac sprue likely from an infectious etiology
- Occurs in inhabitants and visitors of the tropics
- Can be seen several years after exposure

Signs and Symptoms

Symptoms of malabsorption (like celiac sprue)

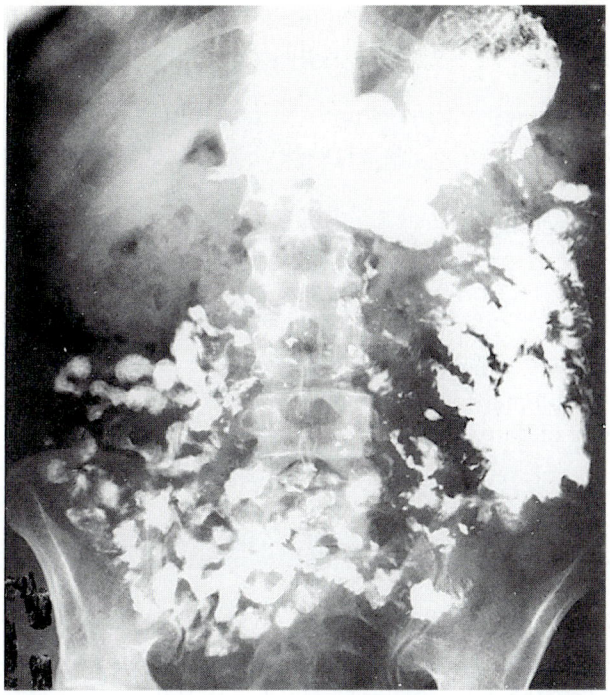

FIGURE 2.3-7. Celiac sprue.

Barium study in a patient with celiac sprue showing dilation of small bowel, lack of mucosal markings, and segmentation and clumping of barium. (Reproduced, with permission, from Fauci et al. *Harrison's Principles of Internal Medicine,* 14th ed. New York: McGraw-Hill, 1998:1622.)

PATHOLOGY

- Mildly flattened intestinal villi
- Jejunal infiltration of **monocytes** (instead of lymphocytes as in celiac sprue)

DIAGNOSIS

- Small bowel biopsy
- Requires malabsorption of at least two nutrients
- Megaloblastic anemia
- Decreased calcium, B_{12}, iron, folic acid, cholesterol, albumin, magnesium

TREATMENT

- Vitamin B_{12} and folate supplementation
- Tetracycline for a few months

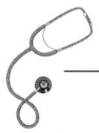

The presence of a normal jejunal biopsy practically excludes the diagnosis of tropical sprue.

▶ LACTASE DEFICIENCY

- Lactase is required to digest lactose, a carbohydrate found in dairy products. Deficiency of lactase results in abdominal symptoms after ingestion of dairy products.

- Congenital deficiency is rare; a milder late-onset form is found in a majority of adult African Americans, Asians, and in 5 to 15% of adult whites.
- Acquired deficiency can occur any time in life.

Signs and Symptoms

- Abdominal cramps
- Flatus
- Diarrhea

Treatment

- Lactase supplementation
- Avoidance of dairy products

Whipple's Disease vs. Sprue
They can have similar symptoms, but Whipple's is far more severe and has more constitutional symptoms, particularly with CNS involvement.

Whipple's is a rare disease that is fatal if untreated, but otherwise completely curable. It is also a favorite on exams.

Typical scenario:
A 54-year-old farmer who has been suffering with diarrhea, weight loss, and arthralgias for the past few months is brought in by his wife for memory deficits that have been occurring for the past 3 weeks.
Think: Whipple's disease.

▶ WHIPPLE'S DISEASE

Definition

- Devastating illness beginning in the GI tract, but spreading systemically
- Profound malabsorption syndrome due to destruction of intestinal lamina propria
- Causative organism is *Tropheryma whippelii*, a gram-negative rod of the *Actinomyces* genus.

Epidemiology

- More common in males (8:1)
- More common in Caucasians
- Peak incidence in 4th to 6th decades

Signs and Symptoms

- Arthralgia
- Abdominal pain
- Malabsorption: Diarrhea, weight loss, steatorrhea, hypoproteinemia, anemia, etc.
- Bacteremia—present but not detectable
- Constitutional symptoms:
  - Low-grade fever
  - Increased skin pigmentation
  - Uveitis
  - Cardiac involvement: Heart failure, endocarditis
  - CNS involvement: Confusion, memory deficits, CN palsies, nystagmus, ophthalmoplegia

Diagnosis

- Demonstration of replacement of intestinal lamina propria by PAS-positive macrophages
- PCR of peripheral blood since *T. whippelii* cannot be cultured

Treatment

- Long-term antibiotic therapy (e.g., TMP-SMZ and tetracycline for 1 year)

- Clinical remission in almost all cases if treated
- Complete histologic reversal has been observed in some cases.

▶ PROTEIN-LOSING ENTEROPATHY

- The GI tract is the primary site for endogenous protein turnover (proteolysis) in the body. During this process, 10 to 20% of the protein is normally lost to the GI lumen.
- Protein-losing enteropathy occurs when plasma proteins (principally albumin) are lost to the GI lumen in excess.

Causes

Myriad causes, most relating to disorders affecting GI mucosa or heart failure

Signs and Symptoms

- Diarrhea
- Edema
- Steatorrhea

Diagnosis

- Alpha-1-antitrypsin is resistant to proteolysis in the gut and, thus, is used to measure protein loss by comparing levels in the serum and stool.
- Lab abnormalities may include low calcium and low B_{12}, in addition to low protein.

Treatment

- Low-fat diet
- Treat underlying cause

MÉNÉTRIER'S DISEASE

Definition

- Protein-losing enteropathy
- Enlarged, tortuous gastric rugae
- Mucosal thickening due to hyperplasia of glandular cells replacing chief and parietal cells
- Low-grade inflammatory infiltrate—*not* a form of gastritis

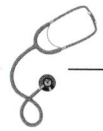

Ménétrier's can look like gastric cancer on barium study.

Signs and Symptoms

- Epigastric pain
- Symptoms of protein-losing enteropathy
- Decreased gastric acid secretion
- Less commonly:
  - Nausea, vomiting
  - Anorexia, weight loss
  - Occult GI bleed

Diagnosis

- Endoscopy with deep mucosal biopsy is definitive.
- Barium swallow will reveal large gastric folds.

Complications

- Gastric ulcer
- Gastric cancer

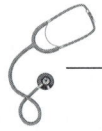

Anticholinergics are thought to reduce the width of tight junctions between gastric mucosal cells.

Treatment

- Anticholinergics, H_2 blockers to reduce protein loss
- High-protein diet
- Treatment of ulcers/CA if present
- Severe disease may require gastrectomy

▶ CONSTIPATION

Definition

Stool frequency < 3 times per week

Etiology

- Low fiber, low fluid intake
- Obstruction
- Disturbed colonic motility
- Medications
- Hypothyroidism
- Diabetes mellitus

Treatment

- Increase fiber to 30 g/day.
- Increase fluid intake.
- Bulk-forming and emollient laxatives

HIGH-YIELD FACTS IN

Hematology–Oncology

Benign Red Blood Cell Disorders

- Iron Deficiency Anemia 149
- Causes of Macrocytosis (MCV > 100) 149
- Folate Deficiency Anemia 149
- Vitamin B_{12} (Cobalamin) Deficiency 150
- Pernicious Anemia 150
- G6PD Deficiency 151
- Aplastic Anemia 152
- Anemia of Chronic Disease 152
- Types of Hemoglobin 153
- α-Thalassemia 153
- β-Thalassemia 154
- Sickle Cell Anemia (SCA) 155
- Immune-Mediated Hemolytic Anemia 156
- Warm Hemolytic Anemia 156
- Cold Hemolytic Anemia 156
- Paroxysmal Cold Hemoglobinuria 156
- Transfusion Reactions 156
- Polycythemia Vera (PV) 158

Coagulation 159

- Coagulation Cascade 159
- Heparin 159
- Warfarin 159
- Activated Partial Thromboplastin Time (aPTT) 160
- Prothrombin Time (PT) 160
- Thrombin Time (TT) 161
- Bleeding Time 161
- Direct Coombs' 161
- Indirect Coombs' 161

Thrombocytopenia 161

- Idiopathic Thrombocytopenic Purpura (ITP) 162

Thrombotic Thrombocytopenic Purpura (TTP) 162
Disseminated Intravascular Coagulation (DIC) 163
Miscellaneous Bleeding Disorders 164
von Willebrand's Disease 164
Hemophilia A 164
Hemophilia B (Christmas Disease) 165
Hematologic Malignacies 165
Acute Leukemia 165
Chronic Myeloid Leukemia (CML) 167
Chronic Lymphocytic Leukemia (CLL) 168
Multiple Myeloma 169
Hodgkin's Lymphoma 169
Non-Hodgkin's Lymphoma 170
Solid Tumor Malignancies 171
Breast Cancer 171
Ovarian Cancer 173
Cervical Cancer 174
Prostate Cancer 174
Testicular Cancer 175
Miscellaneous Metastatic Disease 176
Oncologic Emergencies 177

Benign Red Blood Cell Disorders

▶ IRON DEFICIENCY ANEMIA

Definition

Anemia due to decreased iron stores (iron is needed in hemoglobin synthesis); most common anemia

Etiology

Blood loss (chronic GI bleed or menorrhagia most common)
Malnutrition
Pregnancy

Signs and Symptoms

- Fatigue, exertional dyspnea
- Glossitis
- Angular cheilosis (cracking at the corners of mouth)
- Pallor
- Koilonychia (spoon nails)
- Pica (ingestion of clay, ice)

Diagnosis

- Low hemoglobin/hematocrit
- Low MCV (microcytic)
- Low TIBC, ferritin

Treatment

Oral iron replacement and investigation into underlying cause.

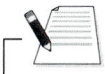

Features of iron deficiency anemia: Fe KAP
"Fe (Iron) **Kap"**
Fatigue
Exercise tolerance ↓
Koilonychia
Angular cheilosis
Pica, **P**allor

▶ CAUSES OF MACROCYTOSIS (MCV > 100)

- Folate deficiency
- Vitamin B_{12} deficiency
- Alcohol abuse
- Liver disease
- Hypothyroidism
- Myelodysplasia

A 38-year-old male with HIV on HAART, with macrocytosis. Cause? AZT

▶ FOLATE DEFICIENCY ANEMIA

Definition

Decreased hemoglobin content of red blood cells due to impaired DNA synthesis. Treatment is oral folate.

Risk Factors

- Alcoholism
- Diet low in folic acid
- Pregnancy
- Malabsorption

Folate deficiency can be differentiated from vitamin B_{12} deficiency by the lack of neurologic abnormalities.

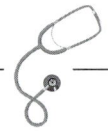

Glossitis is a chronic appearance of the tongue characterized by redness (beefy red), swelling, and loss of papillae.

Signs and Symptoms

- Diarrhea
- Cheilosis
- Glossitis

Diagnosis

Blood smear: Macrocytosis (high mean corpuscular volume [MCV]), basophilic stippling, hypersegmented neutrophils, low reticulocyte count

▶ VITAMIN B_{12} (COBALAMIN) DEFICIENCY

Causes of vitamin B_{12} deficiency
"VITAMIN B"
Vegan
Ileal resection
Tapeworm
Autoimmune (pernicious anemia)
Megaloblastic anemia
Inflammation of terminal ileum
Nitrous oxide
Bacterial overgrowth

Definition

Anemia due to lack of available vitamin B_{12} (used in DNA synthesis); treat with B_{12} replacement (usually IM)

Etiology

- Pernicious anemia (no intrinsic factor)
- Vegan diet (excludes meat, eggs, milk products)
- Fish tapeworm *(Diphyllobothrium latum)*
- Malabsorption (ileal resection, bacterial overgrowth, sprue)

Signs and Symptoms

- Symptoms of anemia
- Neurologic symptoms from subacute combined degeneration of the dorsal columns causing paresthesias, positive Romberg, slowed reflexes, impaired touch and temperature sensitivity, ataxia
- Dementia
- Atrophy of lingual papillae and glossitis

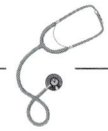

Anemia precedes neurologic symptoms in vitamin B_{12} deficiency.

Diagnosis

- Blood smear shows macrocytosis, basophilic stippling, hypersegmented neutrophils, low reticulocyte count
- Decreased plasma cobalamin levels

▶ PERNICIOUS ANEMIA

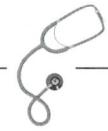

B_{12} replacement can cause hypokalemia. Should see reticulocytes in peripheral smear by 4th day.

Pathophysiology

- Absence of intrinsic factor (IF) causing vitamin B_{12} deficiency.
- Normally, IF and hydrogen ions are both produced by parietal cells of stomach.
- IF binds to vitamin B_{12} and is absorbed in the terminal ileum.
- An autoimmune mechanism is thought to produce antibodies against parietal cells, which destroys them.

Signs and Symptoms

- Same as vitamin B_{12} deficiency; insidious onset
- Associated with vitiligo
- Associated with chronic gastritis

Diagnosis

Schilling test, anti-IF antibody levels

Schilling Test

Purpose: To assess endogenous presence of IF

Steps:

1. Unlabeled vitamin B_{12} is given parenterally (preloading)—this saturates the cobalamin receptors such that a significant proportion of the radioactive vitamin B_{12} is absorbed in intestine and excreted in the urine.
2. Radioactively labeled vitamin B_{12} is administered orally.
3. If the amount of labeled cobalamin measured in an accurately collected 24-hour urine sample is less than 10% of the amount that was administered orally, there is poor absorption of cobalamin in the intestine.

Interpretation:

One may repeat the Schilling test adding intrinsic factor. In cases of pernicious anemia, IF will correct the cobalamin absorption.

Treatment

Usually B_{12} shots IM. However, because a small amount of cobalamin is absorbed even in the absence of IF, oral cobalamin dosages of 300 to 1,000 μg/day have proved adequate.

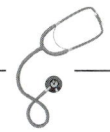

Pernicious anemia is associated with an increased risk of gastric cancer.

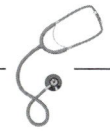

Causes of normochromic, normocytic anemia:

- Bone marrow problems (aplastic anemia, myelodysplastic syndrome)
- Anemia of chronic disease
- Early deficiency in iron, B_{12}, folate

▶ G6PD DEFICIENCY

An X-linked condition that results in reduced glutathione (an antioxidant). Oxidative stresses such as infection, sulfa drugs, quinolones, fava beans, and DKA result in hemolysis. More common in Mediterraneans (Italian, Greek, Arab).

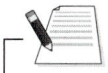

G6PD deficiency is the most common metabolic disorder of red blood cells.

Signs and Symptoms

Acute Hemolysis

- Jaundice, dark urine, acute tubular necrosis due to hemoglobinemia
- Anemia: Pallor, tachycardia, systolic ejection murmur
- Mesenteric and renal ischemia: Abdominal and back pain
- Sudden drop of 3 to 4 g/dL in RBC Hgb

Chronic Hemolysis

- Hepatosplenomegaly

Diagnosis

- Hemolysis:
  - Peripheral smear: Microcytosis, schistocytosis, Heinz bodies

Typical scenario:
A 35-year-old Italian male presents complaining of weakness, back pain, and jaundice. He reports being started on ciprofloxacin 2 days ago for a pneumonia. *Think: G6PD deficiency.*

- CBC/reticulocyte count: Anemia, reticulocytosis
- Haptoglobin: Low
- Direct and indirect Coombs: Negative
- Fractionated bilirubin: Elevated direct and indirect
- Membrane osmotic fragility: Normal
- U/A: Hemoglobinuria, elevated urobilinogen, acute tubular necrosis
- G6PD assay: Requires 3-week wait after acute hemolytic episode to avoid false-negative result from preponderance of younger cells

▶ APLASTIC ANEMIA

Definition

Marrow failure resulting in severe pancytopenia

Pathophysiology

Two mechanisms for are postulated:
- Stem cell defect
- Immune-mediated destruction

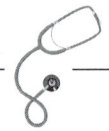

Patients with erythema infectiosum (causative agent: parvovirus B19) should avoid contact with patients with sickle cell anemia due to the risk of aplastic anemia.

Etiology

- Viral hepatitis
- Chloramphenicol (idiosyncratic)
- Parvovirus B19 with sickle cell anemia
- Benzene (dose related), lindane, DDT

Signs and Symptoms

- Weakness, fatigue
- Mucosal bleeding
- Pallor

Diagnosis

- Normochromic, normocytic pancytopenia
- Low reticulocyte count

Treatment

- Bone marrow transplant is treatment of choice, prior blood transfusions can impair success due to sensitization to minor HLA antigens.
- Immunosuppression (steroids, cyclophosphamide)

▶ ANEMIA OF CHRONIC DISEASE

Definition

Anemia observed in patients with infectious, inflammatory, or neoplastic diseases

Etiology

- Tuberculosis
- Malignancies
- Rheumatologic disorders that put body in a state of prolonged inflammation

Pathophysiology

Iron deficiency in the presence of ample iron stores due to impaired iron mobilization

Signs and Symptoms

Signs and symptoms of the underlying disorder

Diagnosis

- Ferritin is normal to increased; serum iron, total iron-binding capacity (TIBC), and transferrin all decreased.
- Erythropoietin appropriately elevated
- Normocytic, normochromic anemia

Treatment

Identification and treatment of underlying disease

► TYPES OF HEMOGLOBIN

- Hemoglobin A: α_2/β_2 globin chains (normal hemoglobin)
- Hemoglobin F: α_2/γ_2 globin chains (fetal hemoglobin)
- Hemoglobin A_2: α_2/δ_2
- Normal distribution of Hb in adults is:
  - 96% Hb A
  - 3% Hb F
  - 1% Hb A_2
- There are two α and one β gene on each chromosome, making a total of four α genes and two β genes in each chromosome pair.

► α-THALASSEMIA

Definition

Genetic defects causing gene deletions of α chains

Epidemiology

$\alpha\alpha/$—thalassemia trait is most common in Asians.
$\alpha-/\alpha-$thalassemia trait is most common in Africans.

Pathophysiology

- Ineffective production of α globin chains causes β globin chains to accumulate.

Signs and Symptoms

Depends on how many of the four foci are deleted or mutated:

- 1/4 foci involved = silent thalassemia
  - Asymptomatic
- 2/4 foci involved = thalassemia trait
  - Mild anemia
- 3/4 foci involved = Hemoglobin H disease
  - Microcytic, hypochromic, hemolytic anemia with marked splenomegaly. Patient may need occasional transfusions.
- 4/4 foci involved = Hemoglobin Barts, hydrops fetalis
  - Incompatible with life

Diagnosis

- Blood smear: Microcytic anemia, hypochromia, target cells, Heinz bodies
- HbH precipitates on staining with brilliant cresyl blue

▶ β-THALASSEMIA

Definition

Gene defects including deletions, abnormalities of transcription and translation, and instability of mRNA in β globin hemoglobin

Pathophysiology

- Ineffective production of β globin chains causes α globin chains to accumulate in the cell.
- The accumulation of α chains form insoluble aggregates that damage cell membranes.
- A partial compensatory increase of the δ and γ chains yields elevated levels of HbA_2 ($\alpha_2\delta_2$) or HbF ($\alpha_2\gamma_2$).

Signs and Symptoms

β-Thalassemia major (Cooley's anemia): Associated with jaundice, hepatosplenomegaly, and jaundice
β-Thalassemia minor: Mild or no anemia

Diagnosis

Elevated HbF and HbA_2 measurements on hemoglobin electrophoresis

Treatment

β-Thalassemia major: Aggressive transfusions, splenectomy to enhance survival of RBCs, bone marrow transplant
β-Thalassemia minor: No treatment indicated.

▶ SICKLE CELL ANEMIA (SCA)

Pathophysiology

- Genetic disease characterized by the presence of hemoglobin S in RBCs.
- Hemoglobin S is formed by substitution of valine for glutamine in the sixth position of the β-hemoglobin chain.
- During periods of high oxygen consumption, this abnormal hemoglobin distorts and causes red blood cell to sickle.
- Sickle cell trait: Heterozygous for sickle gene
- Sickle cell disease: Homozygous for sickle gene

Epidemiology

- More common in blacks than whites.
- Increased incidence in populations from Africa, the Mediterranean, Middle East, and India.

Signs and Symptoms

Acute Crisis

- Symptoms include arthralgias and pain
- Caused by vascular sludging and thrombosis. These vaso-occlusive crises may cause organ failure (secondary to infarction), dehydration, fever, and leukocytosis.
- Acute chest syndrome (hypoxia, chest pain, SOB, infiltrates caused by occlusion of pulmonary vasculature by sickled cells)

Chronic

- Skeletal: Aseptic necrosis of femoral head
- Biliary disease: Pigmented gallstones (increased bilirubin)
- Renal: Chronic hematuria, renal papillary necrosis
- Liver disease: Congestion (heart failure) and viral hepatitis (transfusions)
- Pulmonary: Local infection and vascular occlusions (acute chest syndrome)
- Heart: Enlarged, flow murmur
- Immune: Increased susceptibility to infections, functional asplenism (due to repeated infarction)
- Eye: Ischemic retinopathy
- GU: Priapism

Diagnosis

- Blood smear: Howell–Jolly bodies (cytoplasmic remnants of nuclear chromatin that are normally removed by the spleen), sickled cells
- Blood tests show anemia, increased reticulocyte count, increased indirect bilirubin.
- Hemoglobin electrophoresis will show HbS.

Treatment

- Acute crisis: Analgesia and hydration
- Hydroxyurea acts by increasing amount of fetal hemoglobin.
- *Haemophilus influenzae* and pneumococcal vaccines for prophylaxis
- Acute chest syndrome: Respiratory support, exchange transfusion, and empiric antibiotics for pneumonia

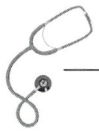

Indications for exchange transfusion in sickle cell disease:
- Stroke/TIA
- Acute chest syndrome
- Priapism
- Third-term pregnancy
- Intractable vaso-occlusive crisis

Signs of SCA: "SICKLE"
Splenomegaly, sludging
Infection
Cholelithiasis
Kidney—hematuria
Liver congestion, leg ulcers
Eye changes

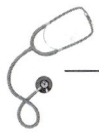

Renal papillary necrosis occurs in SCA because of the very high osmolalities in renal medulla needed to pull the water from the collecting ducts causing the RBCs to sickle.

Patients with SCA are prone to infection with encapsulated organisms. *Salmonella* osteomyelitis is most common among patients with SCA.

▶ IMMUNE-MEDIATED HEMOLYTIC ANEMIA

Presence of autoantibodies to one's RBCs, resulting in hemolysis and splenomegaly

▶ WARM HEMOLYTIC ANEMIA

- Most common form of immune-mediated hemolytic anemia
- IgG antibodies to Rh factor
- Do not usually fix complement
- Active at body temperature
- Treated with steroids
- Seen with lymphomas, leukemias, systemic lupus erythematosus (SLE), and other autoimmune diseases, and drugs. Sixty percent of cases are idiopathic.

▶ COLD HEMOLYTIC ANEMIA

- IgM antibodies
- Active at cool temperatures (dissociate at 30°C) such as in distal body parts
- Fixes complement
- Seen acutely with mycoplasma and infectious mononucleosis (resolve spontaneously) and chronically with myeloproliferative disorders
- Degree of hemolysis is variable.
- Treatment includes keeping warm and corticosteroids.

▶ PAROXYSMAL COLD HEMOGLOBINURIA

- Also called cold hemolysis
- IgG antibodies against P group antigen (Donath–Landsteiner Ab)
- Active at cool temperatures, dissociate at 30°C to cause hemolysis
- Fix complement
- Clinically characterized by acute intermittent massive hemolysis and hemoglobinuria following exposure to cold

▶ TRANSFUSION REACTIONS

Acute Hemolytic Transfusion Reactions

- Life threatening!
- Due to ABO incompatibility
- Host antibodies against one of the ABO major blood groups on donor blood activates complement system and results in immediate intravascular hemolysis.
- Direct Coombs' test is positive (antibodies on RBCs)
- Usually due to human error (improper identification or mislabeling of blood)

Signs and Symptoms

- Begins soon after starting the transfusion
- Usually sudden clinical deterioration:
  - Fever +/– chills
  - Dyspnea
  - Tachycardia
  - Back pain, chest pain, abdominal pain
  - Hypotension
- Sequelae:
  - Death (40%)
  - Acute renal failure
  - Shock
  - Disseminated intravascular coagulation (DIC)

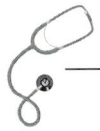

General anesthesia is a frequent setting for blood transfusion. In this setting, immediate hemolytic transfusion reaction should be suspected with:
- Severe hypotension
- Coagulopathic oozing
- Hemoglobinuria

Treatment

- Discontinue transfusion immediately!
- Hemodynamic support/supportive care
- Recheck compatibility of blood with blood bank.

Delayed Hemolytic Transfusion Reactions

- Milder than immediate type
- Predominantly extravascular hemolysis
- Occur 2 to 10 days after transfusion
- Due to anamnestic antibody response
- Pretransfusion antibody level low → screening and crossmatch tests usually negative
- Often has high LDH, high total bilirubin, low haptoglobin

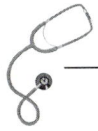

Precipitation of free hemoglobin in the renal tubules is *not* a major contributor to renal failure.

Signs and Symptoms

Most Common
- Fever
- Recurrent anemia
- Asymptomatic

Less Common
- Jaundice
- Hemoglobinemia/hemoglobinuria
- Renal failure → death

Treatment

- Usually no treatment required
- More severe reactions may require hydration, transfusion of properly crossmatched RBCs.

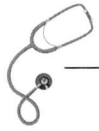

The use of leukocyte-reduced blood products may reduce the incidence of febrile nonhemolytic transfusion reactions.

Febrile Nonhemolytic Transfusion Reactions

- 0.5 to 3.0% of patients receiving transfusions
- Chill followed by fever within a few hours of transfusion; mild
- Lasts only a few hours
- Due to host Ab against antigens on transfused leukocytes and platelets or cytokines from donor leukocytes

Treatment

- Discontinue transfusion (can occur after).
- Rule out acute hemolysis (see Acute Hemolytic Transfusion Reactions on pages 156–157).
- Can give Tylenol and Benadryl as prophylaxis

Allergic Reactions to Plasma

- Incidence of 1 to 3%
- Can get hives, bronchospasm, anaphylaxis
- People with congenital IgA deficiency can have anaphylactic reactions to the IgA in donor blood.

Transfusion-Related Acute Lung Injury (TRALI)

- Sudden severe respiratory distress similar to adult respiratory distress syndrome (ARDS)
- Occurs within several hours of transfusion
- Incidence ~1 in 5,000 transfusions
- Caused by donor Ab against recipient granulocytes → agglutination of granulocytes and complement activation in the pulmonary vascular bed → capillary endothelial damage → fluid leak into the alveoli
- Resolves within 48 to 96 hours without residual effects (interim respiratory support often required)
- Treatment is supportive.

Signs and Symptoms

- Chills/fever
- Chest pain
- Hypotension
- Cyanosis, dyspnea, crackles/rales
- Chest x-ray (CXR) shows diffuse pulmonary edema

▶ POLYCYTHEMIA VERA (PV)

Definition

A myeloproliferative disease that results in increased red blood cells, in addition to mild increases in leukocytes and platelets

Etiology

- **Primary PV:** A primary bone marrow cause (low erythropoietin)
- **Secondary PV** (other causes that result in increased erythropoietin):
  - Hypoxia (high altitudes, lung disease)
  - Smoking (due to carboxyhemoglobin)
  - Renal cell carcinoma

2° polycythemia is associated with hypernephroma, cerebellar hemangioma, hepatoma, and giant uterine myomas.

Epidemiology

- Males more commonly affected
- More common in people > 60
- Associated with high risk of cerebrovascular accidents (hypercoagulation), MIs, and bleeding
- Risk of progression to leukemia or myelofibrosis

Signs and Symptoms

- Pruritus
- Plethora
- Splenomegaly
- Epistaxis
- Neuro symptoms such as vision changes

Diagnosis

- Low erythropoietin in primary
- High erythropoietin in secondary

Treatment

- Serial phlebotomy to decrease blood volume
- Consider hydroxyurea for myelosuppression (in primary)
- Aspirin to prevent thromboses

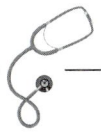

Bone marrow fibrosis is a late complication of polycythemia vera.

Coagulation

▶ COAGULATION CASCADE

Common pathway factors: I, II, V, X (see Figure 2.4-1)

▶ HEPARIN

- Increases partial thromboplastin time (PTT)
- Affects intrinsic pathway
- Acts as cofactor to antithrombin III (antithrombin III inhibits factor Xa and thrombin)
- Low-molecular-weight heparins have 10 times activity against factor Xa.
- Safe in pregnancy
- Adverse effects include bleeding, thrombocytopenia, and osteoporosis.

PiTT = Intrinsic pathway

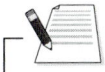

Heparin goes with Intrinsic pathway because H comes right before I.

▶ WARFARIN

- Increases prothrombin time (PT)
- Affects extrinsic pathway
- Decreased vitamin K
- Primarily affects II, V, VII, IX
- Teratogenic
- Risk of initial hypercoagulability due to inhibition of proteins C and S

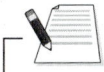

PeT = PT measures extrinsic pathway.

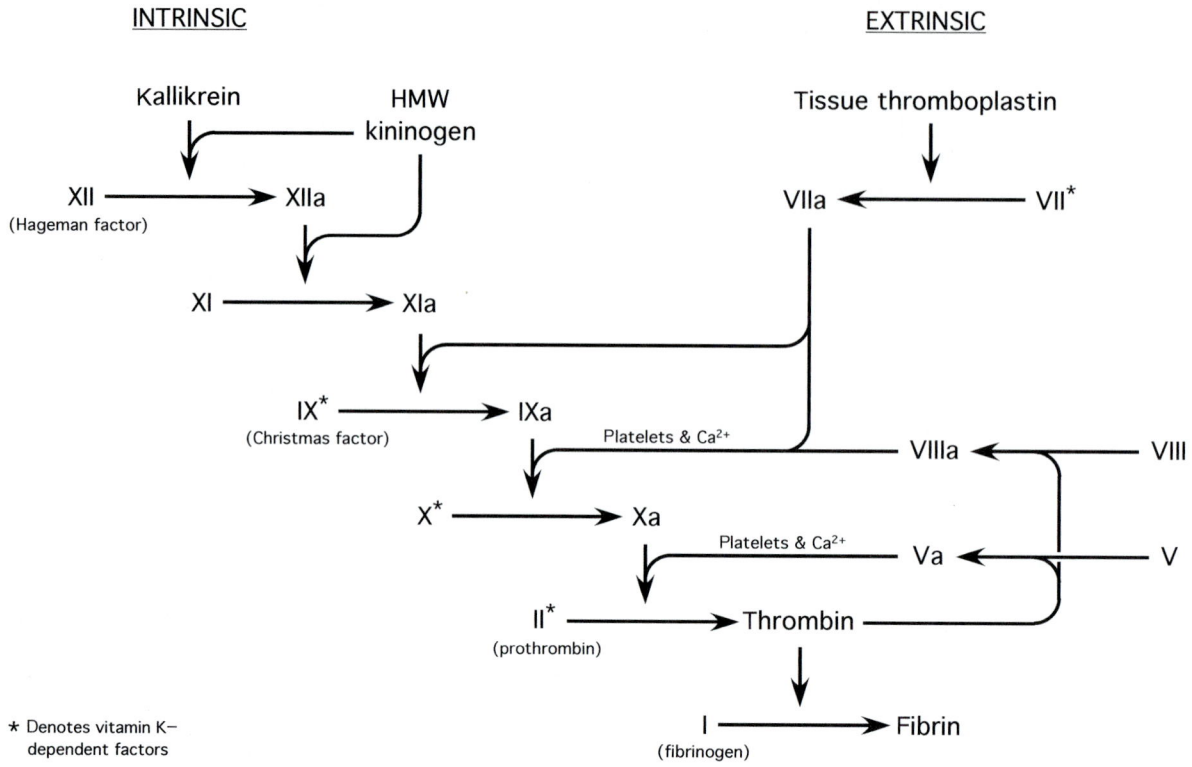

FIGURE 2.4-1. Coagulation cascade.

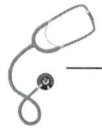

Leafy green vegetables are relatively contraindicated in patients on warfarin therapy due to their high vitamin K content.

ACTIVATED PARTIAL THROMBOPLASTIN TIME (aPTT)

- Tests extrinsic and common pathways
- Isolated elevation of PTT (with normal PT) seen in:
  - Heparin therapy
  - Deficiencies of factors VIII (hemophilia A), factor IX (hemophilia B), factor XI, and factor XII (asymptomatic)
  - Antiphospholipid antibody (prothrombotic state)

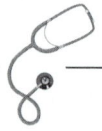

Warfarin has an initial *pro*coagulant effect, taking 48 to 72 hours to become anticoagulant. Concurrent coverage with heparin during this time is needed, and oral warfarin dose is titrated slowly.

PROTHROMBIN TIME (PT)

- Tests intrinsic and common pathways
- Isolated elevation of PT (with normal PTT) seen in:
  - Vitamin K deficiency
  - Warfarin therapy
  - Liver disease (decreased factor production)
  - Congenital (rare)

▶ THROMBIN TIME (TT)

- Measures the time it takes to convert fibrinogen into a fibrin clot
- Elevated in:
  - DIC (consumes fibrinogen)
  - Liver disease (decreased production of fibrinogen)
  - Heparin therapy (inhibits fibrinogen formation)
  - Hypofibrinogenemia (low fibrinogen to start)

▶ BLEEDING TIME

- Measures time from start of skin incision to formation of clot (normal = 3 to 8 min)
- Independent of coagulation cascade
- Elevated in:
  - Thrombocytopenia
  - Qualitative platelet disorders (e.g., renal failure)
  - von Willebrand's disease

▶ DIRECT COOMBS'

- Tests for antibodies on red blood cells
- Elevated in:
  - Drug therapy (α-methyldopa, penicillin, tetracyclines, quinidine, insulin)
  - SLE
  - Autoimmune hemolytic anemia
  - Transfusion reactions

▶ INDIRECT COOMBS'

- Tests for antibodies to red blood cells in the serum (not on the cells)
- Elevated in:
  - Acquired hemolytic anemia
  - Incompatible crossmatched blood
  - Anti-Rh antibodies
  - Drug therapy (mefenamic acid, α-methyldopa)

THROMBOCYTOPENIA

Low platelets can be due to:

- Decreased production (bone marrow problem, as in leukemia)
- Increased consumption (DIC, TTP, ITP)
- Hypersplenism (sequestration of platelets)

Causes of thrombocytopenia:
"PLATELETS"
Platelet disorders: TTP, ITP, DIC
Leukemia
Anemia
Trauma
Enlarged spleen
Liver disease
EtOH
Toxins (benzene, heparins, aspirin, chemotherapy agents, etc.)
Sepsis

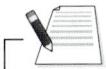

Thrombocytopenia vs. Factor Deficiencies
- Thrombocytopenia presents as oozing from mucosal sites (gums) and petechiae.
- Factor deficiencies (e.g., hemophilia) present with large bleeds (typically hemarthrosis).

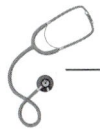

Typically, one transfuses platelets if they drop below 20,000 or if there are signs of bleeding. One unit increases platelets by 10,000.

▶ IDIOPATHIC THROMBOCYTOPENIC PURPURA (ITP)

Typical scenario:
A 27-year-old HIV+ female presents with fever, waxing and waning mental status, and hematuria. CBC shows pancytopenia. *Think: TTP.* Treatment: Plasmapheresis, **not** platelets.

Definition

Immune-mediated thrombocytopenia of unknown etiology

Pathophysiology

Development of antibodies against a platelet surface antigen. The antibody–antigen complexes effectively decrease platelet count by being removed from circulation.

Signs and Symptoms

- Petechiae and purpura over trunk and limbs
- Mucosal bleeding

Classic pentad of TTP:
- Hemolytic anemia
- Thrombocytopenia
- Neurologic changes
- Decreased renal function
- Fever

Diagnosis

- Thrombocytopenia on CBC
- Absence of other factors to explain thrombocytopenia (diagnosis of exclusion)
- Antiplatelet antibodies

Treatment

- Corticosteroids acutely
- May also consider intravenous immunoglobulin for severe cases
- Platelet transfusion if significant bleeding present
- Splenectomy electively to decrease recurrence

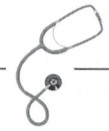

E. coli 0157:H7 is an invasive gastroenteritis resulting in hemolytic uremic syndrome (HUS). HUS differs from TTP in severity and lack of neurologic symptoms.

▶ THROMBOTIC THROMBOCYTOPENIC PURPURA (TTP)

Definition

A hemolytic anemia that results from deposition of abnormal vWF multimers into microvasculature. This is a life-threatening emergency!

Etiology

- Infection (especially HIV and *E. coli* 0157:H7)
- Malignancy
- Drugs (antiplatelet agents, chemotherapy agents, contraceptives)
- Autoimmune disorders
- Pregnancy

Diagnostic pentad for TTP:
"FAT RN"
Fever
Anemia
Thrombocytopenia
Renal dysfunction
Neurologic dysfunction

Signs and Symptoms

- Fever
- Altered mental status (waxing and waning, depending on location and movement of clot)
- Renal dysfunction (hematuria, oliguria)
- Thrombocytopenia—can be mild to severe
- Microangiopathic hemolytic anemia

Diagnosis

- Evidence of hemolysis: Schistocytes on peripheral smear, decreased haptoglobin, elevated LDH, elevated total bilirubin
- Renal failure: Elevated BUN, creatinine
- Fever, confusion
- Normal PT and PTT

Treatment

- **Do not transfuse platelets.**
- Plasmapheresis is mainstay of treatment (given daily, until platelet count rises to normal).
- May give FFP if plasmapheresis not available

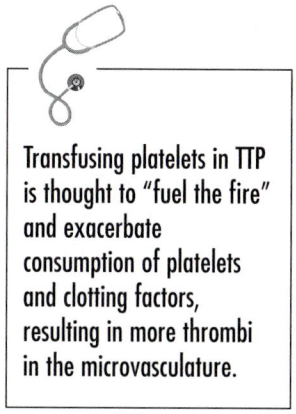

Transfusing platelets in TTP is thought to "fuel the fire" and exacerbate consumption of platelets and clotting factors, resulting in more thrombi in the microvasculature.

▶ DISSEMINATED INTRAVASCULAR COAGULATION (DIC)

Definition

Acquired coagulation defect that results in consumption of coagulation factors I, V, VIII, and XIII, causing bleeding and thrombosis. Can be acute and life threatening or can be chronic, as seen with malignancies.

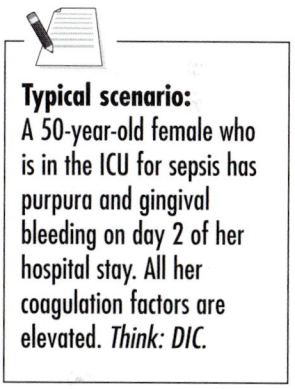

Typical scenario:
A 50-year-old female who is in the ICU for sepsis has purpura and gingival bleeding on day 2 of her hospital stay. All her coagulation factors are elevated. *Think: DIC.*

Etiology

- Obstetric problems (retained dead fetus, abruptio placentae, second-trimester abortion, amniotic fluid embolism)
- Sepsis (particularly with RMSF, HUS, malaria, gram negatives)
- Local tissue damage (snake bites, burns, frostbite)
- Chronic illness: Malignancy, liver disease

Signs and Symptoms

- Petechiae
- Purpura
- Mucosal bleeding
- Patients with chronic DIC may only have laboratory abnormalities.

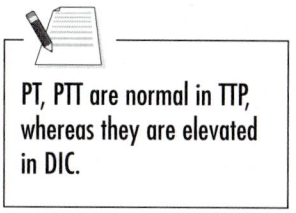

PT, PTT are normal in TTP, whereas they are elevated in DIC.

Diagnosis

- Thrombocytopenia
- Elevated PT, aPTT, and TT
- Decreased fibrinogen
- Presence of fibrin split products (elevated D-dimers)
- Evidence of hemolysis on peripheral smear

Treatment

- Treat underlying cause
- Platelets, FFP, and cryoprecipitate to control bleeding

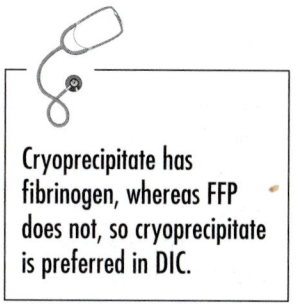

Cryoprecipitate has fibrinogen, whereas FFP does not, so cryoprecipitate is preferred in DIC.

Miscellaneous Bleeding Disorders

▶ VON WILLEBRAND'S DISEASE

Definition

Genetic disease, most commonly autosomal dominant, characterized by lack of a von Willebrand factor (vWF)

Pathophysiology

Three functions of von Willebrand factor:
- Stabilizes factor VIII
- Enhances platelet aggregation and attachment to injured vascular endothelium

Three types of disease:
Type 1: Decrease in amount (quantitative defect) autosomal dominant inheritance
Type 2: Qualitative defect of vWF
Type 3: Virtually total quantitative deficiency

Signs and Symptoms

Epistaxis, menorrhagia in women, severe mucous membrane bleeding, easy bruising; bleeding common after dental extractions or surgery

Diagnosis

- vWF antigen decreased
- Ristocetin aggregation test (measures vWF activity—can distinguish type 2 from others)
- Increase in aPPT due to decrease of factor VIII function.
- Increase in bleeding time due to effects on platelets.

Treatment

- Intermediate purity factor VIII concentrates (contains vWF) or cryoprecipitate
- DDAVP (desmopressin) increases vWF activity

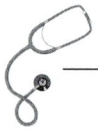

FFP contains all coagulation factors and therefore may be used to treat any coagulation factors deficiency (vWD, hemophilias). FFP is best used when exact defect is unknown. Large volumes of FFP would be needed to correct a particular coagulopathy, whereas specific factor concentrate would correct problem more efficiently.

▶ HEMOPHILIA A

Pathophysiology

Sex-linked recessive disease causing a deficiency of factor VIII

Signs and Symptoms

Dependent on amount of active factor:
- 5 to 25% normal factor VIII activity (mild): Abnormal bleeding when subjected to surgery or dental procedures
- 2 to 5% (moderate) and < 2% (severe) normal VIII activity: Deep tissue bleeding, intra-articular hemorrhages (usually knees), nerve impingement, intracranial bleeding (following trauma)

Diagnosis

- Prolonged aPPT, normal bleeding time
- Clinical picture, family history, and the factor VIII coagulant activity level

Treatment

- Cryoprecipitate
- Recombinant factor VIII
- DDAVP (desmopressin) for patients with mild hemophilia A

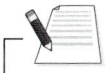

Unlike in vWD, bleeding time in hemophilia A is unaffected because no abnormality with platelets is present.

▶ HEMOPHILIA B (CHRISTMAS DISEASE)

Pathophysiology

X-linked recessive disease that causes a deficiency of factor IX

Clinical

Identical to hemophilia A

Diagnosis

Factor IX assay

Treatment

- Fresh frozen plasma (FFP)
- Recombinant factor IX

Hematologic Malignancies

▶ ACUTE LEUKEMIA

Types

- Acute lymphocytic leukemia (ALL)
- Acute myelogenous leukemia (AML)

Pathophysiology

- Hematopoietic disorder in which progenitor cells have transformed into malignant cells
- These leukemic cells accumulate in the bone marrow to disrupt the differentiation of normal cells.
- Clinical manifestations occur because of the loss of normal bone marrow elements and by infiltration of the body's tissues by malignant cells.

Signs and Symptoms

- Anemia: Weakness, fatigue, pallor, cardiopulmonary compromise
- Neutropenia: Infections, fever

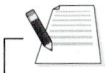

Signs of
"LEUKEMIA"

Light skin (pallor)
Energy decreased
Underweight
Kidney failure
Excess heat (fever)
Mottled skin (hemorrhages)
Infections
Anemia

- Thrombocytopenia: Purpura, hemorrhages
- Marrow infiltration: Bone pain
- Leukemic infiltration: Lymphadenopathy, splenomegaly, hepatomegaly

Diagnosis

- Blasts, anemia, thrombocytopenia on CBC
- Bone marrow biopsy showing > 30% immature cells confirms diagnosis.

Treatment

Three steps of chemotherapy:

- *Induction:* High doses of chemotherapy are used to induce remission.
- *Consolidation:* Chemotherapy is then administered to eradicate residual, undetectable malignant cells.
- *Maintenance:* Ongoing chemotherapy to keep the number of malignant cells low

Complete remission is the goal in cancer patients. This is achieved if normal marrow elements are being produced and less than 5% residual blasts are present in the bone marrow.

Acute Myelocytic Leukemia (AML)

Epidemiology

More common in adults; association with benzene 8 subtypes M0–M7:

- M1–M3 have granulocytic differentiation.
- M4 and M5 are monocytic precursors.
- M6 have predominance of erythroblasts.
- M7 is mainly megakaryocytic.

M_3 = DIC
M_5 = gingival hyperplasia

Signs and Symptoms

- Fatigue, hemorrhage, or bruising (30%)
- Infection of lung, skin (25%)
- Splenomegaly is rare (25%) compared to other types of leukemia.

Adverse effects of chemotherapy agents:
Cisplatin = nephrotoxicity
Bleomycin = pulmonary fibrosis
Vincristine = neurotoxic, palsies
Doxorubicin = cardiotoxic
Tamoxifen = vaginal bleeding

Diagnosis

Specific characteristics:

- M_3: Associated with DIC, Auer rods, t(15;17), add all-*trans* retinoic acid to chemo
- M_5: Associated with gingival hyperplasia
- M_4, M_5: CNS manifestations
- t(8;21) and t(15;17) have better prognosis.

Treatment

- *Induction:* Cytarabine + an anthracycline (daunorubicin)—50 to 80% receive remission
- *Consolidation:* Same chemotherapy as induction
- *Maintenance:* Clinical trials determining best drugs
- Stem cell transplantation is also potentially curative.
- M_3 treated with all-*trans* retinoic acid in addition to cytarabine and daunorubicin.

Acute Lymphocytic Leukemia (ALL)

Epidemiology

Primarily a disease of children, but accounts for 20% of adult leukemias:

- 3 subtypes L1–L3
- L1 occurs in 80% of ALL cases in children.
- Majority of adult cases are L2.
- L3 cell is identical morphologically to the neoplastic cells of Burkitt's lymphoma t(8;14).

Signs and Symptoms

- Symptoms acute at onset often beginning within a few weeks of diagnosis
- Malaise, fever, lethargy, weight loss, bone pain, infection, and hemorrhage
- Lymphadenopathy, splenomegaly, hepatomegaly in about 50%

Diagnosis

- Elevated leukocyte count
- Blasts in peripheral blood
- Absolute neutrophil count, hematocrit, and platelet count decreased
- 25 to 30%: Philadelphia chromosome (chromosome 22) arising from t(9;22)—poorer prognosis
- Periodic acid-Schiff (PAS) reaction will react positive in L1 and L2 subtypes

Treatment

- Patients with Philadelphia chromosome often need bone marrow transplantation.
- *Induction:* Four or five drugs such as vincristine, prednisone, daunorubicin, L-asparaginase, and cyclophosphamide are used.
- *Consolidation:* Cell-cycle phase-specific antimetabolites
- *Maintenance:* Low-dose chemotherapy is standard.
- Post-remission, patients need CNS chemo prophylaxis +/– cranial radiation.

▶ CHRONIC MYELOID LEUKEMIA (CML)

CML is a myeloproliferative disorder (one myeloid precursor clonally proliferates abnormally). It has 25% risk/year of transforming to acute leukemia (blastic transformation).

Signs and Symptoms

- *Chronic phase:* WBC counts increase, spleen and liver enlarge
- *Accelerated phase:* RBC, platelets decrease; symptoms include bone pain, fever, night sweats, and weight loss
- *Blastic phase:* Peripheral blood and marrow are filled with rapidly proliferating leukemic blast cells.

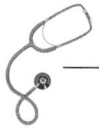

Better prognosis of CML is associated with:

- **Young age (< 40)**
- **No thrombocytopenia**
- **Early stage**
- **Low percentage of blasts**

90% of patients with CML have the Philadelphia chromosome t(9;22).

Diagnosis

- Examining the peripheral blood film shows increased myeloblasts and basophils, white blood cells
- Leukocyte alkaline phosphatase is low in CML cells.
- 90% have Philadelphia chromosome t(9;22).

Treatment

- Allogenic bone marrow transplant treatment of choice for younger patients
- Imatinib (Gleevec) inhibits Philadelphia chromosome and induces indefinite remission (a revolutionary breakthrough!).
- Chemotherapy consists of busulfan and hydroxyurea for those that cannot have BMT (chronic phase) and vincristine and prednisone for those in the accelerated/blastic phase.

▶ CHRONIC LYMPHOCYTIC LEUKEMIA (CLL)

Pathophysiology

- Most common type of leukemia in the Western world
- Malignant clonal disorder of mature lymphocytes which can disrupt normal marrow elements of production
- Since it predominantly affects the B cells, there is an impairment of the humoral immunity
- Generally a chronic disorder that can last for years

Signs and Symptoms

- Lymphadenopathy and splenomegaly often present at discovery of disease
- Infections because of neutropenia, hypogammaglobulinemia
- At later stages of disease, patient may have symptoms of fever, night sweats, weight loss

Diagnosis

- Often suspected or found incidentally on routine CBC (increased lymphocytes)
- Lymph node biopsy
- Usually B cell origin

Stage/Survival

Rai Stage		Survival
0	Lymphocytosis only	> 10 yrs
I	Adenopathy	6–7 yrs
II	Splenomegaly	6–7 yrs
III	Hgb < 10	2–3 yrs
IV	Thrombocytopenia	2–3 yrs

Treatment

- There is no cure, but several treatments are effective; often, just watchful waiting initially.

- Fludarabine (purine analog)
- Rituximab (antibody to CD20)
- Alkylating agent like chlorambucil or cyclophosphamide
- COP: Cyclophosphamide, vincristine, prednisone
- IgG for hypogammaglobulinemia

▶ MULTIPLE MYELOMA

Pathophysiology

Malignant disease of plasma cells that is characterized by:

- Presence of monoclonal immunoglobulin or light chains in the serum and urine
- Bone destruction (lytic lesions) because myeloma cells produce osteoclastic activating factor

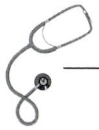

Multiple myeloma: Common triad of back pain, anemia, and renal insufficiency.

Epidemiology

- Median age at diagnosis 68
- Twice as common in blacks than whites

Signs and Symptoms

- Hypercalcemia
- Pathologic fractures/lytic bone lesions
- Renal failure
- Anemia

Typical scenario:
A 60-year-old man with punched out lytic lesions in the skull and mild anemia. *Think: Multiple myeloma.*

Diagnosis

- *Radiography:* Lytic lesions on x-ray
- *Electrophoresis:* Monoclonal elevation of one immunoglobulin
- *Urinalysis:* Free kappa and lambda light chains (Bence Jones proteins)
- *Bone marrow biopsy:* 10 to 20% plasma cells (normal is < 5%)
- *Peripheral smear:* Rouleaux formation

Typical scenario:
A 68-year-old man presents with low back pain, hypercalcemia, anemia, and azotemia. *Think: Multiple myeloma.*

Treatment

There is no cure.

- Chemotherapy:
  - Alkylating agent (melphalan or cyclophosphamide)
  - Thalidomide (antiangiogenesis agent)
  - Prednisone
- Calcitonin, bisphosphonates for high calcium
- Bone marrow transplant is effective.

▶ HODGKIN'S LYMPHOMA

Pathophysiology

Follicular B cells undergo a transformation to malignant cells. Four subtypes based on histology of lymph node and cell type:

1. *Lymphocyte predominant*
2. *Nodular sclerosing:* Most common type; typically presents as cervical lymph node enlargement or mediastinal mass
3. *Mixed cellularity*
4. *Lymphocyte depleted:* Rare, worst prognosis

Epidemiology

- Disease with bimodal distribution having peaks in 30s and 70s
- May have an association with Epstein–Barr virus (EBV)

Clinical

- Presents with asymptomatic lymph node enlargement or CXR showing mediastinal mass
- "B" symptoms may occur in patients with more widespread disease. These include fever, night sweats, weight loss, and shortness of breath.

Diagnosis

- Lymph node biopsy
- Presence of Reed–Sternberg cells is required for diagnosis.

Treatment

Curable depending on stage. Based on staging and pathology, both chemotherapy and radiotherapy are utilized; prognosis is dependent on extension of disease. Generally, if the lesion is small and only on one side of the diaphragm, radiation is used alone. Otherwise, add chemo.

▶ NON-HODGKIN'S LYMPHOMA

Pathophysiology

Most originate from B cells. B cell lymphomas are further classified based on the tissue type origination from lymph node: germinal center, mantle zone, or marginal zone. The working classification is most widely used in the United States. It categorizes lymphoma by low, intermediate, and high grade based on median survival.

Signs and Symptoms/Treatment

- Lymphadenopathy
- Fatigue, weight loss, fever, and night sweats are common symptoms.
- Involvement of mesenteric nodes and extranodal disease is more common.
- Hepatosplenomegaly

Specific Types

Follicular

- A common presentation of the low-grade follicular lymphomas is asymptomatic, painless, diffuse, long-standing lymphadenopathy in a middle-aged individual.
- Bone marrow involvement is present in the majority of patients.

- Treatment includes alkylating agent (cyclophosphamide) and prednisone.
- Least aggressive; median survival is 6 years.

Diffuse Large Cell Lymphoma

- Most common intermediate-grade lymphoma
- Diffuse large cell lymphoma may present in a variety of extranodal sites, particularly the gastrointestinal tract and the head and neck.
- Patients treated with chemotherapy—CHOP (cyclophosphamide, doxorubicin [hydroxydaunomycin], vincristine [Oncovin], prednisone)

Lymphoblastic Lymphoma

- High grade lymphomas derived from thymic T-cells
- Often seen in children
- Associated with a large mediastinal mass and testicular, central nervous system (CNS), and marrow involvement

Burkitt's Lymphoma

- High-grade lymphoma more common in children than adults
- High incidence of bone marrow involvement
- African type has higher association with EBV and jaw involvement than American type.
- Marrow with "starry-sky" appearance
- Treatment includes high-dose cyclophosphamide, methotrexate, and cytarabine and intensive CNS prophylaxis.

Diagnosis

- Lymph node biopsy
- Pathologic subtype (tissue architecture, predominant cell), immunophenotypes, molecular analysis
- Unlike Hodgkin's disease, histology of the nodes is a major predictor of prognosis.

Prognosis

- Depends on histology of malignancy, not spread of disease.
- Generally, prognosis is better if histology is nodular or follicular and cell size is small.
- Prognosis is worse if histology is diffuse and cell size is large.

Solid Tumor Malignancies

▶ BREAST CANCER

Epidemiology

- Second most common cause of **cancer death** in women in the United States (most common is lung CA, as in men). One in eight lifetime risk
- 1% of all breast CA occurs in men
- 10% caused by mutations in one or more of the following genes: p53 (tumor suppressor), BRCA-1, BRCA-2, erbB2 (HER-2/neu)

Most cases of breast cancer are not associated with known gene mutations.

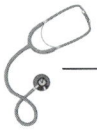

One in eight women who live to age 80 will develop breast cancer.

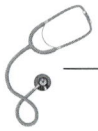

The breasts of young women contain a high proportion of fibrous tissue that is radiopaque, rendering mammograms uninterpretable. As women age, the fiber is replaced by radiolucent fat. At age 35 a woman is still at low risk for breast CA, yet has undergone fatty replacement of a substantial amount of the fiber, making it a good time for the baseline mammogram.

Risk Factors

- Age
- Prior breast CA
- Family history
- Increased estrogen exposure:
  - Early menarche
  - Late menopause
  - Nulliparity/late pregnancy
  - Oral contraceptive pills and hormone replacement therapy **do not** increase risk

Screening

Breast Exams

- Annually by physician (starting at age 20)
- Monthly self-exam (best time is 3 to 5 days after onset of menses)

Mammograms

- Age 35 baseline
- 40 to 49 years, q2y
- 50+, annually

Masses

- Cancer usually painless
- Sonography—differentiate cystic from solid
- Fine-needle aspiration cytology—high false-negative rate, can drain cystic lesions
- Excisional/open biopsy—definitive diagnosis

Prognosis

- Prognosis depends on:
  - TNM staging
  - Axillary lymph node status
  - Tumor grade
  - Tumor size
  - Vascular or lymph invasion
  - Hormone receptor status (better)

Treatment

For nonmetastatic disease:

- Surgical excision
- Breast conservation usually possible, mastectomy required for:
  1. Tumor > 7 cm
  2. Tumor that includes nipple
  3. Extensive intraductal disease
- Adjuvant chemotherapy:
  - Unnecessary in stage I tumors (tumor < 2 cm, no nodes)
  - Battery of standard agents used:
    - Adriamycin, Cytoxan
    - Tamoxifen, an estrogen/progesterone receptor blocker, can be of use in tumors expressing these receptors
    - Postmenopausal women more likely to benefit from tamoxifen
- Radiation reduces the risk of local recurrence but **does not** improve long-term survival.

For metastatic disease:

- Chemotherapy

► OVARIAN CANCER

Epidemiology

Ovarian cancer is the fourth most common cause of death from cancer among women of all ages in the United States.

Signs and Symptoms

- Bloating
- Diffuse abdominal pain
- Ascites
- Dyspareunia
- Irregular vaginal bleeding
- Weight loss

Risk Factors

- Older age at first pregnancy
- Family history

The following appear to lower the risk of ovarian cancer (by prolonging periods of anovulation or suppressing gonadotropin levels):

- Childbearing
- Oral contraceptive use
- Breast-feeding
- Tubal sterilization

FIGO Staging

- Stage I: Ovary only
- Stage II: Ovary + pelvic extension
- Stage III: Ovary + growth outside pelvis
- Stage IV: Metastasis

Screening

There are no currently recommended screening tests.

Prognosis

Despite aggressive treatment, 5-year survival of women with ovarian cancer is only about 40%.

Treatment

- Surgery alone for stages IA and IB
- Surgery (debulking) + chemo (paclitaxel + platinum agent) for more advanced stages

▶ CERVICAL CANCER

Definition

Cervical cancer is an STD associated with human papillomavirus (HPV) types 16, 18, 31, 45, 51, 52, and 53.

Risk Factors

- HPV
- Human immunodeficiency virus (HIV)
- Smoking
- Early age at first intercourse
- Large number of sexual partners

Signs and Symptoms

- Foul-smelling vaginal discharge
- Postcoital and irregular vaginal bleeding
- Pelvic pain
- Dyspareunia
- Enlarged cervix with erosions

Screening

- Yearly Papanicolaou test starting at age 18 or age at first sexual intercourse
- Counsel patients about protective effect of barrier contraceptives.

Treatment

- Colposcopic-directed cervical biopsy for carcinoma-in-situ (stage 0)
- Radical hysterectomy for disease invading cervix (stage I)
- Radiation therapy for disease that invades beyond cervix (stages II–IV)

Prognosis

Stages I and II: 5-year survival is 60%.
Stage III: 5-year survival is 40%.

▶ PROSTATE CANCER

Definition

Adenocarcinoma of the prostatic acini

Epidemiology

- Third most common cause of **cancer** death in men in the United States
- Incidence increases with age; most cases occur after age 50.
- Higher incidence in African Americans

Signs and Symptoms

- Dysuria
- Urinary hesitancy
- Back pain
- Hematuria

Screening

- Begin yearly screening at age 50; start at age 40 for African American men
- Yearly digital rectal exam to look for indurated, nodular prostate
- Yearly screening for prostate specific antigen (PSA) (controversial)
- For PSA > 4.1, transrectal ultrasonography (TRUS) with biopsy of suspicious areas

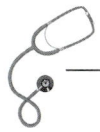

Even advanced prostate CA is often asymptomatic, so screening is important.

Treatment

T1 Disease (Nonpalpable)
- Prostatectomy
- Consider radiotherapy

T2 (Palpable) and T3 Disease (Extracapsular Extension)
- Radical prostatectomy
- Consider androgen deprivation

Metastasis
- Radical prostatectomy
- Androgen deprivation
- Consider chemotherapy

Prognosis

Ten-year survival rates are 75% when the cancer is confined to the prostate, 55% for those with regional extension, and 15% for those with distant metastases.

▶ TESTICULAR CANCER

Definition

Primary germ cell tumors of the testis

Epidemiology

- Common cause of cancer in men aged 20 to 40
- Seen more frequently in whites than in African Americans
- 95% of testicular cancers are germ cell tumors

Typical scenario:
A 23-year-old man presents with gynecomastia, substernal pain, dyspnea, weakness, cough, fever, weight loss. Next step? CXR. Finding? Mediastinal mass = germ cell tumor.

Classification

Germ cell tumors are divided into seminomas and nonseminomas (see Figure 2.4-2).

Findings

- Painless testicular mass or persistent swelling
- Metastases may present as back pain (retroperitoneal) or dyspnea (lung mets).

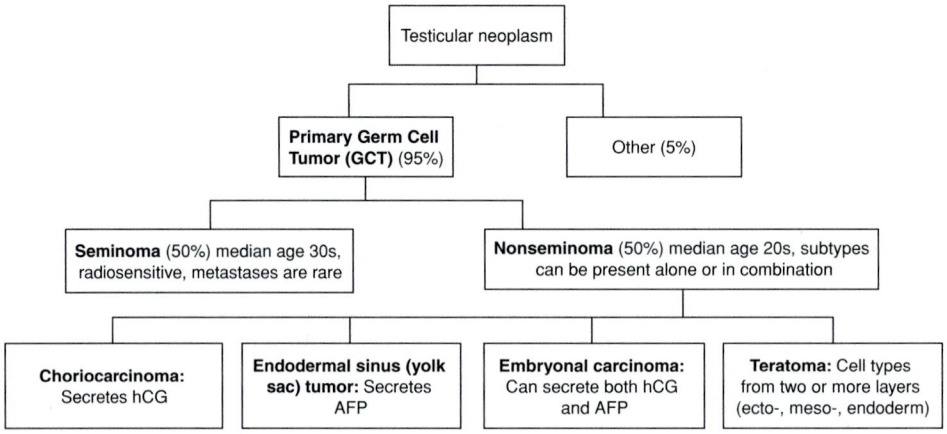

FIGURE 2.4-2. Classification of testicular cancer.

TREATMENT

- Nonseminoma: Orchiectomy, retroperitoneal lymph node dissection (RPLND), chemotherapy for lymph node involvement or metastasis. Patients without lymph node involvement or metastases have a 95% cure rate.
- Seminoma: Orchiectomy, retroperitoneal radiation has 98% cure rate for nonmetastasized seminomas; chemotherapy for metastases.

▶ MISCELLANEOUS METASTATIC DISEASE

Liver Metastasis

- Liver and lung are the most common sites for metastatic disease
- Primary tumors that metastasize to the liver: **Colon > Stomach > Pancreas > Breast > Lung**

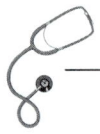

Lots of Bad Stuff Kills Glia
(Origin of brain mets: Lung, Breast, Skin, Kidney, GI)

Bone Metastasis

- Breast and prostate are the most common.
- Kidney, thyroid, testes, lung, prostate, breast
- Lung = Lytic
- Breast = Both lytic and blastic
- Prostate = blastic

Brain Metastasis

- Fifty percent of brain tumors are metastatic lesions.
- Primary tumors metastasizing to the brain: Lung, Breast, Skin (melanoma), Kidney (renal cell carcinoma), GI

Paraneoplastic and Distant Effects of Tumors

Effect	Causes	Associated Neoplasm
Cushing's syndrome	ACTH or ACTH-like peptide.	Small cell lung carcinoma
SIADH	ADH or ANP.	Small cell lung carcinoma and intracranial neoplasms.
Hypercalcemia	PTH-related peptide, TGF-α, TNF-α, IL-2.	Squamous cell lung carcinoma, renal carcinoma, breast carcinoma, multiple myeloma, and bone metastasis (lysed bone).
Polycythemia	Erythropoietin.	Renal cell carcinoma (hypernephroma).
Lambert–Eaton syndrome	Antibodies against presynaptic Ca^{2+} channels at NMJ.	Thymoma, bronchogenic carcinoma.
Gout	Hyperuricemia due to excess nucleic acid turnover (i.e., cytotoxic therapy).	

▶ ONCOLOGIC EMERGENCIES

Hypercalcemia

- The most common metabolic emergency of malignancy
- Symptoms and signs include confusion, nausea, fatigue, decreased PO intake, polyuria, depression, psychosis, nephrolithiasis **(BONES, STONES, GROANS, and PSYCHIATRIC OVERTONES)**
- Can progress to severe confusion and coma
- ECG may show QT interval shortening.
- **Treatment:** Aggressive rehydration with normal saline, furosemide once patient is adequately hydrated, bisphosphonates

Febrile Neutropenia

- Fever in the setting of clinically significant neutropenia (ANC [absolute neutrophil count] < 500)
- **Workup:** Careful history and physical, chest x-ray, pan-culture
- **Treatment:** Antibiotics should be started empirically (usually cefipime + aminoglycoside; add vancomycin if the person has a port or a skin source).

SVC Syndrome

- Caused by obstruction of the superior vena cava by external compression, tumor invasion, or thrombus formation in the SVC lumen
- **Signs/Symptoms:** Dyspnea, facial edema and plethora, cough, neck and arm edema
- **Diagnosis:** CT chest, chest x-ray

- **Treatment:** Chemotherapy, radiation, intubation/tracheal stent for airway compromise, steroids (controversial)

Spinal Cord Compression

- Compression of spinal cord secondary to vertebral collapse or extension of tumor from vertebra
- **Signs/Symptoms:** Back pain, loss of bowel or bladder function, muscle weakness, saddle anesthesia
- **Diagnosis:** Thorough neurologic exam, MRI spine with gadolinium
- **Treatment:** High-dose steroids, radiation therapy, surgical decompression

HIGH-YIELD FACTS IN

Infectious Disease

Definitions 181

Genitourinary Infections 181

- UTI, Cystitis, and Pyelonephritis 181
- Urethritis 183
- Vaginitis 184

Sexually Transmitted Diseases 185

- Syphilis 185
- Balanitis 186
- Genital Herpes 186
- Human Papillomavirus (HPV) 187
- Pelvic Inflammatory Disease (PID) 187
- Prostatitis 188

Pneumonia and Upper Respiratory Tract Infections 189

- Community-Acquired Pneumonias 189
- Hospital-Acquired Pneumonias 191
- Aspiration Pneumonias 191
- Other Respiratory Infections 191

Common Skin Infections 193

Immunity 193

Immunodeficiency 195

- Cell-Mediated Immunodeficiency (CMI) 195
- Humoral Immune Deficiency Disorders 195
- Major Causes of Fever in the Immunocompromised 196
- General Principles of Evaluation and Management 197
- Pulmonary Infiltrate in the Immunocompromised Patient 197

HIV and AIDS 197

Opportunistic Infections and AIDS 202

- *Pneumocystis carinii* Pneumonia (PCP) 202
- Toxoplasmosis 204
- Protozoal Diarrhea 205
- *Mycobacterium avium* Complex (MAC) 205
- Tuberculosis 206

Fungal Infections 206
Viral Infections 207
Neoplastic Disease and HIV 209
Bioterrorism Agents 210
Anthrax 210
Botulism 211
Pneumonic Plague 211
Smallpox 212
Tularemia 213
Tick-Borne Diseases 214
Epidural Abscess 216
Malaria 216

▶ DEFINITIONS

- **Infection:** Microbial process characterized by an inflammatory response
- **Bacteremia:** Invasion of and presence of bacteria in the blood
- **Systemic inflammatory response syndrome (SIRS):** Characterized by two or more of the following:
  - Temperature > 38°C or < 36°C, heart rate > 90, respiratory rate > 20 per minute or $PaCO_2$ < 32, white blood cell count > 12
- **Sepsis:** SIRS and a nidus of infection
- **Severe sepsis:** Sepsis with evidence of organ hypoperfusion
- **Septic shock:** Severe sepsis with hypotension despite adequate fluid resuscitation requiring vasopressors to maintain blood pressure

GENITOURINARY INFECTIONS

UTI, CYSTITIS, AND PYELONEPHRITIS

DEFINITIONS

- A **urinary tract infection (UTI)** is a general term encompassing infection anywhere from urethral meatus to kidneys.
- **Cystitis** is infection of the bladder.
- **Pyelonephritis** is infection involving renal parenchyma.
- **Bacteriuria** is the presence of bacteria in the urine, which may or may not be symptomatic.
- **Pyuria** is the presence of WBCs in the urine, usually associated with bacteriuria.
- **Hematuria** is the presence of RBCs in the urine, often seen with cystitis.

EPIDEMIOLOGY

- More common in women by a ratio of 30:1 from age 1 through 50; beyond age 50 the ratio is 2:1.
- UTI is the most common infectious complication of pregnancy.
- In the elderly, UTI is the most frequently documented infection, the most common cause of sepsis, and the most common nosocomial infection.

RISK FACTORS

Men
- Uncircumsized males
- Prostatic hypertrophy
- Phimosis
- Anal intercourse

Women
- Recent sexual intercourse
- History of prior UTI
- Use of spermicide
- Postmenopausal state

Bugs that cause UTI:
SEEKS PP
S. *saprophyticus*
E. *coli*
E*nterobacter*
K*lebsiella*
S*erratia*
P*roteus*
P*seudomonas* (especially with GU instrumentation)

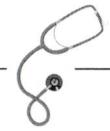

An alkaline urine is suggestive of infection with *Proteus mirabilis* or *Ureaplasma urealyticum.*

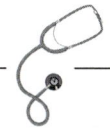

Men with cystitis should be investigated for an underlying causes such at prostatitis or urinary retention.

Both

- Instrumentation (see Table 2.5-1 for common procedures)
- Immunocompromise
- Genitourinary tract abnormalities

Etiology

- *E. coli* is by far the most common pathogen, accounting for 85% of community-acquired UTIs and 50% of nosocomial ones.
- *S. saprophyticus* contributes to ~15% of uncomplicated cases.
- *Klebsiella*, *Proteus*, *Pseudomonas*, and enterococci account for the remainder of cases.
- Group B strep accounts for only ~1% of cases but is a clinically important pathogen in the pregnant patient at term.

TABLE 2.5-1. Common Genitourinary Procedures

Test	Description	Uses
Intravenous pyelography	Contrast is injected into a peripheral vein, followed by radiographs, allowing visualization of the renal parenchyma and the ureters.	▪ Kidney or urethral trauma ▪ Kidney or urethral tumors ▪ Urethral diverticulum ▪ Assessment of renal damage from pyelonephritis

Voiding cystourethrogram	Contrast medium is placed into the bladder via catheter and visualized with x-ray during active micturition.	▪ Congenital abnormalities:
		  ▪ Posterior urethral valves
		  ▪ Ectopic drainage of ureters
		▪ Neurogenic bladder
		▪ Strictures
		▪ Vesicoureteral reflux
		▪ Stress urinary incontinence
		▪ Ureteroceles

Cystometry	Bladder is filled with water via catheter. Bladder is emptied into a measuring device. The pressure is recorded during this whole time.	▪ Benign prostatic hypertrophy ▪ Congenital anomalies ▪ Incontinence
Cystoscopy	Introduction of either a flexible or rigid scope into the urethra	▪ Biopsy ▪ Resection of tumors ▪ Crushing of stones ▪ Catheterization of ureters
Renal ultrasound	Advantage is that it is noninvasive.	▪ Renal calculi ▪ Urinary obstruction ▪ Renal tumors ▪ Renal vein thrombus ▪ Evaluating renal failure—the size of the kidneys give an idea of the chronicity of the failure.

Signs and Symptoms

- **General UTI:** Dysuria, frequency, urgency, nocturia, suprapubic pain, cloudy, malodorous urine, or bloody urine
- **Pyelonephritis:** Spiking fever, shaking chills, costovertebral angle tenderness, nausea, vomiting, anorexia

Diagnosis

- Urine dipstick to look for leukocyte esterase and nitrites is the most widely available and cost-effective test.
- Sensitivities of the test range from 75% to 96%; specifities are better and range from 86% to 97%.
  - Nitrites:
    - False negatives: Bacteria that do not produce nitrite, voided urine that has not remained in the bladder long enough to multiply, ascorbic acid, antibiotics, lack of vegetables in the diet (no nitrate substrate)
    - False positives: Medication color, not fresh urine (skin-contaminating bacteria multiply in the specimen container)
  - Leukocyte esterase results can be seen with > 3,000 and patients already on antibiotics. False-positive leukocyte esterase results are seen with fecal contamination.
    - False positives: Fecal contamination, oxidizing detergents, strong yellow pigments
    - False negatives: Glycosuria, increased specific gravity, oxalic acid, antibiotics
- Urine culture is the definitive test. A positive result is defined as > 100 colony-forming units (CFUs) per millliliter in symptomatic patients, and > 100,000 CFU/mL in an asymptomatic patient. Urine cultures should always be obtained for complicated UTIs, due to high rate of bacterial resistance.
- Imaging is not indicated for uncomplicated UTI.
  - CT scan or renal ultrasound can demonstrate perinephric/intrarenal abscesses, nephrolithiasis, and obstruction. If pyelonephritis does not improve after 48 to 72 hours, these causes should be sought.

Treatment

- Most uncomplicated UTIs are treated with a short course (3–5 days) of oral antibiotics on an outpatient basis.
- Bacteriuria in pregnancy is always treated, regardless of the presence of symptoms, due to high rate of progression to pyelonephritis. Empiric category B antibiotics are nitrofurantoin and ampicillin.
- Consider hospitalization and intravenous antibiotics for high-risk patients: Elderly, immunocompromised, those with indwelling catheters, and patients who are unable to tolerate oral intake.

▶ URETHRITIS

Always treat *Chlamydia* and GC concurrently because coinfection is often present.

Etiology

- *Neisseria gonorrhoeae* and *Chlamydia trachomatis* are the two most common organisms.

When seeing urethritis, consider Reiter's syndrome in the differential.

- *N. gonorrhoeae* (gonococcus [GC]) can cause cervicitis, urethritis, epididymitis, conjunctivitis, PID, pneumonia, and lymphogranuloma venereum.
- C. *trachomatis* can cause cervicitis, urethritis, epididymitis, conjunctivitis, PID, pneumonia, and lymphogranuloma venereum.

Diagnosis

PCR analysis of vaginal or penile swab or urine

The discharge of GC is purulent, whereas with *Chlamydia* it is nonpurulent.

Treatment

- Single-dose therapy:
  - For GC: 125 mg ceftriaxone IM
  - For *Chlamydia:* 1 g azithromycin PO
  - Above combination often given empirically, no compliance issues
- Multiple 7-day combinations exist, if above regimen is not chosen

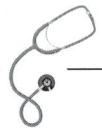

Lactobacilli are used to make yogurt. A Yoplait a day keeps vaginitis away.

▶ VAGINITIS

The normal flora of the vagina creates an acidic environment (pH 3.5 to 4.5) in large part through the colonization of lactobacilli. This protects the vagina from pathogenic organisms. When this environment is disturbed, infections become possible.

Causes

- Bacterial vaginosis (BV)—primarily *Gardnerella*
- *Trichomonas vaginalis*
- Yeast—*Candida albicans*

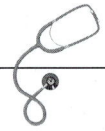

The "whiff" test: Application of KOH to the wet mount will enhance the odor of both *Gardnerella* and *Trichomonas.*

Signs and Symptoms

General

- Vaginal itch and burning sensation
- Abnormal odor
- Increase in discharge:
  - BV: Fishy odor of discharge
  - *Trichomonas:* Fishy odor of discharge, strawberry cervix
  - Yeast: Cheese-like discharge

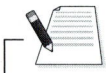

Metronidazole is contraindicated in first-trimester pregnancy. Use clotrimazole instead.

Diagnosis

Seen on wet mount:

- BV: Clue cells (epithelial cells coated with bacteria)
- *Trichomonas:* Motile trichomonads
- Yeast: Pseudohyphae

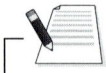

Warn patients against having any alcohol while on metronidazole. It can cause a disulfiram-like reaction when coingested with alcohol.

Treatment

- Metronidazole for BV and *Trichomonas*
- Nystatin for yeast infection
- Treat sexual partners as well in *Trichomonas*.

Sexually Transmitted Diseases

▶ SYPHILIS

Definition and Pathophysiology

- A sexually transmitted or congenital disease with variable clinical manifestations, depending on stage of the disease.
- Syphilis is transmitted primarily through sexual contact but can be spread through any mucosal or epithelial abrasion.
- The causative organism is *Treponema pallidum*, a spirochete.
- Once the spirochete has entered the body, it spreads throughout most organ systems and the disease then progresses through three active stages.

Signs and Symptoms

All patients develop a painless chancre at inoculation site. If untreated, some patients progress to a disseminated (2°) stage, during which the organism is spread throughout the entire body and is highly infectious.

Primary Syphilis

- Appears 3 to 6 weeks after exposure
- A **painless "buttonlike" chancre** with indurated borders develops at inoculation site within 2 to 6 weeks after exposure.
- Usually develop genital chancre, but may have an extragenital lesion.
- Accompanied by regional lymphadenopathy **("bubo")** within 1 week.
- Chancre can last up to 6 weeks if untreated.

Secondary Syphilis

- Appears 4 to 6 weeks after 1° syphilis resolves, lasts for 6 to 8 weeks
- Maculopapular rash (multiple, discrete, firm, "ham-colored" papules scattered symmetrically over trunk, **palms and soles,** and genitals)
- **Condylomata lata**—soft, flat-topped pink papules on anogenital region that are painless wartlike lesions
- Flulike symptoms—fever, malaise, arthralgia, generalized lymphadenopathy, and splenomegaly

Latent Phase

- This stage can last for several years.
- Patients are asymptomatic but remain seropositive.

Tertiary Syphilis

- Develops at any time during the latent phase and continues indefinitely if not treated
- **Gummas**—rubbery granulomatous lesions in subcutaneous tissues of central nervous system (CNS), heart, aorta
- Cardiovascular—vasa vasorum vasculitis, aortic insufficiency
- Neurosyphilis—seizures, personality changes, psychosis, **tabes dorsalis** (posterior column degeneration). The syphilitic pupil is also known as the **Argyll Robertson pupil.**

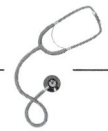

RPR screening is part of dementia workup.

The syphilitic pupil is like a prostitute: It accommodates but doesn't react.

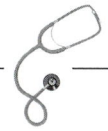

VDRL/RPR false positives are seen in:

- Systemic lupus erythematosus (SLE)
- Infectious mononucleosis
- Hepatitis C

If maternal infection is untreated by 16 weeks' gestation, child may be born with congenital syphilis and is at risk of stillbirth.

Laboratory

- Venereal Disease Research Laboratory (VDRL) and rapid plasma reagin (RPR)—good screening tests but nonspecific
- Fluorescent treponemal antibody-absorption test (FTA-ABS)—done when VDRL or RPR is positive. Good sensitivity and specificity. Remains positive for life, regardless of treatment.
- Darkfield microscopy—smear of exudate from primary chancre or secondary papular lesions reveal a 5 to 20 μm in length spirochete, with kinking and contractile movements but without locomotion.
- *T. pallidum* does not grow in regular blood cultures.

Treatment

Penicillin G

▶ BALANITIS

Definition

Inflammation of the glans penis

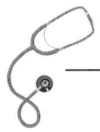

Any patient who presents with balanitis should be screened for diabetes.

Causes

- *Candida albicans*
- Allergic reaction (often to latex condoms)
- Reiter's syndrome

Treatment

- Candidal infections are treated with nystatin.
- Reiter's syndrome is treated with NSAIDs.
- Antichlamydial treatment may also be useful.

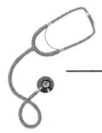

Infections can remain dormant for years, but the herpesvirus is continuously shed and can be transmitted during latent phases.

▶ GENITAL HERPES

Definition

Infection with herpesvirus. Type 1 usually associated with oral lesions, and type II with genital lesions, but not always.

Signs and Symptoms

- **Painful** vesicular lesions on erythematous base
- Local lymphadenopathy
- Neuralgia often precedes an outbreak

Adverse effects of acyclovir:
- **Renal crystals**
- **Allergic interstitial nephritis**

Laboratory

- Tzanck smear test and culture
- Herpes serology

Treatment

Antiviral agents acyclovir, famciclovir, and valacyclovir are not curative but effective in reducing the severity and frequency of outbreak as well as the degree of viral shedding

► HUMAN PAPILLOMAVIRUS (HPV)

Definition

Sexually transmitted disease (STD) caused by the HPV, of which there are many subtypes

Epidemiology

- Most common sexually transmitted disease
- Commonly asymptomatic in men

Signs and Symptoms

- Bowenoid papules on penis
- Condyloma acuminata (papillomatous growths with a soft, macerated surface)
- Warts grow on mucous membrane of penis, perineum, vulva, vagina, and vaginal canal.

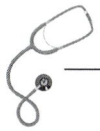

HPV: Mother may infect newborn during delivery, causing **laryngeal papillomatosis.**

Diagnosis

Most HPV warts are flat and invisible to the unaided eye. Coating them with 1% acetic acid turns them white. All white lesions on colposcopy are biopsied for HPV.

Treatment

Lesions are removed via cryosurgery, laser ablation, or chemical ablation (podophyllin).

HPV types 16, 18, 31, 45, 51, 52, and 53 are associated with cervical cancer.

► PELVIC INFLAMMATORY DISEASE (PID)

Definition

Infection of the upper genital structures in women (uterus, oviducts, ovaries), often with involvement of neighboring organs.

Risk Factors

- Younger age at first sexual contact
- Multiple sexual partners
- Use of IUD
- Prior history of PID
- Recent intrauterine instrumentation

C. trachomatis is a predisposing factor for pelvic inflammatory disease (PID) and infertility.

Signs, Symptoms, and Diagnostic Criteria

- Lower abdominal pain
- Tenderness to pelvic exam
- Cervical motion and adnexal tenderness

Plus one or more of the following:

- Fever > 101°F
- Abnormal vaginal/cervical discharge

Typical scenario: A 19-year-old sexually active female presents with left lower crampy pelvic pain for 1 week. Physical exam reveals a temperature of 101°F, cervical motion tenderness, and a mucopurulent vaginal discharge. Laboratory results reveal ESR 65 and WBC 16. *Think: Pelvic inflammatory disease;* check for GC and chlamydia.

- Lab evidence of GC or C. *trachomatis*
- Elevated ESR or C-reactive protein

TREATMENT

Outpatient

- Treat for GC and C. *trachomatis*, major causative organisms.
- Offer HIV testing.
- Remove any infected foreign body.
- Treat all sexual partners.

Criteria for Hospital Admission

- Uncertain diagnosis
- Fever > 102.2°F
- Failure of outpatient therapy
- Pregnancy
- First episode in a nulligravida
- Inability to tolerate PO
- Inability to follow up in 48 hours
- Immunosuppression

▶ PROSTATITIS

Divided into bacterial and nonbacterial

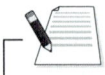

A diabetic patient has a black necrotic parasinus lesion. *Think:* Mucormycosis rhizopus.

Bacterial Prostatitis

DEFINITION

Inflammation of the prostate due to bacteria ascending the urethra and then passing into the prostate through the prostatic ducts.

CAUSES

Most common agents:

- *E. coli*
- *Pseudomonas*

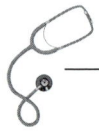

Care must be taken during the rectal exam. Vigorously massaging the prostate can lead to bacteremia.

SIGNS AND SYMPTOMS

- Perineal and suprapubic pain
- Dysuria and urinary frequency
- Fever
- Tender prostate on physical exam

LABORATORY

- Leukocytosis with neutrophil predominance
- Urinalysis (U/A) shows bacteriuria and pyuria.

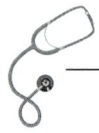

Nonbacterial prostatitis usually causes chronic prostatitis.

TREATMENT

- Outpatient therapy consists of TMP-SMZ or ciprofloxacin for 21 days.
- Indications for hospitalization include severe comorbidities, poor patient compliance, or sepsis.

Nonbacterial Prostatitis

An inflammatory process in the prostate from an unknown etiology. Viral agents or an autoimmune reaction are possible causes.

Signs and Symptoms

- Urinary frequency and dysuria
- Nontender, enlarged prostate on physical exam

Laboratory

- U/A and urine culture are negative.
- Leukocytes can be seen in prostatic secretions.

Treatment

- A trial of antibiotics is often given.
- Anti-inflammatories for symptomatic relief

Pneumonia and Upper Respiratory Tract Infections

▶ COMMUNITY-ACQUIRED PNEUMONIAS

Streptococcus pneumoniae, *Legionella*, *Staphylococcus aureus*, *Haemophilus influenzae*, *Chlamydia pneumoniae*, *Mycoplasma pneumoniae*, and viruses.

Typical Pneumonias

Usually treat with a beta-lactam or fluoroquinolone.

Streptococcus pneumoniae

- **Most common community-acquired pneumonia; typically has lobar consolidation with "rusty-colored" sputum**
- Gram-positive cocci, grows in chains
- Causes multiple infections including acute sinusitis, otitis media, meningitis, septic arthritis, pneumonia, cellulitis, erysipelas, bacteremia, and others
- People with defective complement/antibody function, prior hospitalization, splenectomy, renal insufficiency, diabetes, and other conditions are predisposed to acquired *S. pneumoniae*.
- Treat with beta-lactam antibiotics.

Staphylococcus aureus

- **Consider this in a patient with viral infection ~2 weeks before. "Salmon pink" sputum and cavitary lesions**
- Gram-positive cocci in clusters
- Treat with beta-lactams or vancomycin if MRSA is suspected.

Klebsiella pneumoniae
- "Currant jelly" sputum, "bulging fissure" on chest x-ray (CXR)
- Friedlander's bacillus
- Presents as community-acquired pneumonia, which can progress to empyema and pulmonic abscesses
- May cause biliary or urinary tract infections in hospitalized patients
- Treat with cephalosporin +/– aminoglycoside.

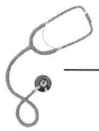

All HIV+ patients should receive the pneumococcal and *H. flu* vaccines.

Haemophilus influenzae
- Gram-negative coccobacilli
- Has many types; the most commonly known is *H. influenzae* type B (HIB)
- Nontypable *H. influenzae* is responsible for sinusitis, otitis media, and community-acquired pneumonia, especially in COPD patients.
- Infection with HIB causes meningitis, especially in children < 3 years of age; currentlly, there is an HIB vaccine to protect against this.
- Treat with third-generation cephalosporin, quinolone, doxycycline.

Moraxella catarrhalis
- Gram-negative coccus
- Mostly in COPD and immunocompromised patients; causes uppre respiratory infections and pneumonia
- Susceptible to penicillin/clavulanic acid, macrolides, and TMP-SMZ

Atypical Pneumonias

Typical scenario: A 21-year-old woman who complains of dry cough, malaise, and low-grade fevers for 2 weeks has a CXR with hazy infiltrates. *Think:* Mycoplasma pneumoniae.

Mycoplasma pneumoniae
- Causes community-acquired pneumonia, "walking" pneumonia, or atypical pneumonia
- Insidious onset with an incubation period up to 3 weeks
- Patients present with fever, pharyngitis, headaches, chills, tonsillitis, arthritis, hemolytic anemia, change in mental status, or erythema multiforme.

Chlamydia pneumoniae
- Common cause of community-acquired pneumonia in children and young adults
- Transmission is person to person.
- Patients often present with fever, nonproductive cough.
- CXR shows segmental infiltrates.
- Treat with quinolone or cephalosporin and macrolide.

Typical scenario: A patient who works in a pet store presents with diffuse, bilateral infiltrate. *Think:* Chlamydia psittaci.

Chlamydia psittaci
- Obligate intracellular parasite
- Host is avian species.
- Transmitted via the respiratory route
- Patient presents with fever, headache, chills, cough, myalgias, abdominal pain, nausea, vomiting.
- On physical exam ~ 70% of patients will have splenomegaly.
- Can be treated with tetracyclines

Legionella pneumophila
- Gram-negative rod, anaerobic
- Source is typically bodies of water.

- Causes Legionnaire's disease, which consists of pneumonia, change in mental status, headaches, diarrhea, abdominal pain, nausea, vomiting, high fever, hyponatremia
- Diagnose with direct immunofluorescent antigen or urinary antigen.
- Treat with macrolides, quinolones, doxycyclines.

Typical scenario: A patient presents with confusion and diarrhea and is found to have a large infiltrate on CXR with a pleural effusion. *Think:* Legionella pneumophila.

▶ HOSPITAL-ACQUIRED PNEUMONIAS

- *Pseudomonas, Enterobacter, Klebsiella pneumoniae, Escherichia coli, Haemophilus influenzae, Staphylococcus aureus*
- **Must always cover for *Pseudomonas;*** use fourth-generation cephalosporin, carbapenem, or piperacillin/tazobactam.

Pseudomonas aeruginosa

- Gram-negative bacillus
- Usually acquired in the hospital
- Most common organism in ventilation-associated pneumonia
- Cystic fibrosis patients can be colonized by *P. aeruginosa,* which correlates with severity of airway disease.

Acinetobacter baumanii

- Small gram-negative coccobacilli
- Often colonize respiratory secretions and endotracheal tubes but also cause nosocomial infections, **particularly ventilator-associated pneumonia**
- Often multidrug resistant
- Treat with a third-generation cephalosporin and an aminoglycoside.

Typical scenario: An elderly patient in the hospital for 3 weeks following an episode of congestive heart failure (or any patient with cystic fibrosis) now has an infiltrate. *Think:* Pseudomonas aeruginosa.

▶ ASPIRATION PNEUMONIAS

- **Patients with a history of losing consciousness (e.g., alcoholic binge, seizures, etc.) present with a right middle lobe infiltrate.**
- Typical organisms are **anaerobes** such as *Bacteroides, Fusobacterium nucleatum, Peptostreptococcus.*
- Treat with anaerobic coverage: Clindamycin (piperacillin/tazobactam and carbapenems have anaerobic coverage as well).

▶ OTHER RESPIRATORY INFECTIONS

Adenovirus

- DNA virus
- Infections occur primarily during the fall and spring seasons.
- Causes upper respiratory tract infection
- Supportive treatment

Epstein–Barr Virus

- DNA virus

- Causes **infectious mononucleosis,** which is characterized by pharyngitis, fever, tender cervical lymphadenopathy, +/– splenomegaly
- **Patients with mononucleosis should not engage in contact sports because their spleen can rupture.**
- Laboratory studies will show abnormal LFTs and lymphocytosis.
- Diagnose with heterophile antibody titers.
- May be associated with hairy leukoplakia
- Supportive treatment

Influenza Virus

- RNA virus
- Three types; A and B constitute one genus, and C makes up the other
- Influenza A periodically undergoes major antigenic changes, known as **antigenic shifts,** causing epidemics.
- Transmission is via areosolized particles.
- Patients present with fever, headache, myalgias, cough, pharyngitis, arthralgias, or lymphadenopathy.
- Influenza may be complicated by a primary viral pneumonia or a 2° bacterial pneumonia caused by *S. aureus*, *S. pneumoniae*, or *H. influenzae*.
- Prophylaxis is with yearly flu vaccinations.
- May treat with amantadine; however, treatment is largely supportive

Typical scenario: A day-care worker presents with arthritis of the hands. *Think: Parvovirus B19.*

Parvovirus B19

- DNA virus
- Causes erythema infectiosum, also known as fifth disease, in children
- Spread through respiratory secretions in people who appear to have the common cold
- In adults, parvovirus B19 presents as acute, symmetric arthritis of the hands, wrists, and knees.
- Treat arthritis with nonsteroidals.

Rhinovirus

- RNA virus
- Causes the common cold, which presents as nasal congestion, rhinorrhea, sneezing, headache, and malaise; self-limited
- Treatment is supportive.

Corynebacterium diphtheriae

- Gram-positive bacillus
- Diphtheria presents as upper respiratory infection (not pneumonia) with low-grade fevers, sore throat, nausea, vomiting
- On exam, may find **grayish exudates that can coalesce to become a pseudomembrane**
- Treat with macrolide or penicillin, diphtheria antitoxin (IV infusion).

Common Skin Infections

Staphylococcus aureus

Overview

- Gram positive, coagulase positive
- Commonly causes infections of skin, septic arthritis, and endocarditis

Syndromes

Toxic Shock Syndrome

- Seen in menstruating women using tampons
- Consists of fever, rash, desquamation of skin, nausea, along with organ failures (kidney, liver)
- Treat by removing foreign body and supportive care (antibiotics are controversial, but clindamycin may decrease toxin).
- Also caused by group A strep

Scalded Skin Syndrome

- The most severe form is toxic epidermal necrolysis.
- Starts as periorbital or perioral erythematous rash and progresses to limbs
- In days, the skin sloughs off.

Streptococcus pyogenes

Overview

- Gram-positive cocci, group A beta-hemolytic
- Causes soft tissue infections such as cellulitis, impetigo, and necrotizing fasciitis
- Also causes pharyngitis, pneumonia, toxic shock–like syndrome
- Treat with penicillin.

Postinfection Sequelae

- **Scarlet fever:** Presents as pharyngitis, strawberry tongue, and a rash that begins on the trunk and spreads to the extremities. Palms and soles have no rash but undergo desquamation.
- **Poststreptococcal glomerulonephritis:** Glomerulonephritis ~2 weeks after strep infection
- **Streptococcal toxic shock syndrome:** Similar to staph

IMMUNITY

Humoral Immunity

- Branch of immune system composed of circulating or cell-bound proteins
- Facilitates and directs cell destruction
- Inactivates toxins

- Two main components:
  - Immunoglobulins: produced by B lymphocytes and plasma cells (see Table 2.5-2)
  - Complement: Produced by the liver

Cellular Immunity

- Branch of immune system composed of cells
- Multiple components:
  - T lymphocytes:
    - Cytotoxic T cells: Kill cells expressing foreign antigens, $CD8^+$
    - Helper T cells: Enhance activity of other T cells, B cells, and macrophages, $CD4^+$
    - Suppressor T cells: Inhibit cellular immune response, $CD8^+$
  - Neutrophils
  - Eosinophils, mast cells
  - Reticuloendothelial system (monocytes, macrophages, histiocytes, Langerhans' cells, Kupffer cells, etc.)
  - Natural killer cells

TABLE 2.5-2. Immunoglobulins and Their Functions

IgG	~70% of total immunoglobulins Predominant antibody in secondary immune response Fixes complement Crosses placenta Four subtypes
IgA	~20% of total immunoglobulins Present in serum, colostrum, saliva, tears, and respiratory and intestinal mucosa Dimer in secretions, monomer in serum
IgM	~10% of total immunoglobulins Predominant antibody in primary immune response Fixes complement best Is a pentamer
IgD	~1% of total immunoglobulins B cell surface receptor
IgE	0.01% of total immunoglobulins Trigger histamine release from mast cells: Immediate hypersensitivity reactions (allergy, anaphylaxis, asthma) Also rises in parasitic infections

IMMUNODEFICIENCY

▶ CELL-MEDIATED IMMUNODEFICIENCY (CMI)

Major Diseases Causing CMI

- AIDS
- Hodgkin's disease and other lymphomas
- Leukemia
- Advanced solid tumors
- Diabetes mellitus
- Sarcoidosis

Iatrogenic CMI

- High-dose corticosteroids
- Cytotoxic chemotherapy
- Radiation therapy

Other Conditions Associated with CMI

- Uremia
- Malnutrition
- Old age

CMI-Associated Infections

- Bacteria: *Listeria*, *Nocardia*, *Mycobacterium tuberculosis*, nontuberculous mycobacteria, *Legionella*, *Salmonella*
- Viruses: Varicella-zoster, herpes simplex, cytomegalovirus (CMV), human papillomavirus (HPV), human herpes virus (HHV)-6, hepatitis B virus (HBV)
- Fungi: *Cryptococcus*, *Candida*, *Histoplasma*, *Coccidioides*, *Aspergillus*, *Pneumocystis carinii*
- Protozoa: *Toxoplasma*, *Cryptosporidium*, *Giardia lamblia*
- Helminths: *Strongyloides stercoralis*

▶ HUMORAL IMMUNE DEFICIENCY DISORDERS

Common Variable Hypogammaglobulinemia

- Can be acquired at any age by men and women
- Low levels of IgG, IgA, and IgM
- Normal numbers of B cells, but are defective
- Patients usually well until 15 to 30 years of age
- Increased susceptibility to infections and autoimmune diseases

Selective IgA Deficiency

- Most common of the selective immunoglobulin deficiencies
- Present with mucous membrane infections (URI, UTI, GI)
- Low-molecular-weight IgM increased in partial compensation
- Serum may contain anti-IgA IgE.
- IgA replacement is useless, may cause anaphylaxis

Other

CLL, multiple myeloma

▶ MAJOR CAUSES OF FEVER IN THE IMMUNOCOMPROMISED

In Cancer Patients

- Fever of unknown origin
- Bacteria: Gram-positive or -negative aerobes, anaerobes at site of mixed infection
- Viruses: Respiratory syncytial virus (RSV), parainfluenza, adenoviruses, herpes simplex virus (HSV), CMV
- Fungi: *Candida*, *Aspergillus*, *Cryptococcus*, *Trichosporon*
- *Pneumocystis carinii* and *Toxoplasma* also seen

In Transplant Patients

Bone Marrow

- Similar causes to cancer patients
- Infection is influenced by time since transplant and type of procedure (allogenic vs. autogenic).

Solid Organ

- Influenced by time since transplant, and type of transplant
- Bacteria: Includes gram positive and negative
- Viruses: CMV, EBV, HBV, hepatitis C virus (HCV), adenovirus
- Fungi: *Aspergillus*, *Pneumocystis carinii*

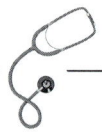

Functionally asplenic patients (sickle cell disease) or postsplenectomy patients (especially from Hodgkin's disease) are at increased risk for infection even if they are not neutropenic.

In Splenectomy Patients

Encapsulated organisms, especially:

- *Streptococcus pneumoniae*
- *Neisseria meningitidis*
- *Haemophilus influenzae*
- *Klebsiella pneumoniae*
- *Salmonella* sp.

Parasites: Malaria, *Babesia*

▶ GENERAL PRINCIPLES OF EVALUATION AND MANAGEMENT

- Determine whether patient is at risk for a systemic or localized infection based on the clinical history:
  - *Pneumocystis carinii* pneumonia (PCP) in HIV+ patients
  - CMV interstitial pneumonitis in allogenic bone marrow transplant patients (30 to 60 days post-transplant)

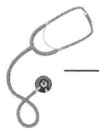

Neutropenic patients are vulnerable to more than one infection at a time. More than one organism may emerge during a single febrile episode. Be aggressive with broad-spectrum antibiotics.

Diagnostic Studies

- Complete blood count (CBC) with manual differential and coagulation studies
- Culture urine and blood.
- CXR regardless of physical exam findings
- Culture sputum with cough or if CXR warrants.
- Culture stool and cerebrospinal fluid (CSF) in AIDS patients, look for cryptococcal antigen.
- In AIDS and transplant patients, obtain CMV antigen.

▶ PULMONARY INFILTRATE IN THE IMMUNOCOMPROMISED PATIENT

DIAGNOSIS

- Infiltrate may represent infection, extension of tumor, chemotherapy complication, fluid overload, pulmonary infarction, or a combination of factors.
- Leukemia patients within 3 days of initiating chemotherapy are very vulnerable to pneumonia, particularly *Pneumocystis carinii*.
- In any cell-mediated immunodeficiency, a pulmonary infiltrate is usually *Pneumocystis carinii*.
- Biopsy should be considered if other diagnostic methods fail, empiric antibiotic therapy is ineffective, or if persistent hypoxia is present.

TREATMENT

Choice of Antibiotic

- Combination therapy (e.g., piperacillin/tazobactam)
- Monotherapy (e.g., third-generation cephalosporins or carbapenem)
- Adjust therapy based on culture results.

HIV AND AIDS

AIDS Definition

Any HIV-infected individual with:

- A CD4 count of < 200/μL, regardless of the presence of symptoms or opportunistic diseases
- An AIDS-defining clinical condition, regardless of CD4 count

Major AIDS-Defining Clinical Conditions

- Candidiasis (pulmonary or esophageal)
- Cervical cancer (invasive)
- Cryptococcus (extrapulmonary)
- CMV retinitis with vision loss
- Encephalopathy, HIV-related
- Herpes simplex (chronic ulcers, pulmonary, or esophageal)
- Kaposi's sarcoma
- Lymphoma (Burkitt's or 1° brain)
- *Mycobacterium avium* complex
- *Mycobacterium tuberculosis*
- Atypical mycobacteriosis
- PCP
- Recurrent pneumonias
- Central nervous system (CNS) toxoplasmosis
- Wasting syndrome due to HIV

Life Cycle of HIV

- HIV gp120 binds CD4 molecule on a $CD4^+$ human leukocytes.
- Fusion with host cell via gp41 molecule on HIV
- HIV RNA internalized into host cell
- HIV reverse transcriptase transcribes HIV RNA into dsDNA.
- DNA translocates to nucleus.
- DNA integrated randomly into host genome by virally encoded integrase
- Activation of host cell needed to transcribe the integrated DNA
- mRNA translated into long HIV polypeptides
- Virally encoded protease cleaves polypeptides at specific sites to generate functional proteins
- New infective virus particle (proteins plus genomic viral RNA) assembles at host cell membrane.
- Budding of new virus particle

Antiretroviral medications work against reverse transcriptase and proteases that cleave the newly formed viral proteins after translation.

Transmission of HIV

- Sexual contact
- Blood products
- HIV^+ mothers to infants intrapartum, perinatally, or via breast milk

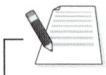

There is no evidence that HIV can be transmitted by casual contact or insects.

Sexual Contact

- Worldwide, HIV is predominantly transmitted by heterosexual sex.
- One-half of U.S. cases are still among homosexual men.
- Incidence of heterosexual transmission in the United States is increasing, mainly among women and minorities.
- HIV is present in infective quantities in seminal fluid and vaginal and cervical secretions.
- Strong association of HIV transmission with receptive anal intercourse.
- Vaginal intercourse: 20-fold greater chance of transmission from man to a woman than woman to a man
- Oral sex: Much less efficient mode of transmission, but cases have been reported.

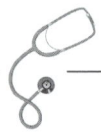

An estimated 10,000 individuals in the United States were infected by contaminated blood products before spring 1985.

- Genital ulceration increases chances of transmission (both infectivity and susceptibility to infection).
- Lack of circumcision is associated with higher risk of infection.

Blood

Common Modes of Blood Transmission
- Sharing contaminated injection drug paraphernalia
- Transfusion of contaminated blood products

Blood Products Capable of HIV Transmission
- Whole blood and packed RBCs
- Platelets and WBCs
- Plasma

Blood Products Incapable of HIV Transmission
- Hyperimmune gamma globulin
- Hep B immune globulin
- Plasma-derived Hep B vaccine
- Rh-immune globulin

Blood Product Screening (United States)
- p24 HIV antigen and HIV antibody by enzyme-linked immunosorbent assay (ELISA), positives confirmed by Western blot
- Self-deferral of donors based on risk behavior
- Screening out of HIV blood based on Hep B or Hep C positivity
- Serologic testing for syphilis

Occupational Transmission
- Transmission risk after skin puncture from blood contaminated sharp object from person with documented HIV infection is 0.3%.
- Transmission for Hep B following similar exposure is 20 to 30%.
- The higher the viral load of the infected patient, the greater the chances of transmission.
- Postexposure prophylaxis and wound cleansing after exposure decrease rate of HIV seroconversion by 79% (to 0.06% for HIV).

Maternal–Fetal Transmission

- HIV can be transmitted from mother to fetus during pregnancy, delivery, or through infected breast milk.
- Transmission rate from untreated mother to newborn is approximately 25% in the United States.
- Zidovudine treatment of HIV-infected pregnant women from the beginning of the third trimester through delivery, with treatment of the infant for 6 weeks after birth, decreases transmission rate to 8%.
- Breast milk transmission (7 to 22%) is most important in developing countries where other means of infant nutrition are not readily available.

Transmission by Other Body Fluids

- HIV can be identified in almost any body fluid.
- Transmission risk via saliva, sweat, tears, and urine is very small.

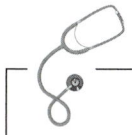

HIV-1 screening of donated blood began in 1985. Risk of infection in the United States from screened blood transfusion is 1 in 450,000 donations.

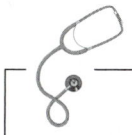

Centers for Disease Control and Prevention (CDC) recommendations for HIV postexposure prophylaxis: Zidovudine, lamivudine, and indinavir for 4 weeks.

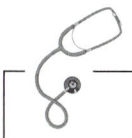

Gamma globulin infusion
- **Pooled serum immunoglobulin G (IgG) from many donors**
- **Half-life 27 days**
- **Very expensive**
- **Slow infusion—risk of anaphylaxis**
- **Used to treat idiopathic thrombocytopenic purpura (ITP) (not thrombotic thrombocytopenic purpura [TTP]), AIDS**

AIDS Epidemiology

AIDS Worldwide

- Approximately 42 million people were infected worldwide as of December 2002.
- In some sub-Saharan African countries, such as Zimbabwe, approximately 30 million are infected.

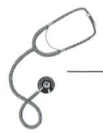

African Americans and Hispanic Americans constitute a disproportionately high number of HIV cases.

AIDS in the United States

Incidence

- AIDS was the fifth leading cause of death in Americans aged 25 to 44 years in 1998.
- The rate of infection is increasing dramatically among heterosexual men and women, especially women and minorities.
- The overall incidence of AIDS has remained stable for the past 8 to 10 years.

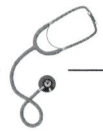

Overall rate of AIDS is declining in the United States. The decline is due in part to the increased rate of HIV reporting and the longer time period from seroconversion to AIDS since effective retroviral therapy has become available.

AIDS Disease

Course

0 to 12 Weeks

- Virus enters bloodstream and is cleared by lymphoid organs or spleen.
- Virus replicates to critical level in lymphoid organs.
- Burst of viremia occurs, disseminating virus throughout body.
- Partial immunologic control of virus replication occurs.

12 Weeks to 8–10 Years

- HIV evades immune system by:
  - Killing off most the HIV-specific cytotoxic T cells with an overwhelming burst of HIV antigen
  - Saturating the antigen presenting cells in lymphoid tissue with HIV antigen (these cells would otherwise help create more virus specific cytotoxic T cells)
- Clinical latency is the disease-free state when opportunistic infections do not occur, but continued decline of CD4 T cells occurs due to viral cytotoxicity.
- CD4 counts fall approximately 50 cells/μL/yr.

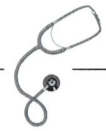

AIDS progression:
- Status of disease: CD4 count
- Rate of progression: viral load (measure of HIV RNA)

More than 10 Years

- CD4 count falls below critical level (usually about 200 cells/μL)
- Patient becomes highly susceptible to opportunistic diseases (see Table 2.5-3).
- CD4 counts may drop to < 10 cells/μL, yet patients can survive for months.
- Patient eventually succumbs to opportunistic infection or neoplasm.

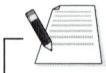

Loss of lymphadenopathy is a marker of disease progression.

Acute HIV Syndrome

- Approximately 60% experience acute viral syndrome within 3 to 6 weeks of primary infection.
- Symptoms (usually last ~1 week):
  - General: Fever, pharyngitis, lymphadenopathy, headache, lethargy, nausea, vomiting, diarrhea

TABLE 2.5-3. Diseases Associated with CD4 Thresholds in AIDS

CD4 Counts			
350	**200**	**100**	**50**
▪ Pneumococcal pneumonia	▪ Kaposi's sarcoma ▪ TB ▪ Oral thrush ▪ Oral hairy leukoplakia ▪ PCP ▪ Lymphoma	▪ Toxoplasmosis ▪ Disseminated *Candida* ▪ Cryptococcosis	▪ MAC ▪ CMV ▪ PML

PML = progressive multifocal leukoencephalopathy (JC virus).

  - Neuro: Meningitis, encephalitis, peripheral neuropathy
  - Dermatologic: Erythematous maculopapular rash and mucocutaneous ulceration
- Ten percent have fulminant course—clinical and immune deterioration immediately after the initial viral syndrome subsides.
- Ninety percent become asymptomatic (clinically latent phase).

Treatment of HIV Infection

General Patient Management

- Disease necessitates patient education about complications, transmission, and prognosis.
- All patients with HIV (especially those with CD4 counts < 200) should designate an individual with durable power of attorney.

Initial and Follow-Up Studies

- Routine chemistry, CBC, and CXR
- CD4 counts
- Two separate HIV RNA levels
- VDRL (Venereal Disease Research Laboratory)
- Anti-*Toxoplasma* Ab titer
- Purified protein derivative (PPD) skin test
- Mini mental status exam

Antiretroviral Therapy

- Major drug classes for HIV therapy are reverse transcriptase inhibitors (nucleoside analogs and non-nucleoside) and protease inhibitors.
- Nucleoside analog reverse transcriptase inhibitors:
  - Zidovudine (AZT):
    - First drug approved for HIV treatment
    - Acts as DNA chain terminator
    - Most appropriately used as part of combination retroviral therapy for patients with CD4 counts < 500
    - Also used as monotherapy for prevention of maternal–fetal transmission of HIV
    - Side effects:
      - Headache, malaise, nausea, fatigue (often subside with extended therapy)

- Macrocytic anemia secondary to low erythropoietin (can be managed with recombinant erythropoietin injections)
- Proximal myopathy
- Lamivudine (3TC):
  - Licensed only for use in combination with AZT
  - Strains of HIV that are resistant to lamivudine are sensitive to zidovudine
  - Toxicities: Pancreatitis, peripheral neuropathies
- Non-nucleoside reverse transcriptase inhibitors:
  - Nevirapine, delavirdine, and efavirenz
  - Bind to reverse transcriptase outside the active site and cause conformational changes that decrease enzyme activity
  - Monotherapy causes rapid resistance
  - Main toxicity is maculopapular rash
- Protease inhibitors:
  - Saquinavir, ritonavir, indinavir, nelfinavir inhibit the activity of HIV protease.
  - Less toxic than the reverse transcriptase inhibitors
  - Monotherapy results in rapid emergence of drug-resistant strains:
    - Indinavir:
      - Main side effects are nephrolithiasis and asymptomatic indirect hyperbilirubinemia
      - Indinavir is potent and well tolerated compared to saquinavir and ritonavir.

Treatment Recommendations

Initiate therapy with two nucleoside reverse transcriptase inhibitors (AZT, 3TC) and a protease inhibitor (indinavir) in any one of these conditions:

- Symptomatic
- Plasma HIV RNA > 20,000 copies/mL
- CD4 count < 500
- Disease is progressing.
- Asymptomatic and CD4 < 200

Opportunistic Infections and AIDS

► *Pneumocystis carinii* Pneumonia (PCP)

- PCP is the initial AIDS-defining illness in 20% of patients.
- Half of patients will have at least one bout of PCP.
- PCP is most common in those with a previous episode of PCP.

Spontaneous pneumothorax complicates PCP in 2% of cases.

Clinical Findings

- Often indolent course
- Nonproductive cough
- Retrosternal pain (worse on inspiration)
- Dyspnea on exertion

- Unexplained weight loss
- Breath sounds are usually clear
- Extrapulmonary manifestations: Acute otitis, retinitis, visceral cystic calcifications, intestinal obstruction, lymphadenopathy, bone marrow involvement, ascites, thyroiditis

Diagnosis

- PaO_2 decreases, a-A gradient increases
- CXR usually normal or shows faint, bilateral interstitial infiltrate
- Lactate dehydrogenase (LDH) is often elevated
- Bronchoalveolar lavage
- Induced sputum sample
- Transbronchial biopsy

Treatment

- Trimethoprim–sulfamethoxazole (TMP-SMZ):
  - Fifty to 60% have side effects including rash, fever, leukopenia, thrombocytopenia, and hepatitis
  - 21-day course
  - Patients get worse before they get better and will not improve until the end of the first week of treatment.
  - May give pentamidine for patients intolerant of TMP-SMZ
- Glucocorticoids:
  - Initiate in any AIDS patient with PCP if $PaO_2 < 70$ mm Hg or a-A gradient > 35 mm Hg
  - Start no later than 36 to 72 hours after starting TMP-SMZ
  - 21-day course (with subsequent taper)
  - Decreases mortality by approximately 50%
- Prophylaxis:
  - TMP-SMZ, dapsone in sulfa-allergic patients.
  - Aerosolized pentamidine for those unable to take systemic prophylaxis

TABLE 2.5-4 Prophylaxis in AIDS

Infection	Prophylaxis	Indication
Pneumocystis carinii pneumonia	Bactrim Dapsone in patients with sulfa allergies	CD4 < 200
Toxoplasmosis	Bactrim Dapsone in patients with sulfa allergies	CD4 < 100
Tuberculosis	Isoniazid	PPD > 5 mm induration (not erythema)
Mycobacterium avium complex	Azithromycin or clarithromycin	CD4 < 100

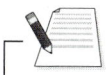

The probability of death from a single incident of PCP has decreased from 50% to 2% since effective treatment has been implemented.

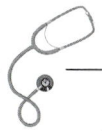

It is advisable to withhold myelotoxic drugs when treating *Pneumocystis* (AZT, ganciclovir).

An HIV patient presents with dry cough ×1 week. He denies fever, night sweats, and chills. His white count is normal. *Likely diagnosis?* Mycoplasma pneumoniae (Lesson: community-acquired pneumonias are still most common, even in AIDS patients.)

An HIV patient with a low CD4 count presents with fever, chest pain, and productive cough. *Likely diagnosis?* Streptococcus pneumoniae *(community-acquired!)*

- HIV+ patients with previous episode of PCP or with CD4 < 200 cells/μL
- Patients with history of oropharyngeal candidiasis
- Unexplained fever (> 100.0°F) for > 2 weeks

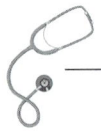

Patients on PCP prophylaxis with TMP-SMZ have a decreased incidence of toxoplasmosis.

▶ TOXOPLASMOSIS

- Most common cause of secondary CNS infection in AIDS
- Seen in 15% of all AIDS patients
- Late complication
- Represents a reactivation syndrome

Clinical Presentation

- Fever, headache, and focal neurological deficits (90%)
- Seizure, hemiparesis, and aphasia also occur.

Diagnosis

- Magnetic resonance imaging (MRI) or head computed tomography (CT) with contrast shows **multiple ring-enhancing lesions** (see Figure 2.5-1)
- IgG antibodies to *Toxoplasma*

Treatment

- Pyrimethamine and sulfadiazine: Leukopenia is the major side effect (treat leukopenia with folinic acid).

AIDS patient with brain lesion:
- Ring-enhancing lesion with mass effect: Toxo
- Periventricular ring: CMV
- Other: CNS lymphoma (associated with EBV)

AIDS patient with diarrhea:
- Cryptosporidia (round)
- *Isospora* (oral)
- Microsporidia

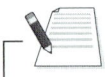

AIDS patient with meningitis:
- Sensation of smell and behavior changes: *Think HSV (temporal lobe involvement).*
- India ink stain with round organisms: *Think* Cryptococcus.

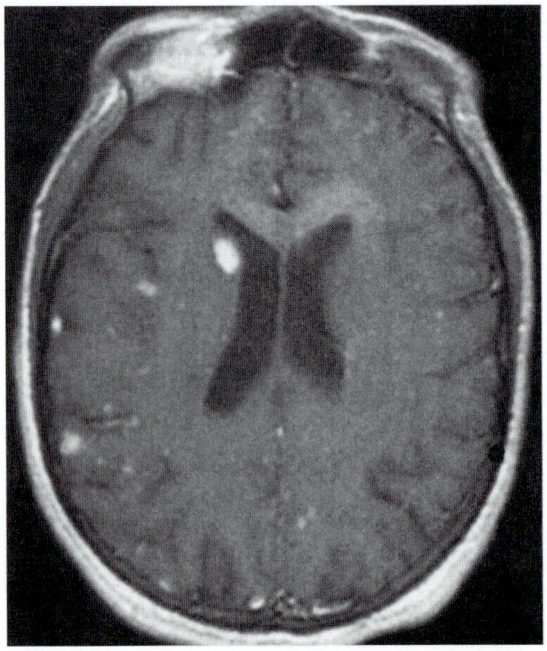

FIGURE 2.5-1. Toxoplasmosis in an AIDS patient. Note ring-enhancing lesions.

(Reproduced, with permission, from Lee SH, Rao K, Zimmerman RA [eds]. *Cranial MRI and CT.* New York: McGraw-Hill, 1999:505.)

- Lifelong treatment for toxoplasmosis is necessary, due to relapse rate of 50% within 6 months.
- No prophylactic regimen with an acceptable side effect profile exists.

▶ PROTOZOAL DIARRHEA

Etiology

Cryptosporidia, microsporidia, and *Isospora belli* are the most common agents.

Treatment

- Cryptosporidia and microsporidia: Paromomycin or erythromycin
- *Isospora:* TMP-SMZ

▶ *MYCOBACTERIUM AVIUM* COMPLEX (MAC)

Epidemiology

- In the United States, disseminated *Mycobacterium avium* is the most common cause of death due to AIDS.
- Median survival after MAC diagnosis is 6 to 8 months.

Symptoms

- Fever
- Weight loss
- Night sweats
- Lymphadenopathy
- Abdominal pain
- Diarrhea

Typical scenario:
A 29-year-old HIV+ patient presents with CD4 count of 100, unexplained fever, and elevated alkaline phosphatase. *Think: MAC.*

Diagnosis

- 85% of MAC patients have mycobacteremia
- Alkaline phosphatase level often elevated
- Long, slender, acid-fast bacilli (AFB) seen in biopsy specimens or sputum
- CXR: 25% have bilateral lower lobe interstitial infiltrate.
- Blood culture confirms diagnosis (turns positive within 2 weeks)

Treatment

- Clarithromycin and ethambutol
- Prophylaxis: Rifabutin when CD4 drops below 100

▶ TUBERCULOSIS

See respiratory chapter for full description.

Epidemiology

- Very common in AIDS patients (approximately 5%)
- HIV increases risk of developing active TB 15 to 30 times.
- HIV disease progresses more rapidly in patients with active TB.

▶ FUNGAL INFECTIONS

Candidiasis

- *Candida* infections are the most common fungal infections in HIV-positive patients, and virtually all patients experience some form of *Candida* infection during their illness.
- Infections occur early: They are often the first sign of immunosuppression.

Thrush

- Very early finding in immunocompromise
- White, cheesy exudates on posterior oropharynx
- Pseudohyphae detectable on wet-mount KOH preps

AIDS-Defining *Candida* Infections

- *Candida* infections of lungs, esophagus, trachea, and bronchi
- Esophagitis is most common:
  - Presents with retrosternal pain and odynophagia
  - Diagnosed with upper GI endoscopy

Treatment

- Oral and vaginal candida: Topical nystatin or clotrimazole troches
- Severe cases can be treated with systemic therapy (oral ketoconazole or fluconazole)

Cryptococcosis

- *Cryptococcus neoformans* is the leading cause of meningitis in AIDS patients.
- 12% of AIDS patients
- Serious, life-threatening infection

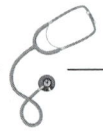

Fluconazole prophylaxis can be given to all patients once CD4 < 100/μL to prevent both cryptococcosis and candidal infections.

Signs and Symptoms

Subacute Meningoencephalitis

- Fever (virtually all patients)
- Nausea and vomiting (40%)
- Altered mental status
- Headache
- Meningeal signs

DIAGNOSIS

- Cryptococcomas: Seen as multiple ring-enhancing lesions on MRI
- Pulmonary disease shows interstitial pattern on CXR.
- CSF or serum cryptococcal antigen
- Identification of organisms on India ink stain of CSF
- Positive culture of C. *neoformans* from any site

TREATMENT

- Amphotericin B for 6 weeks in combination with flucytosine
- Since 50% of patients relapse after therapy is stopped, fluconazole should be given indefinitely.

Aspergillus fumigatus

- **Fungus ball in immunocompromised patient**
- Mold with septated hyphae
- Acquired through inhalation of spores in soil and decay
- Infection in immunocompetent individual can cause a self-limited pneumonitis.
- Invasive aspergillosis is seen in immunocompromised patients and can present as rapidly progressive pulmonary infiltrates, fungus balls.
- Lung biopsy is needed for definitive diagnosis.
- Treat with amphotericin B; some patients may benefit from surgery (removing the fungus ball).

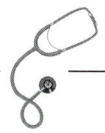

Aspergillus

Invasive aspergillosis: Infection in immunocompromised people often causing a fungus ball.

Allergic aspergillosis: A hypersensitivity reaction in *immunocompetent* people, causing severe obstructive lung disease, wheezing, bronchiectasis. Treat with steroids. **Not** an infection!

▶ VIRAL INFECTIONS

Cytomegalovirus (CMV)

- Ninety-five percent of HIV-positive patients are CMV positive, and clinical syndromes most often represent reactivation of latent infection (see Figure 2.5-2).
- CMV retinitis:
  - 25 to 30% of HIV-positive patients
  - Presents with painless, progressive vision loss; may complain of "floaters"
  - **Diagnosis:** Funduscopy shows perivascular hemorrhage and exudates
  - **Clinical course/complications:** Vision loss is irreversible; may be complicated by retinal detachment
  - **Treatment:**
    - Ganciclovir (ocular implants can be used)
    - Foscarnet
    - Works in 80 to 90% of patients
    - Recurrence is common; maintenance therapy with foscarnet
- CMV also causes esophagitis and colitis.
- CMV Ab–negative patients should receive blood products from CMV-negative donors if at all possible.

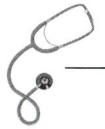

Ganciclovir causes bone marrow suppression and cannot be given with TMP-SMZ or AZT.

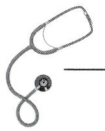

Foscarnet is associated with electrolyte disorders.

Herpes Simplex (HSV)

- HSV in HIV manifests as recurrent orolabial, genital, and perianal lesions.

Typical scenario: An HIV+ patient presents with a painful, poorly healing, perirectal lesion.
Think: HSV.

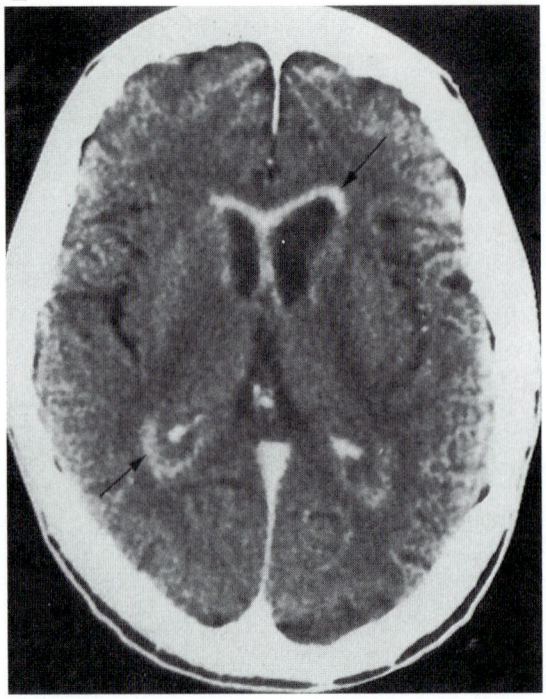

FIGURE 2.5-2. Cytomegalovirus infection in an AIDS patient. Note diffuse periventricular enhancement.

(Reproduced, with permission, from Lee SH, Rao K, Zimmerman RA [eds]. *Cranial MRI and CT*. New York: McGraw-Hill, 1999.)

- Can cause herpetic esophagitis (beefy red and painful esophagus)
- Can cause recurrent herpetic whitlow (painful nodular lesions usually found on fingers)
- Treat with acyclovir, famciclovir, or valacyclovir.

Varicella-Zoster (VZV)

- Shingles:
  - Reactivation of latent infection
  - Usually an early complication of HIV
  - Painful, vesicular skin eruptions
  - Extensive involvement of several dermatomes
  - Treatment with acyclovir may shorten course of disease.
- Primary VZV infection (chickenpox) may be *lethal* in the HIV patient: Treat aggressively with acyclovir and hyperimmune globulin.
- Acute retinal necrosis syndrome:
  - Pain, keratitis, and iritis
  - Associated with trigeminal VZV or orolabial HSV
  - Fundus exam shows widespread, pale gray peripheral lesions
  - Often complicated by retinal detachment

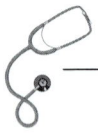

Shingles in any patient under 50 years of age mandates workup for underlying immunodeficiency.

Hepatitis

- Ninety-five percent of HIV+ patients have serologic evidence of HBV or HCV infection.
- Patients with HBV and HIV have less severe inflammatory liver disease because of immunosuppression.

▶ NEOPLASTIC DISEASE AND HIV

Kaposi's Sarcoma

EPIDEMIOLOGY

- Incidence has been decreasing since first recognized as an HIV-associated neoplasm
- Ninety-six percent of HIV-associated cases occur in homosexual men.

CLINICAL FINDINGS

- Multiple vascular nodules appearing in the skin, mucous membranes, and viscera
- Appearance is purplish macular or papular nodule on skin, or discoloration of the oral mucosa
- Lesions often occur in sun-exposed areas.
- Pulmonary involvement can occur; presents as shortness of breath
- May be seen with a normal CD4 count

DIAGNOSIS

Biopsy of suspicious lesion reveals spindle cells, endothelial cells, and extravasation of red blood cells.

TREATMENT

- Indicated when a single or multiple lesions are causing significant pain or discomfort and for lesions in the posterior oropharynx that interfere with swallowing
- Localized irradiation
- Intralesional vinblastine
- Cryotherapy effective in some cases

HIV-associated malignancies:
- **HHV-6,8: Kaposi's sarcoma**
- **HPV: Cervical CA**
- **HBV: Hepatocellular CA**

Lymphomas

EPIDEMIOLOGY

- Six percent of patients develop lymphoma at some point during their disease.
- 120-fold increased incidence in HIV compared with general population
- Three main types occur in HIV:
  - Grade III or IV immunoblastic (60%)
  - Burkitt's lymphoma (20%)
  - Primary CNS lymphoma (20%)

Clinical Presentation

- Dependent on the site of tumor
- Persistent unexplained fever
- Focal seizures
- Rapidly growing mass lesion in the oral mucosa
- 80% have extranodal disease

Treatment

- Standard intensive regimens have been abandoned due to low response rate.
- Patient's with higher CD4 counts do better with chemotherapy than do those with lower counts.
- Primary CNS lymphoma has the poorest prognosis, though none of the HIV-associated lymphomas have favorable prognoses.

Bioterrorism Agents

The following are common agents used in bioterrorism. The inhalational type is expected to be the most common form used in bioterrorism, due to ease of inoculation. Suspected or confirmed cases should be reported to local or state departments of health. Antibiotics are initially given parenterally and then switched to oral once patient improves clinically. In mass casualty situations, parenteral therapy may not be possible; in this situation, oral antibiotics are administered. Antibiotics for treating patients infected in connection with a bioterrorist event are included in the national pharmaceutical stockpile maintained by the Centers for Disease Control and Prevention (CDC), as are ventilators and other emergency equipment.

This information is compiled from the CDC Web site, where the latest surveillance information is available: *http://www.cdc.gov*.

▶ ANTHRAX

Incubation Period

Usually < 1 week

Transmission

- Skin: Direct skin contact with spores; in nature, contact with infected animals or animal products (usually related to occupational exposure)
- Respiratory tract: Inhalation of aerosolized spores
- GI: Consumption of undercooked or raw meat products or dairy products from infected animals
- No person-to-person transmission of anthrax

Signs and Symptoms of Inhalational Anthrax

- Initial phase consists of nonspecific symptoms such as low-grade fever, nonproductive cough, malaise, fatigue, myalgias, profound sweats, and

chest discomfort. Upper respiratory tract symptoms are rare. Physical exam may reveal rhonchi, otherwise normal.
- One to five days after onset of initial symptoms, onset of high fever and severe respiratory distress (dyspnea, stridor, cyanosis) occur. Shock and death occur within 24 to 36 hours. An interim period of a few days of wellness can occur between the two stages, or they may occur in rapid succession.
- Hemorrhagic meningitis can also be seen.

Diagnosis

- Gram-positive bacilli on unspun peripheral blood smear or CSF
- Chest x-ray demonstrates **widened mediastinum with clear lung fields.**
- Aerobic blood culture growth of large, gram-positive bacilli provides preliminary identification of *Bacillus* species.
- Nasal swab for PCR available for epidemiological surveillance; not approved to make individual patient decisions
- A blood test that detects antibodies to a component of the toxin of *Bacillus anthracis* has recently become available, yielding results in 1 hour.

Treatment

- Whenever possible, obtain specimens for culture before initiating antimicrobial therapy.
- Initiate antimicrobial therapy immediately upon suspicion.
- Ciprofloxacin, doxycycline, and amoxicillin are FDA approved for treatment. Duration of treatment is 60 days.
- Supportive care including controlling pleural effusions
- Use standard contact precautions.
- Vaccine available for military personnel and lab workers who handle organism directly

Typical scenario: A group of previously healthy young people develop an acute respiratory illness. CXRs demonstrate a widened mediastinum with clear lung fields.
Think: Anthrax may be a possibility; keep bioterrorism in mind.

▶ BOTULISM

See the neurology chapter.

▶ PNEUMONIC PLAGUE

There are three types of plague: pneumonic, bubonic, and septicemic. The most common form is bubonic, which is not transmitted person to person.

Etiology

Yersinia pestis. Indications that plague had been artificially disseminated would be the occurrence of cases in locations not known to have enzootic infection, in persons without known risk factors, and in the absence of prior rodent deaths.

Incubation

2 to 4 days

Transmission

Via inhalation of respiratory droplets

Typical scenario: A previously healthy 29-year-old banker living in a big city contracts a severe pneumonia characterized by the rapid development of respiratory failure, shock, bleeding, and other signs of the systemic inflammatory response syndrome. Sputum reveals gram-negative bacilli with bipolar staining.
Think: Yersinia pestis.

Typical scenario: A laboratory confirmation of *Y. pestis* is made on autopsy of a healthy 40-year-old living in a big city. There was no history of handling an animal carcass or any travel to an endemic area.
Think: This could be a sentinel event for a bioterrorist attack. Be on the lookout for cases of severe acute respiratory illness in others very shortly.

Signs and Symptoms

- Fever, headache, weakness
- Rapidly developing pneumonia with shortness of breath, chest pain, cough, and sometimes bloody or watery sputum
- Pneumonia progresses for 2 to 4 days and causes respiratory failure and shock.

Diagnosis

- Laboratory analyses may reveal leukocytosis with toxic granulations, coagulation abnormalities, aminotransferase elevations, azotemia, and other evidence of multiorgan failure. All are nonspecific findings associated with sepsis and systemic inflammatory response syndrome.
- Gram stain of sputum or blood may reveal gram-negative bacilli or coccobacilli.
- Wright, Giemsa, or Wayson stain will often show bipolar staining.
- Antigen detection, IgM enzyme immunoassay, immunostaining, and polymerase chain reaction are available at some state health departments, the CDC, and military laboratories.

Treatment

- For optimal survival, antibiotics must be given within 24 hours of first symptoms.
- Streptomycin is drug of choice.
- Other effective agents include gentamicin, tetracycline, doxycycline, and chloramphenicol.
- Isolation of patients using respiratory droplet precautions. Patients are no longer contagious after 24 to 48 hours of antibiotic treatment, although they may still be ill.

Prevention

- Postexposure prophylaxis for people who have had direct, close contact with infected patients (7-day course)
- A plague vaccine is not currently available for use in the United States.

▶ SMALLPOX

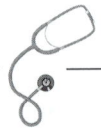

Smallpox may be contagious during the prodrome phase, but is most infectious during the first 7 to 10 days following rash onset.

Incubation Period

7 to 17 days

Transmission

- Generally, direct and fairly prolonged face-to-face contact is required.
- Can be spread through direct contact with infected bodily fluids or contaminated objects such as bedding or clothing
- Rarely, smallpox has been spread by virus carried in the air in enclosed settings such as buildings, buses, and trains.
- Humans are the only natural hosts of variola.

Signs and Symptoms

Prodrome: 2 to 4 Days

- High fever, malaise, head and body aches, and sometimes vomiting
- Patients are acutely ill, in contrast to varicella infection.

Rash

- First emerges as small red spots on the tongue and in the mouth; these subsequently develop into sores that break open and spread large amounts of the virus into the mouth and throat. At this time, the person becomes most contagious.
- Next, rash appears on the skin, starting on the face and spreading to the arms and legs **(centrifugal)** and then to the palms and soles. Usually, the rash spreads to all parts of the body within 24 hours.
- As the rash appears, patient defervesces and may start to feel better.
- By the third day of the rash, the rash becomes raised bumps.
- By the fourth day, the bumps fill with a thick, opaque fluid and often have a depression in the center that looks like a belly button (pustules; characteristic feature of smallpox).
- Fever often will rise again at this time and remain high until scabs form over the bumps.
- The bumps become pustules, which then scab. By the end of the second week after the rash appears, most of the sores have scabbed over.
- The scabs begin to fall off, leaving marks on the skin that eventually become pitted scars. Most scabs will have fallen off 3 weeks after the rash appears.
- Once the scabs have fallen off, patient is no longer contagious.

The rash of smallpox consists of lesions that are all at the same stage of development. In contrast, the lesions of varicella are at all different stages.

Diagnosis

Can be made by PCR, ELISA of throat swab, or culture of fluid from pustules or CSF. Done in specialized laboratories under strict biosafety conditions.

Treatment

- Once the diagnosis is made, patients are quarantined for 17 days or until scabs fall off.
- Treatment consists of fluid replacement and antibiotics for any 2° bacterial infections.
- There is no treatment against the virus itself.

Prevention

A smallpox vaccine is available. It contains the live *vaccinia* virus, a weaker relative of the *variola* virus that causes smallpox. Many first responders and military personnel in the United States have been vaccinated. It is unclear for how long immunity is conferred.

▶ TULAREMIA

Etiology and Transmission

- Bacterial zoonosis caused by *Francisella tularensis*, a small nonmotile, aerobic, non-spore-forming, gram-negative coccobacillus, that survives for weeks at low temperatures in water, moist soil, hay, straw, and decaying animal carcasses
- One of the most infectious pathogenic bacteria known, requiring only as few as 10 organisms via inoculation or inhalation to cause disease
- Occurs mostly in south-central and western United States in summer
- Host reservoirs are rodents. Humans can become incidentally infected through bite of an exposed tick, fly, or mosquito, or by direct contact

with infectious animal (often carcasses) or environment (soil, water, food).
- No person-to-person transmission (no need for patient isolation)

Incubation

Symptoms usually appear at 3 to 5 days, but may be as long as 14 days

Signs and Symptoms

- Sudden onset of high fever, chills
- Headaches
- Diarrhea
- Myalgias, arthralgias
- Cough, coryza
- Progressive weakness
- Inhalation exposures develop hemorrhagic inflammation of airways, pneumonia, and pleuropneumonitis.
- Airborne *F. tularensis* principally causes pleuropneumonitis, ocular involvement, ulcers in broken skin, and oropharyngeal disease.

Adverse effects of tetracyclines:
- **Photosensitivity**
- **Increase preexisting prerenal azotemia**
- **Brown/yellow deposits in teeth and brittle bones (children)**

Diagnosis

- CXR often shows effusions and hilar lymphadenopathy.
- Gram stain, direct fluorescent antibody, or immunohistochemical stains of respiratory secretions and blood
- Culture

Treatment

Streptomycin is drug of choice. Gentamicin, tetracyclines, and chloramphenicol are also effective.

Tick-Borne Diseases

Rickettsia rickettsii

- Gram-negative coccobacillus
- Transmitted by ticks, it causes **Rocky Mountain spotted fever.**
- Patients initially present with fever, nausea, vomiting, and history of recent tick bite.
- After 3 to 4 days of symptoms, rash starts as maculopapular on the distal extremities (wrists and ankles), progresses centrally, and may become petechial.
- Can be fatal if not treated aggressively
- Diagnose with indirect immunofluorescence assay or latex agglutination.
- Treat with doxycycline.

Borrelia burgdorferi

- **Patient presents with Bell's palsy and history of tick bite.**
- Microaerophilic spirochete; transmitted by *Ixodes scapularis* tick
- Causes **Lyme disease**

- Found in the northeastern United States
- **Erythema chronicum migrans** is the pathognomonic skin rash that starts at bite and progresses until there is central clearing.
- **Initial stage:** Fevers, headaches, arthralgias, and myalgias
- **Second stage** (weeks to months): Recurring rash, myocarditis with first, second-, or third-degree heart block; meningitis; cranial nerve palsy; peripheral neuropathy
- **Third stage:** Migratory or oligoarthritis
- **Diagnosis:** ELISA followed by Western blot. If clinical suspicion is high, then treat the patient before checking serologies.
- Treat with doxycycline or amoxicillin if there is no cardiac involvement.
- Treat with penicillin or cephalosporin if there is any cardiac or neurologic involvement.

Ehrlichiosis

- **Etiology:** *Ehrlichia chaffeensis*
- **Presentation:** Similar to Rocky Mountain spotted fever but without the rash
- Fever, headache, leukopenia, thrombocytopenia
- On East Coast of the United States
- Treat with tetracycline or doxycycline.

Typical scenario: A 42-year-old woman who recently camped in the woods of Vermont presents to the ER with one-sided facial droop.
Think: Lyme disease (often presents with Bell's palsy).

Rocky Mountain Spotted Fever

- **Etiology:** By *Rickettsia rickettsii*, gram-negative coccobacillus, found in the southeastern United States
- **Presentation:**
  - **Erythema chronicum migrans** is the pathognomonic skin rash, which starts at bite and progresses until there is central clearing.
  - **Initial stage:** Fevers, headaches, arthralgias, and myalgias
  - **Second stage** (weeks to months): Recurring rash, myocarditis with first-, second-, or third-degree heart block; meningitis; cranial nerve palsy; peripheral neuropathy
  - **Third stage:** Migratory or oligoarthritis
- **Diagnosis:** ELISA followed by Western blot. If clinical suspicion is high, then treat patient before checking serologies.
- **Treatment:** Doxycycline or amoxicillin if there is no cardiac involvement. Use penicillin or cephalosporin if there is cardiac or neurologic involvement.

Babesiosis

- **Etiology:** *Babesia microti*, an intra-RBC parasite (like malaria) transmitted by the *Ixodes* tick in the Northeast and Midwest
- **Presentation:** Fever, chills, myalgias, hemolytic anemia
- **Treatment:** Quinine and clindamycin

Tularemia

- **Etiology:** *Francisella tularensis*, transmitted by tick or flea bites in Arkansas and Oklahoma
- Tick or flea bites
- Arkansas and Oklahoma
- Ulcer at bite site
- **Treatment:** Gentamicin or tetracycline

Epidural Abscess

- Spinal abscesses are most commonly found in the immunosuppressed, IV drug users, and the elderly.
- An abscess can form anywhere along the spinal cord and as it expands, it compresses against the spinal cord and occludes the vasculature.

Etiology

- The infection is generally spread from the skin or other tissue.
- *Staphylococcus aureus*, gram-negative bacilli, and *Tuberculosis bacillus* are the leading organisms involved.

Signs and Symptoms

- Presents with a triad of pain, fever, and progressive weakness.
- The pain develops over the course of a week or two and the fever is often accompanied by an elevated white count.

Diagnosis and Treatment

- Magnetic resonance imaging (MRI) can localize the lesion. Lumbar puncture (LP) is not required unless meningitis is suspected.
- Emergent decompressive laminectomy can prevent permanent sequelae. This should be followed up with long-term antibiotics.

Malaria

Pathophysiology

Vector: *Anopheles* mosquito. Bites human to introduce sporozoites. Merozoites are then released from infected liver cells to infect RBCs.

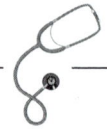

Patients with fever that follows a cyclical pattern every 48 or 72 hours should be considered for malaria.

Epidemiology

- 300 to 500 million malaria cases, with three million deaths, occur annually worldwide.
- *P. falciparum* is responsible for more deaths than the other species and is endemic in Africa.
- *P.vivax* is endemic in India and central America.

Signs and Symptoms

- *P. falciparum* is the most severe because it infects erythrocytes of all ages. It can cause a microvascular blockade that leads to local anoxia affecting the brain (delirium, seizures), kidneys, lungs (pulmonary edema, ARDS), intestines (nausea, vomiting, diarrhea, abdominal pain), liver, and blood.
- *P. vivax* infects mostly younger erythrocytes.
- *P. vivax* and *P. ovale* cause persistent infection in the liver.
- Symptoms of fever and chills occur about 1 to 4 weeks after infection.
- Other symptoms include headache, increased sweating, back pain, myalgias, diarrhea, nausea, vomiting, and cough.

Typical scenario:
A 40-year-old male who recently returned from the Kenyan coast presents with malaise, body aches, and fever. His labs show a normal WBC count, anemia, and elevated LFTs. *Think: Malaria.*

Diagnosis

- Blood smear shows parasites in RBCs (diagnostic).
- Should be considered in any person with febrile illness who immigrates or has traveled to malaria infested region
- Anemia, thrombocytopenia, and elevated liver enzymes may be present.

Treatment

- Chloroquine for *P. vivax*, *P. ovale*, and *P. malariae*. Add primaquine for *P. vivax* and *P. ovale* for hepatic phase.
- If chloroquine resistant, use mefloquine or pyrimethamine/sulfadoxine.
- If very ill, use quinidine.

NOTES

HIGH-YIELD FACTS IN

Nephrology and Acid–Base Disorders

Acid–Base Disorders 221

- General Laboratory Studies 221
- Metabolic Acidosis 222
- Respiratory Acidosis 223
- Respiratory Alkalosis 223
- Metabolic Alkalosis 224
- Interpreting Arterial Blood Gases 224

Electrolyte Disorders 226

- Body Fluids 226
- Hyponatremia 226
- Hypernatremia 229
- Hypokalemia 230
- Hyperkalemia 231
- Hypocalcemia 232
- Hypercalcemia 233
- Malignancy and Hypercalcemia 234
- Primary Hyperparathyroidism 234
- Secondary Hyperparathyroidism/Renal Osteodystrophy 235
- Hypophosphatemia 236
- Hyperphosphatemia 236
- Hypomagnesemia 236
- Hypermagnesemia 236
- General Principles of Electrolyte Disorder Management 236

Acute Renal Failure (ARF) 237

- Tubulointerstitial Diseases 238

Glomerular Disorders 240

- Nephrotic Syndrome 240
- Glomerulonephritis (aka Nephritic Syndrome) 241

Chronic Renal Failure 242
Dialysis 244
Uremic Syndrome 245
Polycystic Kidney Disease 245
Renal Tubular Acidosis 246
Urolithiasis 246

Acid–Base Disorders

▶ GENERAL LABORATORY STUDIES

Serum Electrolytes

- Plasma bicarbonate (HCO_3): Increased in metabolic alkalosis and compensated respiratory acidosis. Decreased in metabolic acidosis and compensated respiratory alkalosis.
- Serum potassium: Increased in acidemia and decreased in alkalemia.
- Serum chloride: Compare with the serum sodium. In dehydration or overhydration they should be increased or decreased proportional to one another. If there is a nonproportionate change, calculate the anion gap later on.

Arterial Blood Gas (ABG)

Normal values:

pH	7.4	(7.35–7.45)
$PaCO_2$	40	(35–45)
PaO_2	90	(80–100)
HCO_3	24	(21–27)
O_2 sat	98	(95–100)
Base excess	0	(–2 to +2)

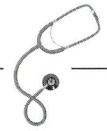

Learn this ABG sequence as these values are frequently reported in this order without labels (e.g., 7.4/40/90/24/98/0).

- **Look for hypoxia** using PaO_2; correlate with the clinical scenario
- **Determine the type of disturbance** using pH, $PaCO_2$, and HCO_3 (see Table 2.6-1)
- **Calculate the degree of compensation:**
  - A change in $PaCO_2$ of 10 mm Hg, up or down, causes pH to increase or decrease by 0.08 units (pH decreases as $PaCO_2$ rises).
  - A pH change of 0.15 is the result of a bicarbonate change of 10 mEq/L.

TABLE 2.6-1. Acid–Base Disturbances

Disorder	Abnormality	Compensation	pH	$PaCO_2$	HCO_3
Metabolic acidosis	Gain H^+/lose bicarb	Increase ventilation	↓	↓	↓
Respiratory acidosis	Hypoventilate	Generate bicarbonate	↓	↑	↑
Metabolic alkalosis	Lose H^+/gain bicarb	Decrease ventilation	↑	↑	↑
Respiratory alkalosis	Hyperventilation	Bicarbonate consumption	↓	↓	

↓ = decreased; ↑ = increased.

Anion Gap

- The concentration of serum anions not measured in routine electrolyte profiles (e.g., lactic and keto acids)
- Anion Gap = Na − (Cl + HCO_3) Normal = 9 − 14 mEq/L

▶ METABOLIC ACIDOSIS

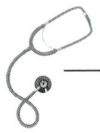

Use Winter's formula to determine if compensation is appropriate in the setting of metabolic acidosis: $1.5 \times (HCO_3^-) + 8 \pm 2 = pCO_2$

DEFINITION

- Decrease in pH with decrease in HCO_3
- Etiology depends on presence or absence of an anion gap

Anion Gap Metabolic Acidosis

See Table 2.6-2 for causes and findings.

Normal Anion Gap Metabolic Acidosis

ETIOLOGY

Renal Losses
- RTA
- Medications (acetazolamide, spironolactone, beta blockers)

GI Losses
- Diarrhea
- Ileostomy

Isopropyl alcohol (rubbing alcohol) does NOT cause acidosis but it is associated with ketonemia. Ketone bodies are not acids.

Causes of anion gap metabolic acidosis:
MUDPILES
Methanol, Metformin
Uremia
DKA
Paraldehyde
INH, **I**ron tablets
Lactic acidosis
Ethanol
Salicylates

TABLE 2.6-2 Causes of Anion Gap Metabolic Acidosis: MUDPILES

CAUSE	FINDINGS/DIAGNOSTIC TOOL
Methanol	Tox screen, vision changes, increased osmolal gap
Uremia	History of renal failure, increased creatinine
DKA	Diabetes, increased serum glucose
Paraldehyde	Tox screen
INH, **I**ron	Medication history
Lactic acidosis	Serum lactate
Ethanol, **E**thylene glycol	Tox screen, history of alcohol abuse
Salicylates	Respiratory alkalosis and metabolic acidosis, tox screen

Therapy for Metabolic Acidosis

- Correct underlying cause
- Often, HCO_3^- is given in IV solution when pH < 7.0, but this practice has **not** been proven to improve mortality.

Typical scenario:
A 47-year-old man was binge drinking EtOH 3 days ago. No alcohol consumption for 3 days. He presents with acidosis and ketonemia. Blood EtOH is zero. *Think: Alcoholic ketoacidosis. Treatment:* Glucose-containing fluids (D_5NS). This stimulates the pancreas to secrete insulin and treats the acidosis.

▶ RESPIRATORY ACIDOSIS

Definition

Hypoventilation from any cause increases the $PaCO_2$ and decreases the serum pH. There is a compensatory increase in bicarbonate.

Etiology

- Pulmonary (chronic obstructive pulmonary disease [COPD], severe alveolar infiltrates, pulmonary edema, interstitial restrictive lung disease)
- Airway obstruction (foreign body, severe bronchospasm, laryngospasm)
- Thoracic disorders (pneumothorax, flail chest)
- Alveolar hypoventilation (myasthenia gravis, severe hypokalemia causing weak muscles of respiration, muscular dystrophy)
- Peripheral nervous system disorders (Guillain–Barré syndrome, botulism, tetanus, organophosphate poisoning)
- Depression of central respiratory drive (narcotic overdose, general anesthesia, increased intracranial pressure [ICP]).

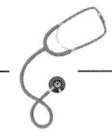

Do not rely on sodium bicarbonate to correct metabolic acidosis. Correct the underlying cause.

Signs and Symptoms

Confusion, encephalopathy, coma

Treatment

- Treat underlying cause.
- Mechanical hyperventilation will decrease the amount of CO_2 retention in severely hypoxic patients.

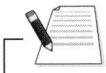

Typical scenario:
A 34-year-old diabetic man with renal insufficiency has normal anion gap. K is high; bicarbonate level is low. *Think: Type IV RTA (hyporeninemic hypoaldosteronism).*

▶ RESPIRATORY ALKALOSIS

Definition

Elevated arterial pH, and hyperventilation resulting in decreased PCO_2 and compensatory decrease in serum bicarbonate

Etiology

- Most commonly caused by anxiety, which provokes hyperventilation
- Other causes: shock, sepsis, pulmonary disease, CVA, pregnancy, liver disease, hyperthyroidism, salicylates

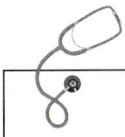

Hyperventilation may be due to tachypnea or hyperpnea.

Signs and Symptoms

- Rapid, deep breathing
- Chest tightness, chest pain, and anxiety
- Circumoral paresthesias, tetany in severe cases

Treatment

- Reassurance
- If patient can be calmed enough, have him or her breathe into a paper bag.
- Decrease the minute volume in the mechanically ventilated patient.

▶ METABOLIC ALKALOSIS

Definition

Elevated pH, increased plasma bicarbonate, and a compensatory increase in $PaCO_2$. Usually seen in cases of volume contraction.

Etiology

Divided into chloride-responsive and chloride-resistant forms:

- Chloride-responsive: Urine chloride < 15 mEq/L:
  - Vomiting or prolonged NG tube drainage
  - Pyloric stenosis
  - Laxative abuse
  - Diuretics
  - Post-hypercapnic states
- Chloride-resistant: Urine chloride > 15 mEq/L:
  - Severe Mg or K deficiency
  - Diuretics (thiazides or loops)
  - Increased mineralocorticoids (Cushing's syndrome, primary aldosteronism, renal artery stenosis)
  - Licorice, chewing tobacco
  - Inherited disorders (Bartter's syndrome)

Signs and Symptoms

- Irritability and neuromuscular hyperexcitability
- Concomitant signs of hypokalemia (muscular weakness, cramping, ileus)
- Suspect metabolic alkalosis when the physical exam suggests hypovolemia and chronic GI volume loss

Treatment

- Mild metabolic alkalosis requires no specific treatment.
- Hydration if cause is volume contraction
- In severe hypokalemia and hypermineralocorticoid states the alkalosis is chloride-resistant and cannot be corrected until potassium is replaced. Specific therapy must address hypermineralocorticoid state.

▶ INTERPRETING ARTERIAL BLOOD GASES

Important Rules

1. There can be only three acid–base disorders at the same time.
2. The body can never overcompensate for the primary acid–base disorder.

Compensations

Respiratory Acidosis
Acute: ↑ in HCO_3 by 1 for every 10 ↑ in CO_2
Chronic: ↑ in HCO_3 by 3 for every 10 ↑ in CO_2
(pH ↓ by .08 for every ↑ in CO_2 by 10 in acute and pH ↓ by .04 for every ↑ CO_2 by 10 in chronic)

Respiratory Alkalosis
Acute: ↓ in HCO_3 by 2 for every ↓ in CO_2 by 10
Chronic: ↓ in HCO_3 by 4 for every ↓ in CO_2 by 10

Metabolic Acidosis
Calculate Winter's formula to determine what the CO_2 should be in a primary metabolic acidosis
A quick way to determine what the CO_2 should be is to look at the last two digits of the pH (i.e., if the pH is 7.28, the CO_2 in a metabolic acidosis should be 28)

Metabolic Alkalosis
CO_2 ↑ by .06 for every ↑ in HCO_3 by 1

Formulas

Winter's: Used to calculate what the CO_2 compensation should be when the primary disorder is metabolic acidosis:

$$1.5\ (HCO_3) + 8 \pm 2 = \text{expected } CO_2$$

Anion gap: Na – (Cl + HCO_3) normally is between 8 and 12; if > 12, go through MUDPILES for underlying cause.
Delta gap: Used to calculate tertiary acid–base disorders. Use only to diagnose non–anion gap metabolic acidosis or metabolic alkalosis. Calculates if the body is excreting bicarbonate properly to compensate for the presence of unmeasurable anions.
Anion gap – 12 (nl gap) = excess anion gap
Excess anion gap + HCO3 = delta gap
If delta gap is > 30, then underlying metabolic alkalosis is present.
If delta gap is < 23, then underlying acidosis is present.
If between 23 and 30, then no tertiary disorder is present.

Putting It All Together

1. Look at pH: If < 7.40, acidosis is present; if > 7.40, alkalosis is present.
2. Next, look at the CO_2. If acidosis is present and the CO_2 is < 40, the primary disorder is metabolic acidosis; if the CO_2 is > 40, the primary disorder is respiratory acidosis. If alkalosis is present and the CO_2 is < 40, the primary disorder is respiratory alkalosis. If the CO_2 is > 40, the primary disorder is metabolic alkalosis.
3. Calculate compensation for the primary disorder using the calculations above to diagnose secondary acid–base disorder.
4. Calculate delta gap to diagnose tertiary acid–base disorder.

Electrolyte Disorders

Major toxins that increase the serum osmolarity: EtOH, methanol, ethylene glycol.

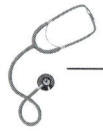

Diarrhea and normal saline hydration (isosmotic volume contraction/expansion) do not change the serum osmolarity.

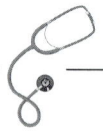

Urine Na^+ can distinguish between renal and extrarenal causes of hypovolemic hyponatremia.
Renal cause: $UNa^+ > 20$ μEq/L
Nonrenal cause: < 20 μEq/L

▶ BODY FLUIDS

Definitions

- Total body water (TBW) is approximately 60% of lean body mass.
- Intracellular fluid (ICF) is two thirds of TBW:
  - The major cations in ICF are K^+ and $Mg2^+$.
  - The major ICF anions are proteins and organic phosphates (ATP, ADP, AMP).
- Extracellular fluid (ECF) is one third of TBW:
  - Consists of interstitial fluid (third space) and plasma
  - The major ECF cation is Na^+.
  - The major ECF anions are Cl^- and HCO_3^-.
- Plasma comprises one fourth of the ECF (one twelfth of TBW). The major plasma proteins are albumin and globulins.
- Interstitial fluid is three fourths of the ECF (one fourth of TBW). The electrolyte composition of interstitial fluid is the same as plasma. However, interstitial fluid contains little protein (ultrafiltrate).

Fluid Shifts Between Compartments

- Water shifts between ECF and ICF so the osmolarities of the two compartments remain equal.
- Solutes that do not cross the cell membranes freely contribute to ECF osmolarity (glucose, sodium, mannitol, IV contrast materials).

Serum Osmolarity

- Normal range: 280 to 300 mOsm/kg
- Serum osmolarity can be estimated with the following formula:

$$\text{Serum osm} = 2(\text{Na} + \text{K}) + \frac{\text{Glucose}}{18} + \frac{\text{BUN}}{2.8}$$

- Elevated in dehydration, hypernatremia, diabetes insipidus, uremia, hyperglycemia, mannitol therapy, toxin ingestion, hypercalcemia, diuretic therapy
- Decreased in syndrome of inappropriate antidiuretic hormone (SIADH), hyponatremia, overhydration with 5% dextrose solution, Addison's disease, hypothyroidism

▶ HYPONATREMIA

Definition

Plasma sodium < 134 mEq/L

Etiology and Classification

Calculate serum osmolarity and determine fluid status of a patient to determine classification of hyponatremia. Hyponatremia is subdivided into three categories based on the serum osmolarity and fluid status:

- Hypotonic hyponatremia is further subdivided into three categories:
  - Isovolemic/hypotonic hyponatremia: Renal failure, SIADH, glucocorticoid deficiency (hypopituitarism), hypothyroidism, and medications
  - Hypovolemic/hypotonic hyponatremia:
    - Loss of both sodium and water
    - Renal losses (diuretics, partial urinary tract obstruction, salt-wasting nephropathies)
    - Extrarenal losses (vomiting, diarrhea, extensive burns, third-spacing (pancreatitis, peritonitis)
  - Hypervolemic/hypotonic hyponatremia: CHF, nephrotic syndrome, cirrhosis
- Isotonic hyponatremia (normal serum osmolarity):
  - SIADH
  - Isotonic infusions (glucose, mannitol)
- Hypertonic hyponatremia (increased serum osmolarity):
  - Hyperglycemia: Each 100 mL/dL increase in serum glucose above normal decreases plasma sodium concentration by 1.6 mEq/L.
  - Hypertonic infusions: mannitol, glucose.

Signs and Symptoms

- Moderate hyponatremia or gradual onset: Confusion, muscle cramps, lethargy, anorexia, nausea
- Severe hyponatremia or rapid onset: Seizures or coma (no exact number, but $Na^+ < 115$ is always severe)

Diagnosis

- Normal osmolarity: Consider pseudohyponatremia and overinfusion of non–sodium-containing isotonic solutions such as glucose and mannitol.
- Low osmolarity: Clinically assess the extracellular fluid volume. Look for tachycardia, hypotension, poor skin turgor (indicative of hypovolemia). Also look for peripheral edema (indicative of hypervolemia). Normal vital signs and no edema usually indicate isovolemia.
- High osmolarity: Measure serum glucose concentration to consider hyperglycemia. Also consider overinfusion of hypertonic, non-sodium-containing solutions (mannitol, glucose, glycine).

Serum Chemistries

See Table 2.6-3.

Pseudohyponatremia

- Simply an error in measurement of sodium due to an increase in other plasma components

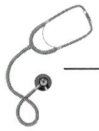

Pseudohyponatremia is suspected if the measured and calculated serum osmolarities are different.

TABLE 2.6-3. Causes of Hyponatremia

		Urine Osm	Urine Sodium
Hypovolemic	Extrarenal: GI losses, skin losses, lung losses, third-spacing (fistula, burns, vomiting, diarrhea, GI suction, edema, pancreatitis)	↑	↓
	Renal: Diuretics, intrinsic renal damage (including acute tubular necrosis), partial urinary tract obstruction	↑	↑
	Adrenal insufficiency (Addison's)	↑	↑
Isovolemic	Water intoxication	↓	↓
	SIADH	↑	↑
Hypervolemic	CHF, liver cirrhosis, and the nephrotic syndrome	↑	↓

↓ = decreased; ↑ = increased.

- Since plasma is 93% water and 7% plasma protein and lipid, and sodium ions are only dissolved in the plasma water, increasing the non-aqueous phase artificially lowers the Na^+ concentration.
- This occurs in multiple myeloma (due to increased plasma protein) or hyperlipidemia.

Treatment—General Rules

- Treatment approach is twofold: Correction of the serum sodium, and treatment of the underlying disorder
- Serum sodium should be corrected only halfway to the lower range of normal within the first 24 hours.
- Never correct sodium faster than 1 mEq/hr. Central pontine myelinolysis (CPM), seizures, and cerebral edema may occur.

Type-Specific Treatment

- **Hypovolemic hyponatremia:** 0.9% NaCl (normal saline) infusion to correct volume deficit. Monitor the serum sodium to prevent complications of rapid correction. Hypertonic saline is rarely indicated.
- **Hypervolemic hyponatremia:** Sodium and water restriction. In CHF, the combination of captopril and furosemide is effective.

Central Pontine Myelinolysis (CPM)

- Sometimes termed osmotic demyelination syndrome, occurs as a treatment complication of severe or chronic hyponatremia (< 110 mEq/L).
- A symmetric zone of demyelination occurs in the basis pontis (and extrapontine areas), leading to stupor, lethargy, quiet and confused delirium, and quadriparesis.
- CPM can be avoided by increasing the serum sodium no faster than 0.5 mEq/hr. Some patients treated symptomatically will recover in 3 to 4 weeks; however, in some, the damage is irreversible.

▶ HYPERNATREMIA

Definition

Serum Na > 145 mEq/L

Etiology and Classification (see Table 2.6-4)

Hypovolemic (most common)

- Loss of water and sodium (water loss >> than sodium loss)
- Renal losses (diuretics, glycosuria); GI, respiratory, or skin losses; adrenal deficiencies

Isovolemic

- Decreased TBW, normal total body sodium, and decreased ECF
- Diabetes insipidus (neurogenic and nephrogenic), skin losses (hyperthermia), iatrogenic causes, reset osmostat

Hypervolemic

- Increased TBW, markedly increased total body sodium, and increased ECF
- Iatrogenic (hypertonic fluid administration)
- Mineralocorticoid excess (Conn's tumor, Cushing's syndrome)
- Excess salt ingestion

Signs and Symptoms

- Fatigue
- Confusion (can progress to coma and seizures)
- Lethargy
- Edema

Treating Hypernatremia

Hypovolemic

- Fluid replacement with normal saline. Correct plasma osmolarity no faster than 2 mOsm/kg/hr.

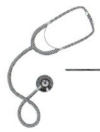

Water deficit (WD) in hypernatremic patients: WD (in liters) = 0.6 × body weight (kg) × (Measured Na/Normal Na) − 1).

TABLE 2.6-4. Causes of Hypernatremia

		Urine Osm	Urine Sodium
Hypovolemic	Renal loss: Osmotic diuresis (glycosuria, urea), acute/chronic renal failure, partial obstruction	N/↓	↑
	Extrarenal loss: Hyperpnea, excessive sweating	↑	↑
	Extrarenal loss: Diarrhea, burns, moderate sweating	↑	↓
	Iatrogenic (bicarbonate, dialysis, salt tablets)	↑	↑
Isovolemic	Diabetes insipidus (from any cause)	↓	↓
Hypervolemic	Mineralocorticoid excess (e.g., Conn's syndrome)	N/↓	N/↓

↓ = decreased; ↑ = increased; N = normal.

Isovolemic

- Fluid replacement with half normal (0.45%) saline. Correct only half of the estimated water deficit in the first 24 hours.
- The correction rate should not exceed 1 mEq/L/hr in acute hypernatremia and 0.5 mEq/L/hr in chronic hypernatremia.
- Vasopressin for central diabetes insipidus

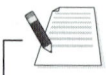

In hypovolemic hypernatremia, always correct fluid deficit with normal saline before anything else.

Hypervolemic

- Fluid replacement with half normal (0.45%) saline (to correct hypertonicity
- Loop diuretic therapy (e.g., furosemide) to increase sodium excretion

▶ HYPOKALEMIA

Periodic paralysis can be associated with either hypokalemia or hyperkalemia. Both forms are autosomal dominant. However, hypokalemic periodic paralysis first presents in the teenage years, whereas hyperkalemic periodic paralysis presents in infancy.

Definition

Plasma potassium < 3.3 mEq/L

Etiology and Classification

- Cellular shift (redistribution) and undetermined mechanisms:
  - Alkalosis (each 0.1 increase in pH decreases serum K^+ by 0.4–0.6 mEq/L.)
  - Insulin (drives K^+ into cells)
  - Vitamin B_{12}
  - Beta-adrenergics
  - Correction of digoxin toxicity with digitalis antibody fragments (Digibind).
- Increased renal potassium excretion:
  - Medications (diuretics, amphotericin B, cisplatin, aminoglycosides, corticosteroids)
  - Renal tubular acidosis type I (distal) or type II (proximal)
  - Hypomagnesemia
  - Osmotic diuresis (mannitol)
  - Bartter's syndrome: JG-cell hyperplasia causing increased rennin/aldosterone, metabolic alkalosis, hypokalemia, muscle weakness, and tetany (seen in young adults).
  - Increased mineralocorticoid activity (1° or 2° hyperaldosteronism), Cushing's syndrome
- GI losses:
  - Vomiting, nasogastric suctioning
  - Diarrhea, laxative abuse
  - Inadequate dietary intake (anorexia nervosa)
- Cutaneous losses from excessive sweating

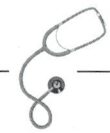

Patients taking digitalis must have their potassium checked regularly because hypokalemia increases the risk and severity of digitalis toxicity.

Signs and Symptoms

- Impaired gastric motility, nausea, and vomiting
- Mild muscle weakness to overt paralysis depending on severity
- Rhabdomyolysis
- Atrial and ventricular dysrhythmias

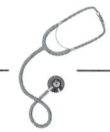

A 20-mEq infusion will raise the serum K by 0.25 mEq/L.

Treatment

Replace potassium (PO or IV, depending on severity). Intravenous infusion of K^+ should not exceed 20 mEq/hr.

▶ HYPERKALEMIA

Definition

Serum K > 5.5 mEq/L

Etiology

- Always consider pseudohyperkalemia (falsely elevated measurement due to homolysis of specimen and leakage of potassium from lysed cells). This is the most common cause of elevated potassium in lab results. Repeat test.
- **Intra- to extracellular potassium shifting** occurs in acidosis, heavy exercise, insulin deficiency, and digitalis toxicity.
- **Increased potassium load** occurs with IV potassium supplementation, potassium containing medications, and increased cellular breakdown.
- **Decreased potassium excretion** occurs with oliguric renal failure, potassium sparing diuretics, beta blockers, angiotensin-converting enzyme (ACE) inhibitors, aldosterone deficiency, and obstructive uropathies.

Signs and Symptoms

- GI: Nausea, vomiting, diarrhea.
- Neuro: Muscle cramps, weakness, paresthesias, paralysis, areflexia, tetany, focal neurologic deficits, confusion
- Respiratory insufficiency
- Cardiac: Arrhythmias, arrest

Diagnosis

ECG Changes

- 6.5 to 7.5 mEq/L: Tall peaked T-waves (see Figure 2.6-1), short QT interval, prolonged PR
- 7.5 to 8.0 mEq/L: QRS widening, flattened P-wave
- 10 to 12 mEq/L: QRS may degrade into a "sine-wave" pattern.
- V-fib, complete heart block, or asystole may occur.

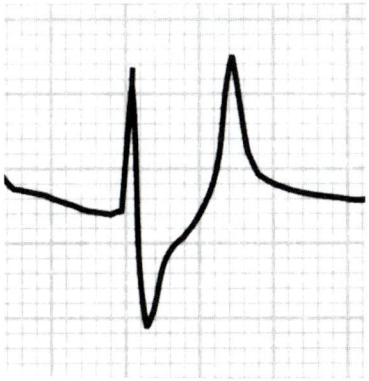

FIGURE 2.6-1. Peaked T-wave due to hyperkalemia.

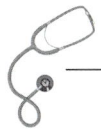

Chronic, slowly developing hyperkalemia is better tolerated than acute changes.

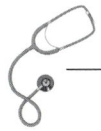

Perform a STAT ECG on patients with moderate to severe hyperkalemia.

Treatments for hyperkalemia:
Calcium
Kayexalate
Insulin and glucose
Dialysis
Bicarbonate
Albuterol

Controlling **K** **I**mmediately **D**iverts **B**ad **A**rrhythmias

Kayexalate is the only treatment of hyperkalemia (other than dialysis) that removes potassium from the body.

Treatment

- Cardiac membrane stabilization (calcium); acts in minutes
  - Contraindicated in patients on digoxin
- Shifting K^+ from ECF to ICF (insulin, albuterol, bicarbonate); acts in minutes
  - This is a temporary fix that wears off after the drugs do.
- Removal of K from the body (cation exchange resin such as Kayexalate, dialysis); takes hours to work

▶ HYPOCALCEMIA

Definition

- Serum Ca < 8.5 mg/dL
- Calcium is found in ionized (bound to serum proteins) and unionized (free) forms. The free fraction is biologically active.

Etiology

- PTH insufficiency
- Pseudohypoparathyroidism (Albrights' hereditary osteodystropy)
- Vitamin D deficiency (intestinal malabsorption, cholestyramine, primidone, renal, or liver disease)
- Toxins: Fluoride, cimetidine, ethanol, citrate, phenytoin
- Sepsis
- Pancreatitis
- Rhabdomyolysis, tumor lysis syndrome (increased serum phosphate)
- Severe magnesium deficiency

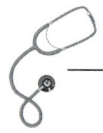

Neck surgery, even long after the procedure, can be associated with postoperative hypoparathyroidism usually due to ischemia of the parathyroid glands.

Parathyroid Hormone (PTH)

Secretion is stimulated by low free calcium and inhibited by increasing free calcium. Three major actions:

- In kidney, PTH facilitates excretion of phosphate and retention of calcium.
- Also in the kidney, PTH stimulates conversion of 25-OH vitamin D to 1,25-dihydroxyvitamin D (active vitamin D). Renal failure results in vitamin D deficiency → low Ca^+ → increased PTH.
- PTH activates bone remodeling.
- Vitamin D causes retention of both calcium and phosphate.

Signs and Symptoms

- Circumoral paresthesia is usually the first symptom.
- **Chvostek's sign:** Facial muscle spasm with tapping of the facial nerve
- **Trousseau's sign:** Carpal spasm after occluding blood flow in forearm with blood pressure cuff.

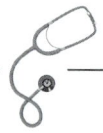

Correcting for hypoalbuminemia:
The measured Ca should be adjusted upward by 0.8 mg/dL for each 1.0 g/dL of albumin below normal.

Diagnosis

ECG findings: Prolonged QT and ST intervals (peaked T-waves are also possible, as in hyperkalemia).

Treatment

- For PTH deficiency: Replacement therapy with vitamin D or calcitriol combined with high oral calcium intake. Thiazide diuretics are used to lower urinary calcium and prevent calcium urolithiasis.
- Repletion of magnesium for hypomagnesemia
- Oral calcium supplementation, dietary phosphate restriction, and calcitriol for chronic renal failure
- Vitamin D and calcium supplementation for pseudohypoparathyroidism
- IV calcium for severe, life-threatening hypocalcemia

Causes of hypercalcemia:
"CHIMPANZEES"
Calcium supplementation
Hyperparathyroidism/ **H**yperthyroidism
Immobility/**I**atrogenic
Metastasis/Milk alkali syndrome
Paget's disease
Addison's disease/ **A**cromegaly
Neoplasm
Zollinger–Ellison syndrome
Excessive vitamin A
Excessive vitamin D
Sarcoidosis

▶ HYPERCALCEMIA

Definition

Serum Ca > 10.2 mg/dL

Etiology

Drugs
- Calcium supplementation (IV)
- Excess vitamin D increases intestinal calcium absorption.
- Antacid abuse
- Thiazides (inhibit renal calcium excretion)
- Lithium

Malignancies
- Colon, lung, breast, prostate (all cause metastasis to bone)
- Multiple myeloma
- Zollinger–Ellison syndrome (as part of MEN I)

Endocrinopathies
- Hyperparathyroidism
- Hyperthyroidism
- Acromegaly
- Addison's disease
- Paget's disease (of bone)

Other
- Immobility (leads to increased bone turnover with increased bone resorption)
- Granulomatous diseases such as sarcoidosis, tuberculosis (1,25-$[OH]_2$-vitamin D production by macrophages within granulomatous tissue)

Primary hyperparathyroidism is the most common cause of hypercalcemia in the outpatient. Malignancy is the most common cause in the inpatient.

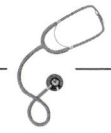

Hypercalcemia is a risk factor for kidney stones.

Signs and Symptoms

- Malaise, fatigue, headaches, diffuse aches, and pains
- Patients are often dehydrated and a vicious cycle ensues. Dehydration decreases renal calcium excretion and patients take in less fluids because of vomiting and nausea.
- Lethargy and psychosis occur when hypercalcemia is severe.
- Metastatic calcifications may occur in skin, cornea, conjunctiva, and kidneys.

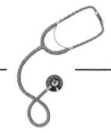

Acute pancreatitis can be precipitated by hypercalcemia.

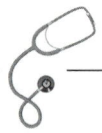

Transient hypoparathyroidism can occur after removal of a parathyroid adenoma because the remaining glands take a few days to begin secreting PTH again.

Treatment

- IV fluids +/– Lasix
- Calcitonin
- Bisphosphonate derivatives (decrease osteoclastic activity)
- Parathyroidectomy if hyperparathyroid is cause

▶ MALIGNANCY AND HYPERCALCEMIA

Definition

Humoral hypercalcemia of malignancy: From tumor production of PTH-related peptide. Stimulates bone resorption and renal calcium reabsorption. PTH-related peptide is not detected by the usual PTH immunoassay. Specific immunoassay exists for PTH-related peptide.

Local osteolytic hypercalcemia: Malignant cells in multiple myeloma or solid tumors with bone metastases may cause osteoclast stimulation. Osteoclast-activating factors (OAFs) are interleukins, transforming growth factors, and other cytokines.

Management of Severe Hypercalcemia

- Rehydration with normal saline to initiate calciuresis.
- IV infusion of **Pamidronate** (bisphosphonate) should be initiated simultaneously.
- May also use calcitonin.
- May also use furosemide to increase diuresis once patient is hydrated

▶ PRIMARY HYPERPARATHYROIDISM

Hyperparathyroidism: "Stones, bones, groans, and psychiatric overtones"

Definition

- Elevated parathyroid hormone and elevated serum calcium.
- May occur in conjunction with MEN I or MEN IIa (all glands are hyperplastic).
- Usually, only one parathyroid gland is enlarged, and hypercalcemia suppresses the function of the remaining glands.

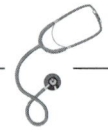

Hypercalcemic crisis is an uncommon manifestation of 1° hyperparathyroidism. It presents with severe hypercalcemia, volume depletion, and altered mental status.

Epidemiology

More common in middle-aged to elderly women.

Signs and Symptoms

- Usual presentation is asymptomatic hypercalcemia noted on routine laboratory examination.
- Patients may also have nonspecific complaints like fatigue, weight loss, depression, abdominal pain, or arthralgias.

- Hypercalciuria from the kidneys' inability to reabsorb the large calcium load may lead to nephrocalcinosis or renal calculi.
- Elevated PTH levels lead to bone remodeling and decreased bone mass.

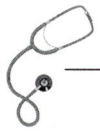

In patients with underlying cardiac failure consider furosemide to maintain diuresis and pulmonary artery pressure monitoring to avoid volume overload.

Diagnosis

- Hypercalcemia
- PTH level in the high-normal range
- Hypophosphatemia
- Hypercalciuria

► SECONDARY HYPERPARATHYROIDISM/RENAL OSTEODYSTROPHY

Pathophysiology

- Nephron loss reduces phosphate excretion, causing hyperphosphatemia
- This lowers serum calcium (increasing PTH secretion) and impairs calcitriol formation.
- Decreased calcitriol formation (also due to nephron loss) reduces intestinal calcium absorbtion.
- This provides further stimulation for PTH secretion.

Etiology and Classification

Three types of bone lesions are associated with secondary hyperparathyroidism:

1. Osteitis fibrosa cystica: Normal bone is replaced by fibrous tissue, primitive woven bone, and cysts.
2. Osteomalacia: Associated with vitamin D deficiency, characterized by defective osteoid mineralization.
3. Adynamic bone disease: Cause is unknown.

Signs and Symptoms

- Bone pain
- Proximal muscle weakness
- Pruritus
- Soft-tissue ulcerations
- Diffuse soft-tissue calcifications

Treatment

Goal is to normalize the calcium–phosphate balance:

- Reduce intestinal absorption of phosphate with aluminum-containing antacids.
- Vitamin D with calcitriol to increase serum calcium and reverse some of the bone changes
- Subtotal parathyroidectomy may benefit patients who do not respond to medical therapy.
- Renal transplant in selected patients

▶ HYPOPHOSPHATEMIA

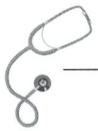

A common cause of high phosphate serum values is *in vitro* hemolysis. Most labs will report that the specimen was hemolyzed, however.

- Serum phosphate < 2.5 mg/dL
- Usually alcoholism or malnutrition is cause. Also seen with DKA
- Symptoms are neuro (mental status change, agitation) and muscle weakness.
- Severe hypophosphatemia (< 1 mg/dL) can result in rhabdomyolysis or seizures.
- Treat with phosphate supplementation.

▶ HYPERPHOSPHATEMIA

Hungry-bone syndrome is the rapid transfer of calcium into bones following removal of a hyperactive parathyroid nodule.

- Plasma phosphate > 5 mg/dL
- **Etiology:** Renal failure (particularly acute tubular necrosis [ATN]), tumor lysis syndrome (rapid necrosis of tumor after chemotherapy), iatrogenic (excessive amounts given IV or PO)
- **Treatment:** Oral calcium carbonate (binds phosphate in gut and decreases absorption)

▶ HYPOMAGNESEMIA

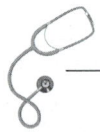

When supplementing calcium or potassium, always check for hypomagnesemia. The calcium and potassium levels will not elevate if magnesium is low.

- Serum magnesium < 1.8 mg/dL
- **Etiology:** Drugs (loop diuretics, amphotericin, gentamicin), insulin, hungry bone syndrome
- Low magnesium causes hypokalemia and hypocalcemia refractory to replacement
- ECG changes similar to hypokalemia
- Treat with oral or IV supplementation

▶ HYPERMAGNESEMIA

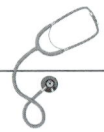

IV magnesium infusion:
- Cardiac monitor
- Vitals q 10 min
- Monitor deep tendon reflexes
- Monitor urine output

- Serum magnesium > 2.3 mg/dL
- **Etiology:** Iatrogenic (during treatment of eclampsia/preeclampsia), magnesium-containing drugs (some laxatives, antacids) if given to a patient with renal failure
- **Treatment:** IV fluids, calcium if there are ECG changes; dialysis if refractory

▶ GENERAL PRINCIPLES OF ELECTROLYTE DISORDER MANAGEMENT

- Always check the other electrolytes—isolated electrolyte abnormalities are uncommon.
- Abnormal calcium level is meaningless without an albumin level in an asymptomatic patient.
- Redraw labs if *in vitro* hemolysis is a possibility.

- If severe, place patient on continuous ECG monitoring.
- Neurological exam soon after treatment begun—focus on level of consciousness, presence of confusion, and deep tendon reflexes. Serial neuro exams during treatment can guide therapy while labs are pending.

Acute Renal Failure (ARF)

Definition

Clear-cut definition does not exist. Usually rapid onset of oliguria with increasing BUN and creatinine. Often occurs in the hospitalized patient.

Classification

Prerenal, postrenal, or intrinsic renal failure

General Approach

- Renal failure suspected from oliguria or increasing BUN/creatinine
- Prerenal (due to decreased blood to kidney):
  - BUN rising out of proportion to creatinine (> 20:1)
  - Volume depletion from hemorrhage, dehydration, surgery
  - CHF causing decreased cardiac output and secondary renal hypoperfusion
  - Third-spacing from cirrhosis, nephrotic syndrome, sepsis, burns
  - Most common cause of inpatient renal insufficiency due to decreased renal perfusion
  - Exacerbated by NSAIDs and ACE inhibitors
- Postrenal (due to obstruction of urinary excretion):
  - Bilateral ureteral obstruction: Urothelial tumor, benign prostatic hypertrophy (BPH), cervical CA
  - Urethral obstruction: Bladder CA
  - Renal sonogram: May show bilateral hydronephrosis, retrograde ureterogram is more sensitive
  - Reversible if obstruction removed in time
  - Postobstructive diuresis: Frequent temporary sequela of obstruction removal. Postobstructive diuresis is overdiuresis by kidneys, resulting in dehydration and electrolyte disturbance. If present, hydrate and follow electrolytes.
- Intrinsic renal failure:
  - Acute tubular necrosis (ATN) due to: Medications (aminoglycosides, cisplatin, pentamidine, lithium, amphotericin), rhabdomyolysis, IV contrast
  - Acute allergic interstitial nephritis (AIN)
  - Vascular disorders and atheromatous emboli
  - Glomerular disorders (nephrotic and nephritic syndromes)

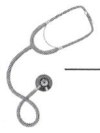

Oliguria: Urine output < 400 mL/day. Minimum volume needed to excrete daily production of metabolites and waste products.

Urinary Sodium

- Prerenal failure has low urine sodium (< 15 mEq/L) and high urine osmolarity (> 500 mOsm/L). The urine specific gravity is usually around 1.020.

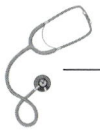

Dopamine, diuretics, mannitol, and saline confound use of fractional sodium excretion in finding etiology of renal failure.

- Intrinsic renal failure has high urine sodium (> 15 mEq/L) and low urine osmolarity (< 400 mOsm/L).
- The fractional sodium excretion (FE Na^+) is the best discriminator between prerenal and intrinsic renal failure:

$$\text{FE } Na^+ = \frac{(\text{Urine Na/Plasma Na})}{(\text{Urine creatinine/Plasma creatinine})} \times 100\%$$

Prerenal failure: < 1.0% Intrinsic renal failure: > 1.0%

Urinary Sediment

Intrinsic renal disease shows large amounts of protein and an "active" sediment (blood, protein, and red and white cell casts) that often will point toward the underlying cause of the renal disease:

- Acute glomerulonephritis: Red blood cell casts with hematuria and proteinuria and low urine specific gravity
- Acute tubular necrosis: Many renal epithelial cells and pigmented granular casts

Serologic Testing

Serologic testing can further delineate the cause of the failure:

- Antiglomerular basement membrane Ab in Goodpasture's syndrome
- Antineutrophil Ab (ANCA) in microscopic polyarteritis nodosa or Wegener's syndrome
- Antinuclear Ab (ANA) in SLE

▶ TUBULOINTERSTITIAL DISEASES

- Most common cause of intrinsic ARF
- Include ATN and interstitial nephritis
- Tubulointerstitial causes of renal failure are the most common in the hospital and have the best outcomes if recognized early.

Acute Tubular Necrosis

Definition

Acute necrosis of renal tubules due to ischemic or toxic insult

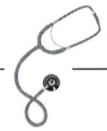

Peripheral neuropathies and renal osteodystrophy are features of the uremic syndrome not seen in ATN.

Etiology

- Ischemic: Shock, trauma, sepsis, hypoxia
- Toxic: IV contrast media, aminoglycosides, rhabdomyolysis, and tumor lysis

Course

- Patients present with dramatic renal failure
- Most survive and recover normal renal function.
- Severity correlates with survival.

- Failure lasts 1 to 2 weeks, during which intensive care is required.
- ~50% have normal urine output (less severe).

Diagnosis

- Muddy brown granular casts
- High urine sodium
- FE Na is > 1%.

Prevention

- Monitor creatinine in patients receiving nephrotoxic substances.
- Maintain adequate intravascular volumes in patients going to or recovering from surgical procedures.
- Maintain good cardiac output.

Treatment

- Normal saline for volume replacement
- IV diuretic therapy is frequently used in the early stages of ATN to promote urine flow—there is little evidence that this prevents progression of ATN.
- Match fluid and salt intake to the daily outputs.
- Discontinue precipitating cause (e.g., meds).
- Manage electrolyte disturbances (particularly high potassium).

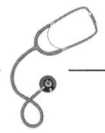

NSAIDs usually do not cause interstitial nephritis, but by inhibiting prostaglandin synthesis they decrease the GFR, which can precipitate renal failure in a patient with underlying renal problems.

Acute Interstitial Nephritis

Definition

Inflammation of the renal parenchyma

Etiology

- Systemic diseases: Sarcoidosis, Sjögren's syndrome, lymphoma
- Systemic infections: Syphilis, toxoplasma, CMV, EBV
- Medications: Beta-lactam antibiotics, diuretics, and NSAIDs

Clinical and Lab Findings

- Clinical and lab findings similar to ATN
- Drug-induced interstitial nephritis is associated with eosinophils in the urine as well as other signs of systemic hypersensitivity reaction.

Treatment

- Address underlying cause.
- Manage renal failure as for ATN.

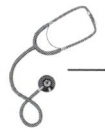

Allergic interstitial nephritis is characterized by WBCs, eosinophils, and white cell casts in the urine. Treat with steroids and stop offending agent.

GLOMERULAR DISORDERS

▶ NEPHROTIC SYNDROME

DEFINITION

Glomerular lesion causing proteinuria > 3 g/day. It indicates a defect in the glomerular filtration barrier.

"Maltese crosses" seen in polarized light examination of urinary sediment are indicative of cholesterol in the urine.

PATHOPHYSIOLOGY

- Loss of glomerular impermeability to plasma proteins resulting in proteinuria and loss of albumin (hypoalbuminemia)
- Severe decrease in serum proteins and oncotic pressure, resulting in edema and serosal effusions
- Hypercholesterolemia also common
- Hypercoagulability due to loss of proteins C and S and antithrombin III

COMMON CAUSES OF THE NEPHROTIC SYNDROME

- **Minimal change disease (nil disease,** lipoid nephrosis):
  - Usually idiopathic, usually found in children
  - Electron microscopy shows loss of epithelial foot processes, but light microscopy shows no change.
  - Usually responds to steroid therapy
  - Recurs frequently
  - Does not progress to chronic renal failure (unlike the other causes of nephrotic syndrome)
- **Focal glomerulosclerosis:**
  - Glomerular scarring involving limited number of glomeruli
  - Immunoglobulin and complement deposition detected by immunofluorescence
  - Most commonly seen in intravenous drug abusers and HIV patients
  - Leads to hypertension and chronic renal failure
  - Steroids usually not helpful
- **Membranous glomerulonephritis:**
  - Common cause of adult nephrotic syndrome
  - Caused by immune complex deposition
  - Idiopathic, or associated with SLE, hepatitis B, or solid tumors
  - Treat with steroids and cytotoxic agents (chlorambucil)
  - Rule of thirds
- **Systemic causes:**
  - Sickle cell anemia (papillary damage due to sickling in hyperosmotic medullary interstitium)
  - Diabetic glomerulopathies (diffuse glomerulosclerosis, nodular glomerulosclerosis). Most common secondary cause of nephrotic syndrome
  - Multiple myeloma (Bence Jones proteinuria from immunoglobulin light chains or their breakdown products)

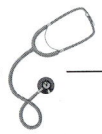

Rule of thirds for membranous glomerulonephritis: One third progress to CRF; one third have spontaneous remission; one third remain nephrotic but do not progress.

▶ GLOMERULONEPHRITIS (AKA NEPHRITIC SYNDROME)

Definitions and Terminology

- Indicates inflammation and glomerular damage
- Nephritic syndrome: Involves abrupt-onset hematuria with RBC casts, mild proteinuria; often includes hypertension, edema, and azotemia
- Acute glomerulonephritis (AGN): Nephritic syndrome (synonym)

Poststreptococcal Glomerulonephritis (PSGN) (aka Postinfectious Glomerulonephritis)

- Associated with group A, beta-hemolytic streptococcus (usually associated preceding with pharyngitis or impetigo)
- Immune complex deposition with complement (IgG, C3, C4) in a granular pattern leads to glomerular damage.
- Presents approximately 14 days after infection with dark urine and edema
- Usually reversible but occasionally progresses (more in adults than in children)
- **Labs:** Nephritic sediment (RBC casts), low complement
- **Treatment:** Treat underlying infection. Immunosuppressive drugs are ineffective.

IgA Nephropathy (aka Mesangial Proliferative)

- Most common glomerulonephritis
- Presents as hematuria during a viral infection or after exercise
- Has immune complex deposition of IgA and C3 in mesangial matrix ("mesangial hypercellularity")
- No effective treatment

Membranoproliferative

- Associated with hepatitis C and cryoglobulinemia
- Immune deposits on basement membrane cause basement membrane to look double layered; also mesangial proliferation
- Labs: Nephritic sediment and low complement
- Frequently progresses to renal failure
- Treat adults with ASA and dipyridimole. Treat children with steroids.

Other Diseases Associated with Acute Nephritic Syndrome

Secondary (Multisystem-Associated) Glomerular Diseases

- Collagen vascular disorders:
  - Polyarteritis nodosa
  - Systemic lupus erythematosus (SLE)
  - Wegener's granulomatosis
  - Henoch–Schönlein purpura (HSP)
- Hematologic disorders:
  - Thrombotic thrombocytopenic purpura (TTP), hemolytic–uremic syndrome
  - Serum sickness

If a patient presents with hematuria immediately after an infection, think IgA nephropathy.
If a patient presents 2 weeks after infection, think postinfectious glomerulonephritis.

RBC casts are pathognomonic of any glomerulonephritis.

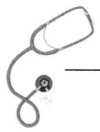

Antimicrobial therapy of the initial streptococcal infection does NOT prevent the onset of PSGN (as opposed to rheumatic fever).

Glomerulonephritis can also occur after other bacterial infections, viral infections, and parasitic infections.

- Glomerular basement membrane diseases:
  - Alport's syndrome
  - Goodpasture's syndrome
  - Thin basement membrane disease

Rapidly Progressive Glomerulonephritis (RPGN)

Definition

- Any glomerulonephritis that progresses can subsequently become this.
- Also called crescentic GN because biopsy shows epithelial cell proliferation (crescents) in glomeruli
- Characterized by fulminant renal failure with proteinuria, hematuria, and RBC casts
- Uncommon

Classification (Three Categories)

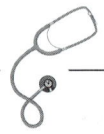

In 60 to 90% of patients, the anti-GBM Ab cross-react with pulmonary alveolar basement membranes.

1. Pauci-immune RPGN:
   - 50% of RPGN
   - No immune complex or complement deposition
   - ANCA is serologic marker for pauci-immune RPGN associated with systemic vasculitis.
   - Examples: Churg–Strauss, Wegener's (c-ANCA positive), polyarteritis nodosa (p-ANCA positive)
2. Immune complex RPGN:
   - 40% of RPGN
   - Can be associated with certain medications, syphilis, some malignancies
   - Examples: Postinfectious glomerulonephritis, lupus nephritis, IgA nephropathy
3. Anti–glomerular basement membrane Ab disease:
   - 10% of RPGN
   - Anti-GBM Ab present in blood—can be seen on GBM with immunofluorescent microscopy
   - Cytotoxic T-cells may contribute to the pathogenesis.
   - Example: Goodpasture's disease

Prognosis and Treatment

- Eighty percent of untreated patients progress to end-stage renal disease in 6 months.
- Treat with steroids and cyclophosphamide.

Chronic Renal Failure

Definition

Slowly progressing loss of renal function, usually over years, at a constant rate

Etiology

- Diabetes mellitus: Diffuse glomerulosclerosis, nodular glomerulosclerosis (Kimmelstiel–Wilson lesions)

- Idiopathic failure
- Hypertension: Nephrosclerosis
- Chronic glomerulonephritis: Red blood cell casts
- Chronic tubulointerstitial diseases: Sodium wasting, no proteinuria, prolonged obstructive uropathies
- Polycystic kidney disease

Pathophysiology

- Nephrons are lost and remaining healthy nephrons compensate by increasing their GFR. This process damages the healthy nephrons causing disease progression.
- Loss of renal endocrine function: Decreased synthesis of activated vitamin D, ammonia, and erythropoietin

Renal Function in CRF

- Usually asymptomatic until GFR less than 50% of baseline
- Water and sodium balance:
  - Initially: Decreased urine concentrating ability, easy dehydration, sodium wasting
  - Later: volume overload after the kidneys are unable to excrete dietary sodium
- Potassium: Once GFR becomes markedly diminished the ability to excrete dietary potassium is lost. The distal tubule compensates for the loss of excretory function until there is oliguria.
- Acid–base balance: When GFR is < 50% of baseline the tubular excretion of H^+ is impaired because renal production of ammonia is impaired, causing anion gap metabolic acidosis.
- Calcium and phosphate:
  - Hypocalcemia, hyperphosphatemia
  - Decreased activation of vitamin D due to loss of 1-hydroxylase activity
  - Secondary hyperparathyroidism
  - Severe bone resorption
  - Ectopic calcifications
- Serum creatinine increases (creatinine clearance decreases with decreased GFR).
- BUN increases, but to a lesser extent than the creatinine.

Signs and Symptoms

- Uremic syndrome, nephrotic syndrome (see individual sections)
- Ultrasound often reveals shrunken kidneys with cortical thinning.
- Rule out urinary tract infection (UTI) with urine culture.

Treatment

- ACE inhibitors may slow progression.
- Treat reversible causes.
- Diet: Modest protein restriction with near normal caloric intake decreases nitrogen intake and avoids catabolism.
- Dialysis (see below)

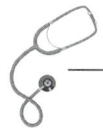

Renal biopsy should be performed before end-stage renal disease occurs because at that point the biopsy is unlikely to uncover a specific cause.

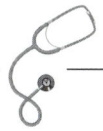

Anion gap increases because sulfates and phosphates are retained as well as H^+.

Creatinine is neither secreted nor reabsorbed by the nephron, it is only filtered. Therefore, the creatinine clearance is directly proportional to the GFR.

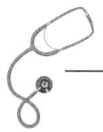

GFR and creatinine clearance:
For each doubling of the serum creatinine, the GFR has decreased by 50%.

Large kidneys are seen on sonogram in diabetes, amyloidosis, polycystic kidney disease.

▶ DIALYSIS

Chronic hemodialysis (HD) is the mainstay of therapy for chronic renal failure, but chronic ambulatory peritoneal dialysis (CAPD) is also an alternative. There is no absolute lab value that requires dialysis. The decision is clinical and based on a constellation of factors.

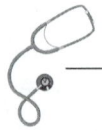

Patients on chronic medications (cardiac meds, warfarin, chemotherapy, etc.) dramatically drop their serum drug levels during dialysis. The timing and dosing of doses must be decided with the dialysis schedule in mind.

Absolute Indications for Dialysis

- Uremic pericarditis with or without cardiac tamponade
- Progressive motor neuropathy
- Intractable volume overload
- Life-threatening and intractable hyperkalemia or acidosis
- Toxins (e.g., ethylene glycol)

Clinical Findings Responding to Dialysis (Relative Indications)

- Fluid and electrolyte imbalances
- Volume-dependent hypertension
- CNS abnormalities
- Anemia and bleeding diatheses
- Anorexia, nausea, and vomiting
- Glucose intolerance
- Weight loss
- Pruritus and ecchymoses

Hemodialysis

- The two most commonly used vascular access sites are arteriovenous fistulae (usually in the forearm) and artificial shunts inserted between an artery and a vein. Dialysis needles are placed directly into the shunt.
- Dialysis patients are frequently instrumented and combined with the dialysis patient's impaired immunity, infection is common. Subacute bacterial endocarditis may occur if the infections are not recognized early and treated correctly.
- Viral hepatitis is also a risk of hemodialysis because of the frequent necessity of transfusion.

Chronic Ambulatory Peritoneal Dialysis

- Permanent catheter is inserted into the peritoneum allowing dialysis to be undertaken by the patient outside the hospital.
- Approximately 2 L of dialysis fluid is infused rapidly and allowed to remain in the peritoneal cavity for 4 to 6 hours. The fluid is then drained and new fluid is immediately infused.
- Peritoneum acts as a dialysis membrane.
- Infusion of hypertonic glucose solution allows for concurrent volume reduction.
- Bacterial peritonitis is more common than with HD.
- Hypoalbuminemia, hypertriglyceridemia, and anemia are common.

▶ UREMIC SYNDROME

Definition

Uremia is a syndrome associated with chronic renal failure that affects multiple organ systems.

Signs and Symptoms

- Appearance: Pale complexion, wasting, purpura, excoriation
- Complaints: Pruritus, polydipsia, nausea, anorexia, vomiting
- Urinalysis: Isosthenuria, proteinuria, abnormal sediment with tubular casts

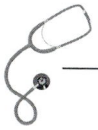

Isosthenuria: Inability of kidney to concentrate urine; fixes specific gravity at 1.010.

Systemic Effects

- CNS: Foot drop, carpal tunnel syndrome, clonus, asterixis, seizures
- Cardiac and pulmonary:
  - Hypertension leading to left ventricular hypertrophy (LVH) and diastolic dysfunction
  - Accelerated atherosclerosis, development of ischemic heart disease
  - Pleuropericardial inflammation (pericarditis with effusion and tamponade)
  - Calcification of mitral and aortic valves
  - Pulmonary edema and pleural effusions
- Hematologic:
  - Normochromic, normocytic anemia due to decreased erythropoietin synthesis, among other reasons
  - Defective platelet function—prolonged bleeding time
  - White cell function and absolute counts are reduced, resulting in increased likelihood of infection.
- GI: Mild GI bleeding, nausea/vomiting, anorexia
- Metabolic: Elevated triglycerides, insulin resistance with impaired glucose tolerance is common.

▶ POLYCYSTIC KIDNEY DISEASE

- Autosomal dominant
- Kidneys are enlarged and have multiple cysts.
- Patients typically present in their 30s or 40s with flank pain.
- Approximately 50% of patients will develop end-stage renal disease by the age of 60.
- Associated extrarenal manifestations are berry aneurysms (subarachnoid hemorrhage), hepatic cysts, and diverticula in the large intestine.
- Complications of polycystic kidneys are hypertension, recurrent urinary tract infections, and kidney stones (calcium oxalate and uric acid stones).
- Diagnose via ultrasound or CT scan.

Renal Tubular Acidosis

Definition

Defect in renal tubular function that results in metabolic acidosis with a normal anion gap

Etiology (see Table 2.6-5)

- There are three types: 1, 2, and 4 (there is no type 3).
- May be inherited or acquired via medications or disease states
- Types 1 and 4 occur in the distal tubules.
- Type 2 occurs in the proximal tubule.

Pathophysiology

- Type 1 is caused by a defect in hydrogen secretion causing acidosis and hypokalemia.
  - Can be caused by SLE, sarcoidosis, medication (lithium, amphotericin B)
  - Patients may also get renal stones due to hypercalcemia.
- Type 2 is caused by a defect in bicarbonate reabsorptin (aka bicarbonate wasting).
  - Can be caused by multiple myeloma, heavy metals, medication (acetazolamide)
  - Potassium can be low to normal.
- Type 4 is caused by a defect in aldosterone secretion (acts similar to spironolactone) and ammonium excretion.
  - Patients usually have low renin and aldosterone levels.
  - Caused by diabetic nephropathy, renal transplant, obstructive uropathy
  - Usually associated with hyperkalemia

Urolithiasis

Definition

Calculi in the urogenital system

TABLE 2.6-5 RTA Types

	Defect	Plasma Bicarbonate Level	Urine pH	Plasma K^+
Type 1 RTA	Impaired acidification of urine	Low	> 5.3	Low
Type 2 RTA	Decreased bicarbonate resorption	12–20	> 5.3	Low to normal
Type 4 RTA	Decreased aldosterone	Typically > 17	< 5.3	High

Epidemiology

- One of the most common diseases of the urinary tract
- Two to 5% of the population will form a urinary stone at some point in their lives.
- Majority of stones form between the ages of 20 and 50.
- Male-to-female ratio of 3:1
- Familial tendency in stone formation
- Tendency for recurrence—36% of patients with a first stone will have another stone within 1 year.

Types of Stones

Calcium Oxalate Stones (75%)

- Strongly radiopaque
- Treat with thiazides.
- Increased incidence in inflammatory bowel disease (increased oxalate), hypercalcemia (hyperparathyroidism), decreased citrate (forms stable soluble complex with calcium), uricosurea (small urate crystals serve as nidi for larger calcium stones)

Struvite ($Mg\ NH_4\ PO_4$) Stones (15%)

- Moderately radiopaque
- Common in *Proteus* UTIs due to high urinary pH (*Proteus* makes urease, which cleaves urinary urea yielding two molecules of ammonia—the conjugate base of ammonium ion)
- Treat by lowering urine pH.

Uric Acid Stones (< 1%)

- Radiolucent
- Increased incidence in myeloproliferative diseases and gout (due to increased purine turnover)
- Treat by raising urine pH.

Cystine Stones (< 1%)

- Moderately radiopaque
- Seen in congenital cystinuria (*not* homocystinuria)
- Hexagonal crystals, positively birefringent
- Treat by raising urine pH.

Predisposing Factors

- Dietary history—large calcium and alkali intake
- Prolonged immobilization
- Residence in hot climate
- History of urinary tract infections
- History of calculus in the past and in family members
- Drug ingestion (analgesics, alkalis, uricosuric agents, protease inhibitors)
- Prior history of gout
- Underlying gastrointestinal disease (Crohn's, ulcerative colitis, PUD)

Typical scenario:
A 39-year-old man presents with severe back pain and hematuria. He is writhing around, unable to find a comfortable position, and is nauseous.
Think: Renal colic due to urolithiasis.

Signs and Symptoms

- Severe, abrupt onset of colicky pain which begins in the flank and may radiate toward the groin. In males, the pain may radiate toward the testicle. In females, it may radiate toward the labia majoris.
- Nausea and vomiting are almost universal with acute renal colic.
- Abdominal distention from an ileus
- Gross hematuria

Diagnosis

Urinalysis (see Table 2.6-6)

- Vast majority of patients (about 85%) will have RBCs in the urine. However, its absence does not rule out renal stones.
- Urinary pH can aid in differentiating the type of stone present. Normal urinary pH is about 5.85. If the pH is > 6, one should suspect the presence of urea-splitting organisms (proteus). A low urine pH (≤ 5) suggests uric acid stones.

TABLE 2.6-6. Interpretation of the Urinalysis

Finding	Significance
Color	▪ Red or brown indicates presence of hemoglobin, myoglobin (as with rhabdomyolysis), or red food (beets).
Clarity	▪ Normal urine should be clear. ▪ Turbidity or cloudiness can be caused by excessive cellular material or protein, or precipitation of salts.
pH	▪ Normal pH ranges from 4.5 to 7.5. ▪ Alkaline urine indicates type 1 RTA or UTI with *Proteus* or *Ureaplasma.* ▪ Acidic urine can be seen with ASA overdose or type 2 RTA.
Specific gravity	▪ Normal specific gravity is 1.002 ot 1.035. ▪ High (> 1.010) indicates dehydration. ▪ Inability to concentrate urine in the setting of dehydration indicates renal disease.
Protein	▪ Proteinuria indicates glomerular dysfunction. ▪ Microalbuminuria is a marker for early diabetic nephropathy. ▪ Protein loss in urine of > 3 g/day is nephritic syndrome.
Glucose	▪ Glucose in urine can indicate hyperglycemia.
Ketones	▪ Seen in DKA, isopropyl alcohol intoxication, and starvation ketosis
Nitrite	▪ Normal is negative. ▪ Positive nitrite indicates bacteria present in the urine, usually gram-negative rods.
Leukocyte esterase	▪ Positive findings indicate the presence of white cells and infection.

TABLE 2.6-6. Interpretation of the Urinalysis (continued)

FINDING	SIGNIFICANCE
Red blood cells	▪ Present in glomerulonephritis, tumor, trauma, renal stones, renal infarct, malignant hypertension (also often erroneously positive in menstruating females)
White blood cells	▪ Also called pyuria; seen in UTIs, prostatitis, vaginitis
Eosinophils	▪ Seen in allergic interstitial nephritis (AIN)
Squamous epithelial cells	▪ From the skin surface or outer urethra; a measure of contamination
Casts	▪ Urinary casts are formed in the distal convoluted tubule and the collecting duct. ▪ RBC casts: Glomerulonephritis ▪ WBC casts: Pyelonephritis or glomerulonephritis ▪ Muddy brown granular casts: ATN ▪ Hyaline casts: Prerenal azotemia
Crystals	▪ Renal stones, ethylene glycol intoxication
Bilirubin	▪ Extravascular hemolysis
Hemoglobin	▪ Intravascular hemolysis

- WBCs or bacteria may suggest underlying urinary tract infection and should be aggressively treated.

Radiographic Studies (see Table 2.6-7)

- Plain abdominal film (KUB) will reveal only radiopaque stones (60 to 70%)
- Renal ultrasound is useful to detect hydronephrosis and is easy, cheap, and doesn't require subjecting the patient to intravenous contrast. It misses small stones
- Noncontrast renal computed tomography (CT) is most useful to diagnose small stones. It can accurately locate stones in the renal system and detect the presence of hydronephrosis. Overall sensitivity is about 95%.
- Intravenous pyelogram has been the gold standard for the diagnosis of renal and ureteral calculi. It can clearly outline the entire urinary system making it easy to see hydronephrosis and the presence of any type of stones. In addition, an intravenous pyelogram (IVP) can demonstrate renal function and allow for verification that the opposite kidney is functioning properly.

TREATMENT

- Analgesia
- Hydration

TABLE 2.6-7. Common Genitourinary Procedures

Test	Description	Uses
Intravenous pyelography	Contrast is injected into a peripheral vein, followed by radiographs, allowing visualization of the renal parenchyma and the ureters.	▪ Kidney or urethral trauma ▪ Kidney or urethral tumors ▪ Urethral diverticulum ▪ Assessment of renal damage from pyelonephritis

Voiding cystourethrogram	Contrast medium is placed into the bladder via catheter and visualized with x-ray during active micturition.	▪ Congenital abnormalities:
		  ▪ Posterior urethral valves
		  ▪ Ectopic drainage of ureters
		▪ Neurogenic bladder
		▪ Strictures
		▪ Vesicoureteral reflux
		▪ Stress urinary incontinence
		▪ Ureteroceles

Cystometry	Bladder is filled with water via catheter. Bladder is emptied into a measuring device. The pressure is recorded during this whole time.	▪ Benign prostatic hypertrophy ▪ Congenital anomalies ▪ Incontinence
Cystoscopy	Introduction of either a flexible or rigid scope into the urethra	▪ Biopsy ▪ Resection of tumors ▪ Crushing of stones ▪ Catheterization of ureters
Renal ultrasound	Advantage is that it is noninvasive.	▪ Renal calculi ▪ Urinary obstruction ▪ Renal tumors ▪ Renal vein thrombus ▪ Evaluating renal failure—the size of the kidneys give an idea of the chronicity of the failure.

Passage of Stones

- Ninety percent of stones < 5 mm will pass spontaneously.
- Fifteen percent of stones 5 to 8 mm will pass.
- Five percent of stones > 8 mm will pass.

For Stones Unlikely to Pass Spontaneously

- Extracorporeal shock lithotripsy has been effective for stones located in the kidney with 85% success rate.
- Percutaneous nephrolithotomy, which establishes a tract from the skin to the collecting system, is used when stones are too large or too hard for lithotripsy.

HIGH-YIELD FACTS IN

Pulmonology

Basics 253

- Hypoxia 253
- Lung Physical Exam 253
- Pleural Effusion 254
- Pulmonary Function Tests (PFTs) 255

Lung Infections 257

- Pneumonia 257
- Tuberculosis 259

Obstructive Disorders 262

- Chronic Obstructive Pulmonary Disease (COPD) 262
- Asthma 263
- Obstructive Sleep Apnea (OSA) 266

Upper Respiratory Tract Problems 266

- Acute Cough 266
- Chronic Cough 266
- Postnasal Drip Syndrome 267
- Sinusitis 268
- Pertussis (Whooping Cough) 269

Miscellaneous Lung Disorders 270

- Adult Respiratory Distress Syndrome (ARDS) 270
- Bronchiectasis 270
- Hemoptysis 271
- Pulmonary Embolism 272
- Pneumothorax 273

Mediastinum 274

- Mediastinitis 275
- Pneumomediastinum 275

Interstitial Lung Disease 275
Examples of Environmental Lung Disease **276**
Lung Cancer 276

BASICS

▶ HYPOXIA

- **V/Q mismatch:** Due to perfusion of poorly ventilated alveoli, or due to alveoli not being perfused. Responds to supplemental oxygen. Examples: Chronic obstructive pulmonary disease (COPD), congestive heart failure (CHF), pulmonary embolism (PE), pulmonary fibrosis, asthma
- **Right-to-left shunt:** Intrapulmonary due to perfusion of nonventilated lung, or extrapulmonary, such as congenital heart disease
- **Anemia:** Decreased hemoglobin decreases oxygen carrying capacity, has a normal PaO_2, decreased PvO_2
- **Improper oxygen utilization:** Cytochrome impairment due to cyanide poisoning, diphtheria toxin, etc.
- **Low inspired oxygen:** At high altitude or other low-oxygen environment
- **Carbon monoxide poisoning:** CO-Hgb "carboxy-Hgb" is unavailable for oxygen transport, O_2 unloaded at lower oxygen tensions. CO poisoning does not cause cyanosis. At highly toxic levels, it can cause a "cherry red" discoloration of lips and nails.
- **Diffusion defect:** Gas exchange compromised due to defect in alveolar interface. Example: interstitial lung disease
- **Hypoventilation:** Occurs with apnea, neuromuscular disorders (Guillain–Barré, myasthenia gravis, amyotrophic lateral sclerosis [ALS])

The most important determinant of the amount of oxygen delivery to tissues is *hemoglobin.*

Arterial oxygen content = $PaO_2 \times 0.0031 + 1.38 \times Hb \times SaO_2$

Typical scenario:
A married couple comes to the hospital complaining of "flulike" symptoms, including headache, nausea, vomiting, and disorientation. The wife thinks they caught the virus from a neighbor when they borrowed his home generator. *Think: Carbon monoxide poisoning.*

▶ LUNG PHYSICAL EXAM

Tactile Fremitus

Performed by placing ulnar side of hand or palm against the patient's posterior chest wall and having the patient say "ninety-nine." Vibrations are felt through the chest wall and can be compared from one side to the other.

- Increased tactile fremitus = increased density of the lung (consolidation)
- Decreased tactile fremitus = excess subcutaneous tissue on the chest, air or fluid in chest cavity (pneumothorax, pleural effusion) or overexpansion of lung

Percussion

Tapping the body to determine underlying structure. The sound produced depends on the air–tissue ratio of the structure involved.

- **Dull** = increased density, such as fluid in the lungs or lung cavity or consolidation, or solid organ (liver)
- **Flat** = large muscle mass (thigh)
- **Tympanic** = hollow air-containing structure (stomach)
- **Resonant** = structure of air within tissue (lung)
- **Hyperresonant** = decreased density and more air, such as in emphysema, dull with represents

TABLE 2.7-1. Lung Auscultation

Term	Mechanism	Causes
Crackle (rale)	Excessive airway secretions	Bronchitis, pneumonia, pulmonary edema, atelectasis, fibrosis
Wheeze	Rapid airflow through obstructed airway	Asthma, pulmonary edema, bronchitis
Rhoncus	Transient airway plugging	Bronchitis
Pleural rub	Inflammation of the pleura	Pneumonia, pulmonary infarction

Auscultation (see Table 2.7.1)

- **Crackles (rales):** Short, discontinuous nonmusical sounds heard mostly during inspiration
- **Wheezes:** Continuous, musical, high-pitched sounds heard mostly during expiration
- **Rhonchi:** Lower-pitched lung sounds
- **Pleural rub:** Grating sound produced by motion of pleura, heard best at end of inspiration/beginning of expiration

Egophony

Spoken words by the patient are increased in intensity and take on different quality during auscultation. Patient says "eeee" and will be heard as "aaaa" in areas of consolidation and in areas of **consolidation** and in areas of **compressed lung above a pleural effusion.**

▶ PLEURAL EFFUSION

Definition

Pleural effusion is classified as a transudate or exudate depending on origin.

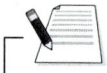

Transudates:
- CHF
- Cirrhosis
- Nephrosis

Transudative pleural effusions are due to:

- Increased hydrostatic pressure
- Decreased oncotic pressure

Exudative pleural effusions are due to:

- Increased capillary permeability

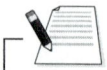

Exudates:
- Tumor
- Trauma
- Infection

Diagnosis

Light's criteria: The effusion is an *exudate* if one or more of the following is present:

- Ratio of pleural to serum protein > 0.5
- Ratio of pleural to serum lactic dehydrogenase (LDH) > 0.6
- Pleural fluid LDH > ⅔ upper normal limit

Common Associations

The effusion is *parapneumonic* if:
- Pleural fluid leukocyte count > 10,000/mm^3 with high PMNs
- Parapneumonic effusions are always exudates.
- WBC > 100,000 = empyema

Gross blood in pleural fluid is associated with:
- Tumor (breast cancer, lung cancer, lymphoma)
- Trauma
- Pulmonary infarction
- Aortic dissection

Low glucose in pleural fluid is associated with:
- Empyema
- Rheumatoid arthritis (glucose extremely low)
- Tumor
- Tuberculosis

High amylase in pleural fluid is associated with:
- Pancreatitis
- Renal failure
- Tumor
- Esophageal rupture

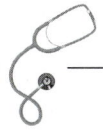

Empyema (pus in pleural space), positive cultures, or loculated effusion always require chest tube.

▶ PULMONARY FUNCTION TESTS (PFTs)

Spirometry measures the rate at which the lung changes during forced breathing.
- Forced vital capacity (FVC): Patient inhales maximally, then exhales as rapidly andd completely as possible. The exhalation and subsequent inhalation are recorded as a flow volume curve.
- FEV_1: The volume of air exhaled in the first second of the FVC maneuver
- FEV_1, FVC, and the ratio between them (FEV_1/FVC) are used to determine lung disease and severity.
  - Normal FEV_1 = > 80%
  - Normal FVC = > 80%
  - Normal FEV_1/FVC ratio = > 0.7

Normal Spirometry	Obstructive Lung Disease	Restrictive Lung Disease
FVC normal	FVC normal or decreased	FVC decreased
FEV_1 normal	FEV_1 decreased	FEV_1 normal or decreased
FEV_1/FVC > 0.7	FEV_1/FVC < 0.7	FEV_1/FVC > 0.7
	Lung volume normal or increased	Lung volume always decreased

Obstructive lung disease patterns are seen with chronic bronchitis, emphysema, asthma.

Restrictive lung disease patterns are seen with interstitial lung diseases, neuromuscular diseases (ALS, myasthenia gravis, Guillain–Barré), chest wall disorders (obesity, kyphoscoliosis).

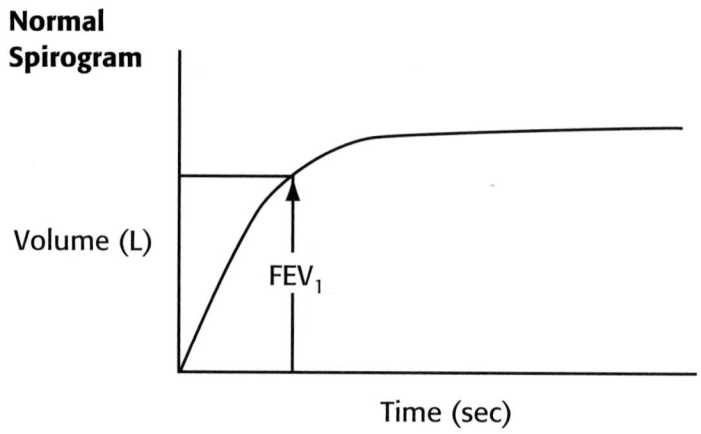

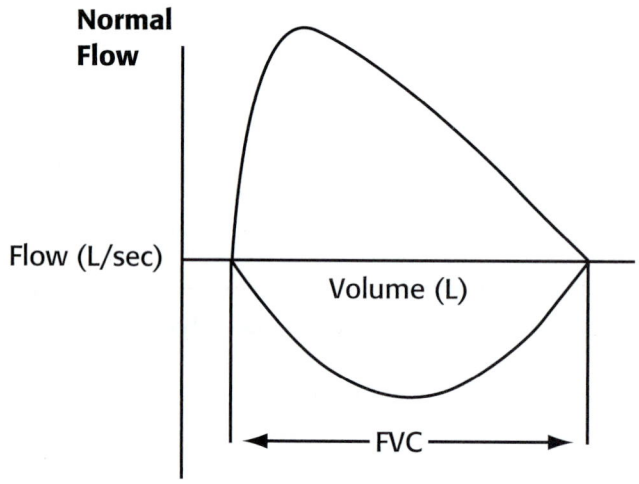

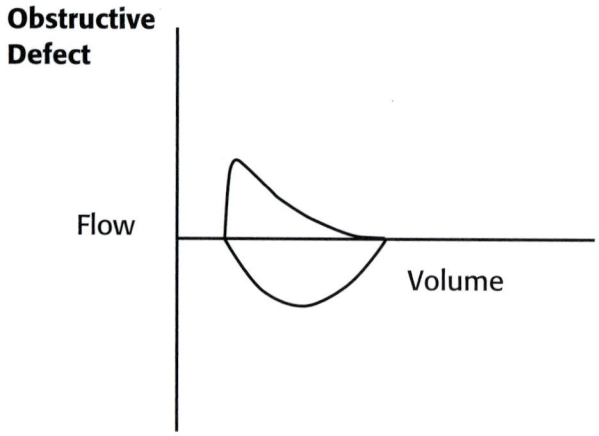

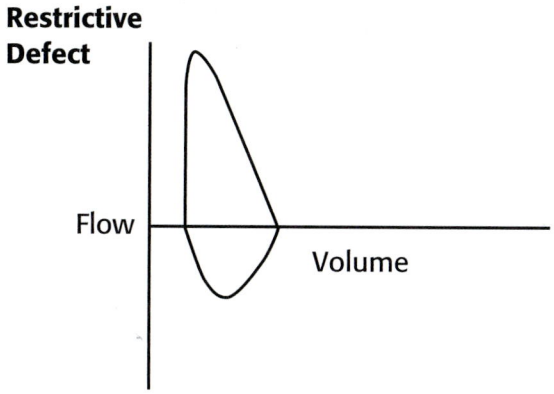

LUNG INFECTIONS

▶ PNEUMONIA

DEFINITION

Infection of the lung parenchyma by any microorganism

ETIOLOGY

See Table 2.7-2 for organisms affecting immunocompetent host and Table 2.7-3 for those affecting immunocompromised hosts.

PATHOPHYSIOLOGY

- Aspiration of nasopharyngeal, oral, or gastric contents
- Hematogenous spread
- Direct inoculation (stab wounds, endotracheal tube)

SIGNS AND SYMPTOMS

Patients with pneumonia may have few signs or symptoms, or may be extremely ill.

Typical Symptoms
- Fever
- Cough with sputum production
- Pleuritic chest pain

Atypical Symptoms
- Dry cough
- Headache
- Malaise
- Gastrointestinal (GI) symptoms

Physical Exam
- Dullness to percussion
- Rales

Typical scenario:
A 27-year-old patient has pneumonia, bullous myringitis, and a chest film that looks worse than expected. *Think:* Mycoplasma pneumoniae.

A patient comes to the ER with consolidation and pleural effusion on CXR. What is the most important test to determine admission/treatment? Thoracentesis

Typical scenario:
A patient with HIV who has a CD4 count of 52 does not take antiretroviral medications or TMP-SMX, is hypoxic on room air, and has a diffuse bilateral infiltrate on chest film. *Think:* Pneumocystis carinii *pneumonia (PCP).*

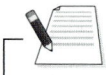

Typical scenario:
An elderly man presents with pneumonia, gastrointestinal symptoms, bradycardia, and hyponatremia. *Think: Legionella.*

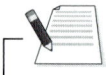

If you see *currant jelly sputum,* think *Klebsiella.*

If you see *rusty sputum,* think *Pneumococcus.*

If a patient develops a *post-influenza pneumonia,* think *Pneumococcus.*

If you see *bulging fissure* on film, think *Klebsiella.*

If there are no bacteria on Gram stain, consider *Legionella* and *Mycoplasma.*

If *serum LDH* is high, think *PCP.*

TABLE 2.7-2. Likely Organisms Causing Pneumonia

Community acquired, typical 1. *S. pneumoniae* 2. *H. influenzae*
Community acquired, atypical 1. *Chlamydia pneumoniae* 2. *Legionella pneumophila* 3. *Mycoplasma pneumoniae*
Hospital acquired 1. *Pseudomonas aeruginosa* 2. *S. aureus* 3. Enteric organisms

TABLE 2.7-3. Causes of Pneumonia in Immunocompromised Hosts

IMMUNOCOMPROMISED HOSTS, HIV ORGANISM	CD4 COUNT/dL
M. tuberculosis	< 500
Pneumocystis carinii	< 200
Histoplasma capsulatum	< 200
Cryptococcus neoformans	< 200
M. avium-intracellulare	< 50
Cytomegalovirus	< 50
Immunocompromised hosts, neutropenia 1. *P. aeruginosa* 2. Enterobacteriaceae 3. *S. aureus* 4. *Aspergillus*	
Immunocompromised hosts, splenectomy, sickle cell anemia Encapsulated organisms	
Immunocompromised hosts, chronic steroid use 1. *M. tuberculosis* 2. *Nocardia*	
Alcoholics 1. *S. pneumoniae* 2. *H. influenzae* 3. *Klebsiella pneumoniae* 4. *M. tuberculosis*	

- Tactile fremitus in consolidated lobe or segment
- Egophony (E to A changes) with stethoscope

Diagnosis

Chest X-Ray

Most patients with pneumonia will have an infiltrate on film corresponding to a lobe or segment. More specific findings may include:

- Upper lobe *(Mycobacterium tuberculosis, Klebsiella)*
- Small cavities without air-fluid levels *(M. tuberculosis)*
- Large cavities with air-fluid levels (*Staph* sp., anaerobes, gram-negatives, coccidioidomycosis, nocardiosis)
- Diffuse bilateral infiltrate (PCP, *Mycoplasma)*

Gram Stain

An adequate sputum sample should contain:

- < 10 epithelial cells per low-power field (the fewer the better)
- > 25 leucocytes per low-power field

If you see *small gram-negative rods with a halo* on Gram stain, think *H. flu.*

Loeffler's pneumonia is idiopathic eosinophilic pneumonia.

Criteria for Admission

Most patients with community-acquired pneumonia do well as outpatients. Factors crucial to determining admission to hospital are:

- Age > 50
- Nursing home residents
- Underlying chronic disease
- Change in mental status
- Tachypnea, tachycardia, or hypotension
- $PaO_2 < 60$
- Pleural effusion

Pneumonias causing relative bradycardia (slower than expected heart rate for temperature or disease, but above 60 bpm):

- *Legionella*
- *Salmonella*
- *Chlamydia psittaci*

Treatment

The best choices for empiric coverage until cultures are completed are:

Community-acquired (cover for both typicals and atypicals):

- No risk factors: Macrolide (erythromycin, azithromycin)
- Risk factors present (CHF, diabetes, etc.): Macrolide and 2nd-/3rd-generation cephalosporin or extended-spectrum quinolone alone

Hospital-acquired: Add *Pseudomonas* coverage (e.g., cefixime or piperacillin–tazobactam).

Immunocompromised: Add PCP coverage (trimethoprim–sulfamethoxazole ([TMP-SMZ])

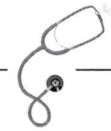

Steroid administration in PCP prevents respiratory failure and improves survival.
Give for:

- A-a gradient > 35
- $PaO_2 < 75$

▶ TUBERCULOSIS

Tuberculosis is a leading cause of death worldwide. In the United States, the incidence of tuberculosis decreased every year until 1984, but then rose again until 1993.

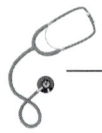

Sites of TB disease:
- **Lungs (85% of all cases)**
- **Central nervous system (TB meningitis)**
- **Lymphatics**
- **Genitourinary system**
- **Bones (Pott's disease)**
- **Disseminated TB (miliary)**

Pathophysiology

Transmission occurs by inhalation of droplet nuclei produced by the cough or sneeze of a patient with pulmonary TB disease. Particles may remain suspended in air for several hours:
- 5% of those infected will develop TB disease in 2 years.
- 5% more will develop TB disease in their lifetime.
- 90% will remain infected but disease free.

Epidemiology

High-Prevalence Groups
HIV-infected persons
Close contacts of persons with TB disease
IV drug users
Immunocompromised persons (non-HIV)
Foreign-born persons
Residents of medically underserved communities
Prisoners
Homeless

High Risk for TB Once Infected
HIV-infected persons
IV drug users
Immunocompromised persons (non-HIV)
Abnormal chest film

Symptoms

- Productive cough
- **Night sweats**
- **Hemoptysis**
- Anorexia
- Weight loss
- Fever, chills, fatigue
- Chest pain

Diagnosis

Findings
- Positive PPD
- Infiltrate or granuloma in upper lobes of lungs
- Acid-fast bacilli (AFB) on sputum microscopy

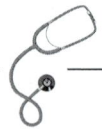

Anergy (does not mount response) can be screened by planting the common antigens *mumps* and *Candida*. If no response, PPD is useless.

How to Use the TB Skin Test

1. Screen patients in high-prevalence groups.
2. Gives a positive reaction 2 to 10 weeks after infection
3. Plant 0.1 mL of PPD intradermally on volar aspect of the forearm.
4. Read 48 to 72 hours after placement.
5. Measure induration, not erythema (see Table 2.7-4).

False Positives
- Bacillus Calmette–Guérin (BCG) vaccinated
- Nontuberculous mycobacterial infection

TABLE 2.7-4. Interpretation of PPD Skin Test

Measured Induration		
15 mm or Greater	**10 mm or Greater**	**5 mm or Greater**
All patients are considered infected.	Considered infected if: IV drug user Foreign born Medically underserved Nursing home resident Prisoner Child under age 4 Health care worker Other medical problems	Considered infected if: HIV Close contact Abnormal chest film Immunocompromised

False Negatives

- Ten to 25% of patients with TB infection have negative skin tests.
- The two-step TB skin test is used in high-prevalence patients who have a negative first test: The first test boosts the immune response to a second skin test, which will turn positive in infected patients.

Treatment

Latent TB

- INH daily for 9 months (may be given twice weekly if directly observed therapy [DOT] is used)
- Rifampin daily for 4 months if in contact with people with INH-resistant TB
- Close contacts with negative PPD should be retested in 10 weeks.
- Pregnant women should wait until after delivery for treatment unless high risk (e.g., HIV).

Active TB

- Standard regimen: 2 months of INH, rifampin, pyrazinamide, and ethambutol followed by 4 months of INH/rifampin followed by 7 months of INH/RIF
- Pregnant with TB: 2 months of INH, rifampin, and ethambutol followed by INH and rifampin (no ethambutol) for 7 more months.

Infectivity

- People are considered no longer infectious when they are undergoing appropriate therapy, improving clinically, and have had three consecutive sputum smears on different days negative for TB

Toxicity of TB Medication

INH

- Peripheral neuropathy (can be prevented with administration of pyridoxine)
- Seizures in overdose: These can be very difficult to break with standard measures—remember to give pyridoxine!
- Hepatitis (check liver function tests each month)

Typical scenario:
A patient is brought in by ambulance in status epilepticus. The patient's family member says he has no medical history except tuberculosis. *Think: INH toxicity.* Treat with pyridoxine.

Rifampin

- Induces hepatic microsomal enzymes
- Is excreted as a red-orange compound in urine, stool, sweat, and tears; will discolor contact lenses

Ethambutol

- Optic neuritis and impaired color vision are related to cumulative dose.

Obstructive Disorders

▶ CHRONIC OBSTRUCTIVE PULMONARY DISEASE (COPD)

Definition

Chronic bronchitis and emphysema are forms of chronic obstructive pulmonary disease. COPD is defined by a chronic obstruction to expiratory airflow, accompanied by a decrease in FEV_1.

Chronic bronchitis: Chronic expiratory airflow obstruction accompanied by chronic productive cough (and excess secretions) for 3 or more months in each of 2 successive years

Emphysema: Chronic expiratory airflow obstruction accompanied by permanent enlargement of the airspace distal to the terminal bronchioles due to destruction of alveolar septa

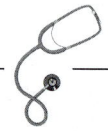

The term *COPD* is preferred to describe both chronic bronchitis and emphysema, as many patients have elements of each disease.

Pathophysiology of Emphysema

- **Centrilobular** emphysema affects the respiratory bronchioles.
- **Panlobular or panacinar emphysema** occurs in patients with alpha-1-antitrypsin deficiency. Alpha-1-antitrypsin protects against the degradation of lung elastin.
- **Distal acinar emphysema** is associated with spontaneous pneumothorax.

Pink puffers
(emphysema)

- **Barrel-shaped chest**
- **Thin and wasted**
- **Low PCO_2, normal to low PO_2**

Epidemiology

- Higher prevalence in men
- Mortality rates are higher in whites.
- Only 15% of smokers develop COPD.

Blue bloaters
(chronic bronchitis)

- **Right heart failure**
- **Polycythemia**
- **High PCO_2, low PO_2**

Risk Factors

- Smoking
- Alpha-1-antitrypsin deficiency (autosomal recessive inheritance, more common in Mediterraneans)

Diagnosis/Findings

- Chest x-ray: Hyperinflated lungs, flattened diaphragm
- Physical exam: Barrel chest
- Pulmonary function tests (PFTs): Irreversible obstructive pattern (low FEV_1)

- Electrocardiogram (ECG): Right-sided strain; often multiple atrial tachycardia
- Computed tomography (CT): Shows loss of alveolar walls in emphysema

Symptoms

- Cough
- Dyspnea on exertion
- CO_2 retention (chronic bronchitis)
- Weight loss (emphysema)
- Tachypnea

Treatment

- Smoking cessation
- Oxygen has also been shown to improve COPD patients' IQ, exercise tolerance, and mortality! Oxygen should be given to:
  - Patients with a resting PaO_2 of < 55 mm Hg
  - Patients with PaO_2 of 55 to 59 who have cor pulmonale, erythrocytosis, or who desaturate during exercise
- Maintain vaccination against influenza and *S. pneumoniae*.
- Beta agonists and ipratropium bromide improve FEV_1 modestly.
- Steroids improve FEV_1 by > 20% in about 11% of patients.
- Antibiotics for COPD exacerbations reduce the duration of COPD exacerbation symptoms by 20% and decrease hospital admissions by 50%.
- Lung reduction surgery improves FEV_1 by 100% and decreases residual volume by 40%; done less frequently now due to the fact it is no longer reimbursed.

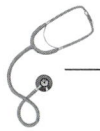

Supplemental oxygen is the only therapy for COPD proven to extend life.

▶ ASTHMA

Definition

A chronic condition characterized by airway inflammation, bronchoconstriction, and hypersecretion, which is reversible (typically with bronchodilators)

A 54-year-old male with pancreatitis goes into respiratory failure. CXR shows bilateral infiltrates. Diagnosis? ARDS (sepsis is the most common cause of ARDS)

Pathophysiology

- The early phase of asthma is immunoglobulin **E** (IgE) mediated, associated with histamine release from mast cells.
- The late phase is associated with cytokine release and is improved by steroids.

Triggers

- Exposure to pets, dust, smoke, carpets
- Aggravation by exercise, hot or cold weather
- Seasonal changes

Signs and Symptoms

The airflow obstruction associated with asthma that produces expiratory wheezing in mild disease progresses to both inspiratory and expiratory wheezing in moderate disease, and then diminished breath sounds and no wheezing in severe disease:

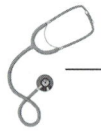

Cough-variant asthma: Cough is the patient's only symptom. The diagnosis of asthma is demonstrated by response to asthma-specific treatment.

- Chest tightness
- Wheezing
- Shortness of breath
- Cough (especially at night)

Differential diagnosis of wheezing:

- Reactive airway disease (usually from postnasal drip syndrome)
- Congestive heart failure (CHF)
- Foreign body aspiration (most often in children)
- Asthma

Physical Exam

- Wheezing on exhalation
- Decreased air entry, increased expiratory phase
- Decreased peak flow and FEV_1
- Retractions of sternocleidomastoids
- Intercostal muscle use for breathing
- Oxygen saturation < 95%
- Inability to speak full sentences

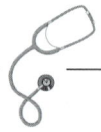

MDIs deliver smaller particles than nebulizers and therefore reach the smallest airways better. Nebulizers are favored for hospital treatment because of ease of use.

Treatment (see Table 2.7-5)

Beta-2 Agonists (Rapid Onset)

- Delivered by metered dose inhaler (MDI) or nebulizer
- Promote bronchodilation
- *Note:* Beta-2 agonists cause an intracellular shift of potassium and can be used as temporary treatment of hyperkalemia.

TABLE 2.7-5. Asthma Classification and Treatment

Classification	Frequency of Symptoms	Treatment
Mild intermittent	1–2 episodes per month	**PRN:** Short-acting beta-2 agonists as needed
Mild persistent	> 2 per week but < 1 per day	**PRN:** Short-acting beta-2 agonists as needed **Maintenance:** May add inhaled/oral steroids or cromolyn or leukotriene modifier
Moderate persistent	Daily	**Maintenance:** Inhaled or oral steroids and long-acting beta-2 agonist; may also use cromolyn or leukotriene modifier **PRN:** Short-acting beta-2 agonist as needed
Severe persistent	Continuous	**Maintenance:** Inhaled or oral steroid + long-acting beta-2 agonist **PRN:** Short-acting beta-2 agonist

Ipratropium Bromide (Rapid Onset)
- Delivered by nebulizer or MDI
- Dry up bronchial secretions
- Effects of beta agonists and ipratropium bromide are additive.

Steroids (Take 6 Hours to Work)
- Reduce inflammation
- Delivered by MDI for asthma prevention
- Oral or IV use for acute exacerbations

Preventative Medications
- Leukotriene modifiers such as zafirlukast
- Mast cell stabilizers such as cromolyn

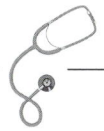

Permissive hypercapnia is the practice of allowing a patient to have high CO_2 while intubated in order to increase expiratory phase and prevent breath-stacking.

Methylxanthines such as theophylline are no longer regularly used for asthma due to the narrow therapeutic window and the frequency of adverse effects, including nausea, vomiting, headache, and, in severe toxicity, seizures and arrhythmias.

Allergen removal: Common environmental triggers should be addressed, including smoking, dust, pets, carpets, cockroaches and seasonal allergens.

Frequent visits to the PMD with review of medications and teaching can prevent acute attacks.

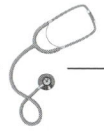

CO_2 is reduced by raising the patient's minute ventilation (tidal volume × respiratory rate).

Intubation of Asthmatics

Patients with asthma may need to be electively or emergently intubated. The key indicator for intubation is the declining clinical status of the patient, including:
- Severe tachypnea
- Dyspnea
- Hypoxia
- Mental status changes or inability to communicate

Arterial blood gases **(ABGs)** can aid assessment of how sick the patient is but should never delay intubation in a patient who requires respiratory assistance.

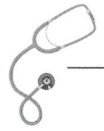

High tidal volumes and high rates can lead to barotrauma and are thought to contribute to ARDS.

Ventilation techniques in an intubated asthmatic include:
- Keep respiratory rate at 12 to 14/min.
- Keep tidal volume at 6 to 8 mL/kg.
- Prolong expiratory time to prevent stacking breaths.
- Do not try to overventilate to "blow off" CO_2 (this can lead to barotrauma).

Interpretation of Arterial Blood Gases in Asthma

The notation for arterial blood gases is: pH/P_{CO_2}/PO_2/calculated HCO_3/calculated Sa_{O_2}

Sample ABGs
- Normal: 7.4/40/98
- Mild asthma: 7.48/30/60 (acute respiratory alkalosis)
- Severe asthma: 7.40/40/55 (the "normalization" of the pH and P_{CO_2} in the presence of continued symptoms and hypoxia indicate that the patient is getting fatigued and is no longer able to blow off CO_2)

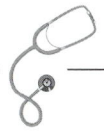

If an asthmatic in respiratory distress has a normal pH and normal PCO_2, *beware of impending respiratory failure: intubate (he is tiring out).*

▶ OBSTRUCTIVE SLEEP APNEA (OSA)

Definition

Brief periods of breathing cessation (apnea) or marked reduction in tidal volume (hypopnea) occurring during sleep due to occlusion of upper airways.

Signs and Symptoms

Snoring, persistent daytime sleepiness, drowsiness while driving, morning headache, obesity, hypertension, large neck circumference

Differential Diagnosis

Simple snoring, central sleep apnea, other disorders causing daytime sleepiness (insufficient sleep, circadian rhythm disturbances, narcolepsy, periodic limb movement disorder)

Diagnosis

Made with polysomnography (sleep study). OSA is defined by ≥ 5 episodes of apnea and hypopnea per hour of sleep (apnea–hypopnea index).

Treatment

- Lateral sleeping position, avoidance of alcohol or sedative medications, weight loss
- Continuous positive airway pressure (CPAP) during sleep
- Surgery (tonsillectomy, uvulopalatopharyngoplasty, tracheostomy)

Upper Respiratory Tract Problems

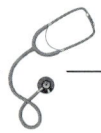

Most common causes of chronic cough:
- **Postnasal drip**
- **Asthma**
- **GERD**

▶ ACUTE COUGH

Definition

Cough is a common presenting complaint of patients. Acute cough, or cough of less than 3 weeks' duration, is most commonly caused by the postnasal drip associated with the common cold. See Table 2.7-6 for causes of acute cough.

Smoker with chronic cough: Always instruct to quit smoking first. Chest x-ray is the first step in workup of any cough.

▶ CHRONIC COUGH

Definition

Cough of > 3 weeks' duration

Etiology

- Postnasal drip (PND)
- Asthma
- Gastroesophageal reflux disease (GERD)
- See Table 2.7-7 for a complete list of causes.

TABLE 2.7-6. Causes of Acute Cough

Prevalence	Cause
Very common	Postnasal drip (due to common cold, acute bacterial sinusitis, allergic rhinitis, environmental irritant rhinitis)
Common	Pertussis Chronic obstructive pulmonary disease (COPD) exacerbation
Less common	Asthma Congestive heart failure Pneumonia Aspiration syndromes Pulmonary embolism

▶ POSTNASAL DRIP SYNDROME

Definition

Postnasal drip is thought to be the single most common cause of both acute and chronic cough.

Etiology

All causes of rhinitis can cause postnasal drip and cough.

Pathophysiology

The mechanical action of secretions dripping into the hypopharynx triggers the cough reflex.

Postnasal drip syndrome, asthma, and GERD account for nearly 100% of causes of chronic cough in nonsmokers with normal chest films, who are not on angiotensin-converting enzyme (ACE) inhibitors.

TABLE 2.7-7. Causes of Chronic Cough

Prevalence	Causes
Common	Postnasal drip syndrome (PNDS) Asthma Gastroesophageal reflux disease (GERD)
Less common	Chronic bronchitis Bronchiectasis Postinfectious cough (pertussis)
Uncommon	Bronchogenic carcinoma ACE inhibitors
Rare in adults	Psychogenic cough

Signs and Symptoms

- Cough
- Nasal discharge or nasal obstruction
- Dripping sensation or tickle in the throat
- Drainage may be present on the posterior pharyngeal wall.

Treatment

Postnasal drip syndrome (PNDS) due to the common cold is treated with a first-generation antihistamine and a decongestant. Nonsedating antihistamines have been shown to be ineffective in this case.

PNDS due to allergic rhinitis is treated with nasal corticosteroids, nasal cromolyn, or nonsedating antihistamines.

Treatment of PNDS due to sinusitis is addressed below.

► SINUSITIS

Definition

- Sinusitis is a common cause of PNDS and cough.
- Acute sinusitis is a bacterial infection that usually involves an obstructed maxillary sinus. Chronic sinusitis is the persistence of sinus inflammation for 3 or more months.
- Also associated with:
  - Allergic rhinitis
  - Dental infections
  - Foreign body or tumor
  - Cystic fibrosis
  - Asthma

Signs and Symptoms

- Purulent nasal discharge
- Sinus pain worse on bending forward
- Fever
- Tenderness to percussion over sinuses

Diagnosis

- Transillumination findings are inconsistent.
- Computed tomography (CT) scan is extremely sensitive but is not specific to sinusitis, and many false positives occur. CT scan should be reserved for hospitalized patients, or for the diagnosis of chronic sinusitis.

Treatment

- Acute sinusitis: Amoxicillin or trimethoprim–sulfamethoxazole (TMP-SMZ) or amoxicillin–clavulanic acid for 1 to 2 weeks, although some evidence suggests that a 3-day course of TMP-SMZ produces the same results
- Persistent chronic sinusitis: May require subspecialist involvement

Complications of Untreated Chronic Sinusitis

- Preseptal or periorbital cellulitis
- Orbital cellulitis
- Epidural, subdural, or cerebral abscess
- Meningitis
- Dural sinus venous thrombosis

▶ PERTUSSIS (WHOOPING COUGH)

Definition

Caused by *Bordetella pertussis*, a gram-negative coccobacillus

Epidemiology

Whooping cough is thought to be a common cause of cough in adults. Although only about 4,000 cases of pertussis are reported each year, seroprevalence studies indicate that pertussis is the cause of persistent cough in adults in 12 to 30% of cases.

Immunization

- Before routine immunization, whooping cough was a common cause of infant death.
- DTP (killed whole-cell) or DTaP (acellular) at 2, 4, 6, 18 months, and 4 to 6 years

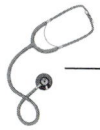

Immunity to pertussis is lost 12 years after the last immunization.

Signs and Symptoms

Catarrhal Stage
- Lasts 1 to 2 weeks
- Characterized by mild upper respiratory infection (URI) symptoms

Paroxysmal Stage
- Lasts 2 to 4 weeks
- Characterized by prolonged paroxysmal cough
- Often worse at night

Convalescent Stage
- Characterized by gradual improvement of symptoms

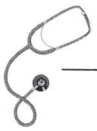

The classic "whoop" caused by rapid air inspiration against a closed glottis is rarely seen in adults.

Diagnosis

Nasopharyngeal swab and culture

Treatment

Macrolide antibiotics, such as erythromycin, will reduce the severity of the disease if started within 8 days. Identification and treatment of adult patients is important to help prevent transmission to unimmunized or incompletely immunized children.

Miscellaneous Lung Disorders

▶ ADULT RESPIRATORY DISTRESS SYNDROME (ARDS)

The first step in asthma treatment is to remove the offending agent.

- Condition that results from increased permeability of alveolar capillaries causing fluid to fill alveoli
- O_2 treatment does not improve condition due to effective AV shunting.
- Etiologies include shock, DIC, septicemia, trauma, and near drowning.
- Chest x-ray shows diffuse bilateral fluffy infiltrates.
- Treatment usually involves mechanical ventilation with positive end-expiratory pressure (PEEP).
- Diagnosis: (1) ratio of $PaO_2/FiO_2 \leq 200$, (2) bilateral fluffy infiltrates, (3) no CHF

▶ BRONCHIECTASIS

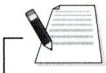

Most common organisms to colonize bronchiectatic lung:
H. influenzae
S. aureus
Pseudomonas aeruginosa

Definition

Bronchiectasis is a chronic condition characterized by pathological dilatation of the medium-sized airways. It is usually caused by an abnormal inflammatory response to an initial infectious or toxic insult.

Etiology

- Cystic fibrosis
- Immotile cilia syndromes (Kartagener's)
- Frequent infection (from hypogammaglobulinemia or other immunocompromise)

Pathophysiology

The resulting airway damage allows bacterial colonization, buildup of secretions, and continued bronchial destruction. Bronchiectasis is the cause of chronic cough in about 4% of cases.

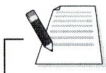

Tuberculosis is the most common cause of **hemoptysis.**

Signs and Symptoms

- Chronic cough
- Hemoptysis
- Wheezing
- Failure to thrive

Diagnosis

High-resolution CT scan will detect bronchial dilatation and destruction in 60 to 100% of cases. Patients with cystic fibrosis will have abnormal pancreatic function and an abnormal sweat test.

Treatment

- Chest physiotherapy
- Antibiotics

- Bronchodilators, mucolytics
- Uncommon treatments: Local resection, bronchial artery embolization for hemoptysis, lung transplantation

▶ HEMOPTYSIS

Definition

Coughing up of blood due to bleeding from the lower respiratory tract. See Table 2.7-8 for a list of causes.

Massive hemoptysis is bleeding > 600 mL in 48 hours, or bleeding causing clinical impairment of respiratory function.

Workup

Chest x-ray, high-resolution CT, bronchoscopy

Treatment

- Supplemental oxygen
- Place patient with bleeding side down.
- Suppress cough reflex (i.e., codeine).

Patients with massive hemoptysis usually require surgical involvement. Initial therapy includes:

- Intubation of the good lung
- Endobronchial cold saline or epinephrine
- Bronchial artery embolization

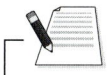

Typical scenario:
A patient with hemoptysis, sinusitis, and glomerulonephritis. *Think: Wegener's granulomatosis.*

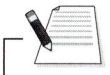

Typical scenario:
A patient with dyspnea, hemoptysis, and acute renal failure. *Think: Goodpasture's syndrome.*

TABLE 2.7-8. Causes of Hemoptysis

Incidence	Cause
Common	TB Bronchiectasis Lung cancer Bronchitis Pneumonia Unknown
Uncommon	Coagulopathy Congestive heart failure Pulmonary embolism Wegener's Goodpasture's
Rare	Systemic HTN, pulmonary HTN, trauma, vasculitis, foreign body, collagen vascular disease, pulmonary arteriovenous malformation

▶ PULMONARY EMBOLISM

Definition

Pulmonary thromboembolism results from disruption of a deep venous thrombosis or local stasis, causing blockage of pulmonary blood flow beyond the embolus. Very large PEs that impede blood flow in both the right and left pulmonary arteries are called saddle emboli.

Risk Factors

- Immobilization
- Leg fracture or leg surgery
- Hypercoagulable state (malignancy, pregnancy, genetic)
- Proximal leg deep venous thrombosis
- Stroke

Symptoms/Signs

- Tachycardia
- Dyspnea, cough
- Tachypnea
- Pleuritic chest pain
- Hemoptysis
- Hypoxia

Findings/Tests

- ECG: S in lead I, Q and inverted T waves in lead III, or may show diffuse ST changes, and tachycardia
- Chest film: May show an infiltrate or may be normal
- ABGs: Usually reveal hypoxemia, hypocapnia, and respiratory alkalosis
- D-dimer: Measures products of fibrin degradation (will be elevated)
- Leg ultrasonography (venous duplex): To detect DVT
- Ventilation–perfusion scan (V/Q scan): To look for perfusion defects at site of PE
- Helical (spiral) CT: To look for embolus in the pulmonary vasculature. Does not detect small emboli.
- Pulmonary angiogram: The gold standard for detection of PE. Invasive test.

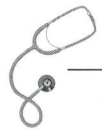

Diagnosis of PE is difficult, and a high clinical suspicion should be maintained.

How to Use Tests to Diagnose PE

Multiple algorithms have been constructed, but most share the following principles:

1. Determine your level of clinical suspicion based on history, physical exam, ECG, and chest film as high, intermediate, or low risk.
2. Patients with a low risk of PE can be ruled out with a negative D-dimer test (sensitive but not specific).
3. Patients can be ruled in and treated after a positive leg sonogram to look for DVT or a high-probability V/Q scan.
4. Low- and intermediate-risk patients with a normal V/Q scan are ruled out.
5. Intermediate-probability V/Q scans are not helpful and require further testing, either spiral CT or angiogram.

S_1-Q_3-T_3 on ECG is the classic ECG finding for PE, but the most frequent rhythm is sinus tachycardia (see Figure 2.7-1).

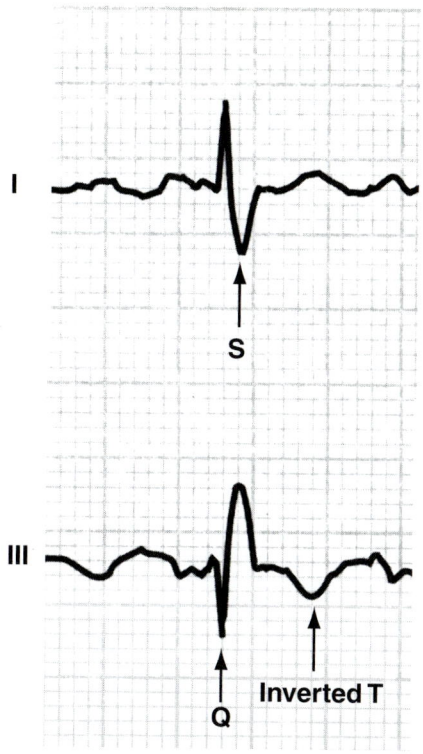

FIGURE 2.7-1. Pulmonary embolism. S_1-Q_3-T_3 pattern.

Angiography is the gold standard in the diagnosis of:

- Deep venous thrombosis
- Dissecting aortic aneurysm
- Ischemic bowel syndrome
- Pulmonary embolism

TREATMENT

Acute treatment of PE includes:

1. Most common choice is anticoagulation with heparin or low-molecular-weight heparin
2. Thrombolysis if hemodynamically unstable or echo shows right ventricular strain
3. Interventional pulmonary angiography: Mechanical disintegration or local thrombolysis
4. Surgery: Embolectomy

Prolonged treatment:

1. Patients with DVTs are orally anticoagulated for 6 months.
2. Patients with PEs are orally anticoagulated for 1 year.

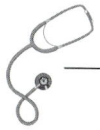

PIOPED study showed that when applying data from a V/Q scan, the clinical probability of PE must be taken into account in determining whether or not to treat.

▶ PNEUMOTHORAX

DEFINITION

Air in the pleural space

Typical scenario:
A 20-year-old tall man arrives complaining of sudden onset of severe shortness of breath and pleuritic chest pain. *Think: Primary spontaneous pneumothorax.*

Epidemiology

- Spontaneous pneumothorax affects approximately 20,000 persons per year, usually from rupture of a subpleural bleb or pleural necrosis due to lung disease.
- Primary spontaneous pneumothorax occurs in an otherwise healthy person, while secondary spontaneous pneumothorax occurs in patients who have underlying lung disease.

Etiology

Primary Spontaneous Pneumothorax
- Male smokers
- Patients tall for weight

Secondary Spontaneous Pneumothorax
- COPD
- Cystic fibrosis
- Pneumonia
- Cancer

Signs and Symptoms

- Chest pain
- Dyspnea
- Hyperresonance of affected side
- Decreased breath sounds of affected side
- Tracheal deviation *away* from affected side (in tension pneumothorax)

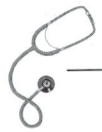

Expiratory chest film is more sensitive for pneumothorax than inspiratory chest film.

Diagnosis

- ECG: ST segment changes possible
- Upright chest x-ray is ~83% sensitive, demonstrates an absence of lung markings where the lung has collapsed.

Treatment

- Oxygen
- For pneumothoraces > 20%: Tube thoracostomy to remove air
- Pleurodesis to adhere the visceral and parietal pleura

Mediastinum

Masses

Anterior (4 Ts)
- Thymoma
- Teratoma
- Thyroid
- Terrible lymphoma

Middle
- Vascular lesions
- Lymph nodes

Posterior
- Neurogenic tumor

▶ MEDIASTINITIS

Causes of Mediastinitis
- Esophageal perforation
- Post-median sternotomy
- Inhalation anthrax (hemorrhagic mediastinitis)
- Tuberculosis, histoplasmosis (chronic)

Symptoms
- Initial symptoms similar to viral syndrome
- After 1 to 3 days, fever, dyspnea, hypoxia, hemorrhagic mediastinitis, and death occur.

Treatment
- High-dose penicillin, ciprofloxacin, or doxycycline is recommended.

▶ PNEUMOMEDIASTINUM

Causes
- Rupture of alveolus, bronchus, or trachea
- Esophageal rupture
- Dissection of cervical (neck) or abdominal free air into mediastinum

Treat underlying cause.

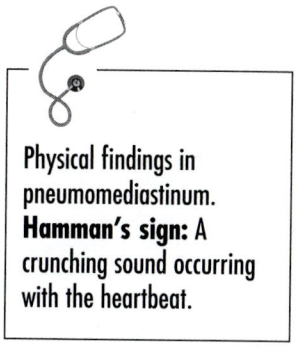
Physical findings in pneumomediastinum. **Hamman's sign:** A crunching sound occurring with the heartbeat.

INTERSTITIAL LUNG DISEASE

A group of diverse disorders involving the parenchyma of the lung which cause alveolitis, interstitial inflammation, and fibrosis or a granulomatous response. There are known and unknown etiologies.

ETIOLOGY

Known
Environmental/occupational (dusts, fumes)
Drugs (amiodarone, gold)
Radiation
Infections
Hypersensitivity pneumonitis
Pulmonary edema
Neoplasms (lymphatic carcinoma, lymphoma)

Unknown
Sarcoidosis
Idiopathic pulmonary fibrosis
Collagen vascular disease
Goodpasture's
Alveolar proteinosis
Amyloidosis
Bronchiolitis obliterans with organizing pneumonia
Neurofibromatosis, tuberous sclerosis
Lymphangioleiomyomatosis
Eosinophilic pneumonias
Lymphocytic interstitial pneumonia

Clinical Manifestations

Dyspnea (chronic, progressive), exercise intolerance, nonproductive cough, tachypnea, end-inspiratory crackles, clubbing of digits, pulmonar hypertension)

Diagnosis

Usually requires biopsy. Workup initially includes CXR (may show diffuse bilateral reticular infiltrates), high-resolution CT, PFTs (mostly demonstrate restrictive abnormalities).

Treatment

Removal/cessation of exposure to known environmental causes. Often, there is no effective treatment.

- Supplemental oxygen as needed
- Steroids (possibly in combination with cyclophosphamide or azathioprine)
- Lung transplant

▶ EXAMPLES OF ENVIRONMENTAL LUNG DISEASE

Asbestosis: A diffuse interstitial lung disease caused by dusts of mineral silicates. Asbestos exposure is associated with an increased risk of squamous cell CA, adenocarcinoma, and mesotheliomas.
Silicosis: Nodular fibrosis of the lung caused by exposure to silica flour, sand blasting, or the manufacture of abrasive soaps. These patients are at a greater risk of developing pulmonary TB disease.
Coal workers' pneumoconiosis: An occupational hazard of ~50% of all coal miners; they develop progressive massive fibrosis.
Byssinosis (cotton dust exposure): Patients experience "chest tightness" with an associated decrease in FEV_1 with exposure to cotton dust. Treatment is to wear protective equipment and to use bronchodilators.
Farmer's lung: A *hypersensitivity pneumonitis* caused by exposure to spores of thermophilic actinomycetes. Thought to be associated with a suppressor T-cell defect, is IgG mediated. Symptoms include fever, chills, cough, and dyspnea, and episodes occur more frequently during wet weather. Treat with steroids, and avoid exposure. Long-term complications include pulmonary fibrosis and weight loss.

Typical scenario:
A farmer presents with fever, cough, and difficulty breathing after several days of filling his silo with grain. *Think: Hypersensitivity pneumonitis.*

Lung Cancer

Small cell lung cancer has a rapid mitotic rate and therefore is sensitive to chemotherapy. Surgery is not indicated.

Types

Small Cell Lung Cancer
- Central location
- Sensitive to chemotherapy
- Surgery is not indicated.
- Poor prognosis (2 to 4 months from diagnosis to death)

Non–Small Cell Lung Cancer

- Includes squamous, large cell, and adenocarcinoma
- Poor response to chemotherapy
- Treated with surgery if early stage
- Prognosis varies with stage.

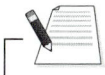

Two types of cancer share a "s"entral location:
- Small cell
- Squamous cell

Epidemiology

- Leading cause of cancer death in both men and women in the United States
- Cases have been decreasing in men, but increasing in women.
- Smoking is by far the most important causative factor in the development of lung cancer.

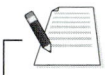

Bronchoalveolar cancer, a type of adenocarcinoma, is not linked to smoking and is more common in women.

Etiology

- Smoking
- Passive smoke exposure
- Radon gas exposure
- Asbestos
- Arsenic
- Nickel

Chronic cough is the most common symptom of lung cancer.

Signs and Symptoms

- Cough
- Hemoptysis
- Dyspnea

TABLE 2.7-9. Syndromes Associated with Lung Cancer

Horner's syndrome	Sympathetic nerve paralysis produces enophthalmos, ptosis, miosis, amd ipsilateral anhidrosis.
Pancoast's syndrome	Superior sulcus tumor injuring the 8th cervical nerve and the 1st and 2nd thoracic nerves and ribs, causing shoulder pain radiating to arm
Superior vena cava syndrome	Tumor causing obstruction of the superior vena cava and subsequent venous return, producing facial swelling, dyspnea, cough, headaches, epistaxis, syncope. Symptoms worsened with bending forward and on awakening in the morning
Syndrome of inappropriate antidiuretic hormone (SIADH)	Ectopic antidiuretic hormone (ADH) release in the setting of plasma hyposmolarity, producing hyponatremia without edema. Seen in small cell lung cancer
Eaton–Lambert syndrome	Presynaptic nerve terminals attacked by antibodies, decreasing acetylcholine release. Treated by plasmapheresis and immunosuppression, 40% associated with small cell lung CA, 20% have other CA, 40% have no CA.
Trousseau's syndrome	Venous thrombosis associated with metastatic cancer
PTH-like hormone	Results in high calcium, low phosphate; seen in squamous cell lung cancer

TABLE 2.7-10. Distinction Between Small and Non–Small Cell Lung Cancer

Characteristic	Small Cell Lung Cancer	Non–Small Cell Lung Cancer
Histology	Small dark nuclei scant cytoplasm	Copious cytoplasm, pleomorphic nuclei
Ectopic peptide production	Gastrin, ACTH, ADH, calcitonin, ANF	PTH
Response to radiotherapy	80–90% will shrink	30–50% will shrink
Response to chemotherapy	Complete regression in 50%	Complete regression in 5%
Surgical resection for	Not indicated	Stages I, II, IIIA
Included subtypes	Small cell only	Adenocarcinoma, squamous cell, large cell, bronchoalveolar
5-year survival rate all stages	5%	11–83%

ACTH, adrenocorticotropic hormone; ADH, antidiuretic hormone; ANF, atrial natriuretic factor; PTH, parathyroid hormone.
Note: ADH is also known as arginine vasopressin (AVP).

Paraneoplastic Syndromes in Lung Cancer
Small cell: SIADH, Eaton–Lambert syndrome, ectopic ACTH
Squamous cell: PTH-like hormone, often cavitates

- Hoarseness (recurrent laryngeal nerve paralysis)
- Postobstructive pneumonia
- Dysphagia
- Associated (paraneoplastic) syndromes (see Table 2.7-9)

Treatment

The two main types of lung cancer, small cell and non–small cell cancer, have different responses to radiotherapy, chemotherapy, and surgery (see Table 2.7-10). Generally: small cell—always chemo, never surgery; non–small cell—surgery if cancer is local, chemo only if there are mets.

HIGH-YIELD FACTS IN

Rheumatology

Lower Back Pain 280

- Leading Causes of Lower Back Pain 280
- Lumbar Disk Herniation 281
- Vertebral Compression Fracture 281
- Spinal Metastasis and Cauda Equina Syndrome 282
- Osteoarthritis (OA) 283

Connective Tissue Disorders 284

- Rheumatoid Arthritis (RA) 284
- Systemic Lupus Erythematosus (SLE) 286
- Drug-Induced Lupus (DIL) 288
- Scleroderma (aka Systemic Sclerosis) 289
- Sarcoidosis 289
- Sjögren's Syndrome 291
- Polymyositis and Dermatomyositis 292

Seronegative Arthritides 293

- Ankylosing Spondylitis 294
- Reiter's Syndrome and Reactive Arthritis 295
- Behçet's Syndrome 296
- Gonococcal Septic Arthritis 296

Vasculitis 296

- Polyarteritis Nodosa (PAN) 296
- Churg–Strauss Disease 297
- Wegener's Granulomatosis 297
- Takayasu's arteritis 298
- Temporal Arteritis 298

Joint Disorders 298

- Gout 298
- Pseudogout 300
- Nongonococcal Septic Arthritis 300
- Avascular Necrosis (AVN) of the Hip 301
- Costochondritis 302
- Carpal Tunnel Syndrome 302

Rheumatology is a broad discipline covering diseases of the joints, connective tissue, and certain immunological disorders. Also covered in this chapter are conditions that are not typically classified as rheumatology but nonetheless affect the musculoskeletal system. Table 2.8-1 discusses laboratory data commonly used in rheumatology.

Lower Back Pain

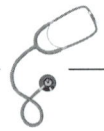

Leading causes of low back pain: **ACTIONS**

▶ LEADING CAUSES OF LOWER BACK PAIN

- Arthritis (RA, OA)
- Congenital anomalies (not covered here)
- Trauma (strains, sprains, fractures, and lumbar disk herniation)
- Infection

TABLE 2.8-1. Laboratory Data Commonly Used in Rheumatology

Finding	Significance
Erythrocyte sedimentation rate	Determined by filling a tube with whole blood and measuring the rate of sedimentation of red cells—changes in the rate are seen with increased plasma proteins. Certain proteins called *acute-phase reactants* (negatively charged proteins) are produced at an increased rate during an inflammatory response. These proteins cause RBCs to adhere to one another like stacks of coins called rouleaux, which fall through the plasma faster than free RBCs. This is a very nonspecific test. An increased ESR is seen in infections, tissue infarctions, malignancies, collagen-vascular diseases, and states of increased physiologic stress (pregnancy, extreme exercise).
Antinuclear antibodies	Found in many rheumatologic disorders, such as: ■ SLE ■ Rheumatoid arthritis ■ Scleroderma ■ Polymyositis and dermatomyositis
Rheumatoid factor	This is an IgM antibody directed against the Fc portion of IgG. Found mainly in rheumatoid arthritis but also in vasculitides
Complement levels	Complement levels drop when there is decreased production in the liver or increased loss—either through the formation of immune complexes or from glomerular disease. Complement levels can be low with: ■ Liver disease (viral hepatitis) ■ SLE nephritis ■ Glomerulonephritis (C3 is the most reduced) ■ Bacterial endocarditis ■ Serum sickness ■ Rheumatoid arthritis with vasculitis

- Osteoporosis
- Neoplasms
- Spinal stenosis

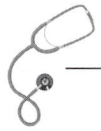

Osteoarthritis can lead to osteophytes and hypertrophy of spinal facets, which can compress nerve roots.

► LUMBAR DISK HERNIATION

Definition

- Disk herniation is a common cause of chronic lower back pain.
- L4–L5 and L5–S1 are the most common sites affected.
- Herniation occurs when the nucleus pulposus prolapses through the annulus fibrosis.
- More common in men

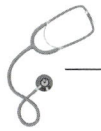

The nucleus pulposus is a thick gel. Herniation of the nucleus pulposus is like toothpaste being squeezed out of the tube.

Signs and Symptoms

- Limited spinal flexion
- Pain and paresthesia with a dermatomal distribution
- Specific signs depend on nerve root involved:
  - L4: Decreased knee jerk, weakness of anterior tibialis
  - L5: Weakness of extensor hallucis longus, decreased sensation over lateral aspect of calf and first web space
  - S1: Decreased ankle jerk, decreased plantar flexion, decreased sensation over lateral aspect of foot

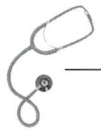

Remember:
L3–L4 herniation affects L4 nerve root
L4–L5 affects L5
L5–S1 affects S1

Treatment

- Nonsteroidal anti-inflammatory drugs (NSAIDs) for symptomatic relief
- Advise smoking cessation.
- Surgical treatment is indicated only for severe cases.

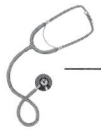

Cigarette smoking is associated with an increased risk of herniation.

VERTEBRAL COMPRESSION FRACTURE

- This is the most common manifestation of osteoporosis.
- It is also seen in patients on long-term steroids and in patients with lytic bony metastases.
- The thoracic spine is the most common site affected (see Figure 2.8-1).

Signs and Symptoms

- Height loss
- Sudden back pain after mild trauma
- Local radiation of pain—the extremities are rarely affected (unlike a herniated disk).

Diagnosis

Plain radiographs of LS will not show compression fracture until there is loss of 25 to 30% bone height. MRI and CT are more sensitive.

Treatment

- Symptomatic relief with NSAIDs
- Vertebroplasty:
  - Usually reserved for fractures with > 50% loss of bone height
  - Consists of an orthopedic cement (polymethylmethacrylate) that is injected into the vertebral body
  - Restores height and relieves pain
- Prevention of osteoporosis:
  - Weight-bearing exercises
  - Estrogen replacement therapy
  - Calcium supplementation to increase bone mass
  - Calcitonin to inhibit bone resorption
  - Bisphosphonates to inhibit osteoclast activity

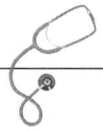

Bisphosphonates such as alendronate (Fosamax) irritate gastric mucosa, so advise patients to eat beforehand and stay upright for 30 minutes after taking it.

▶ SPINAL METASTASIS AND CAUDA EQUINA SYNDROME

- Metastatic lesions invade the spinal bone marrow, leading to compression of the spinal cord.
- Typically involves the thoracic spine
- Cauda equina syndrome occurs when the compression occurs below spinal cord (which typically ends at around L1) at the lumbar and sacral nerve roots.
- The most common primary tumors involved include breast, lung, prostate, kidney, lymphoma, and multiple myeloma.

Signs and Symptoms

- Back pain
- Lower extremity weakness

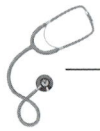

Spinal cord compression is an emergency. Missed diagnosis can lead to permanent paralysis.

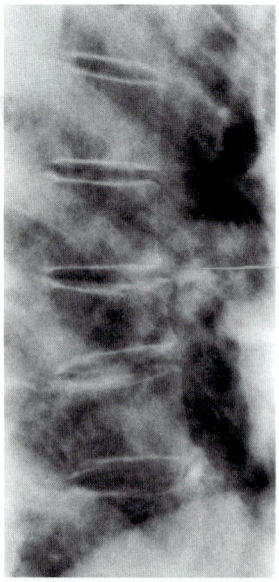

FIGURE 2.8-1. Compression fracture of osteoporosis. Note the anterior collapse of the vertebra.

(Reproduced, with permission, from Wilson FC, Lin PP. *General Orthopedics.* New York: McGraw-Hill, 1997:489.)

- Hyperreflexia
- Upward Babinski sign
- Urinary incontinence
- Decreased rectal sphincter tone
- Cauda equina syndrome classically has saddle anesthesia and bladder/bowel incontinence.

Diagnosis

MRI is the preferred imaging technique.

Treatment

Glucocorticoids are used to reduce inflammation and edema. Radiation therapy should be started as soon as possible. Surgery is indicated only if radiation fails to improve the symptoms or if compression is due to actual bone fragment (radiation will not shrink bone).

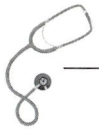

Any cancer patient who develops back pain should be investigated for spinal metastases.

Common causes of spinal cord compression:
- **Multiple myeloma**
- **Lymphoma**
- **Metastatic lung, prostate, and breast cancer**

▶ OSTEOARTHRITIS (OA)

Definition

Degeneration of articular cartilage followed by new and abnormal bone formation; more common in women

Etiology

- *Primary disease:* No known cause
- *Secondary disease:* Known underlying etiology such as trauma, metabolic (hemachromatosis, Wilson's disease), endocrine (acromegaly), or congenital (congenital hip dislocation)

Signs and Symptoms

- Joint pain relieved with rest
- Morning stiffness that resolves within 30 minutes
- Painless nodules on the hand (see Figure 2.8-2):

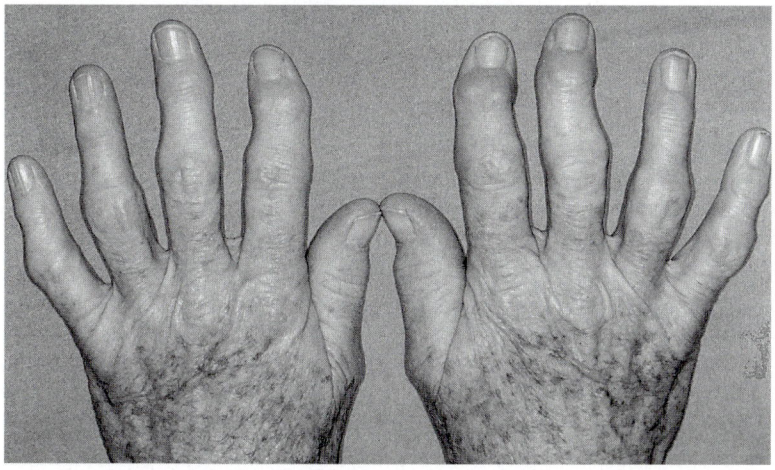

FIGURE 2.8-2. Heberden's and Bouchard's nodes of osteoarthritis.

(Reproduced, with permission, from Wilson FC, Lin PP. *General Orthopedics.* New York: McGraw-Hill, 1997:413.)

- **Heberden's nodes** at the DIPs
- **Bouchard's nodes** at the PIPs
- Loss of range of motion (e.g., decreased internal rotation of hip)
- Joint effusions

Saddle anesthesia: Loss of sensation over the buttocks, perineum, and thighs. Seen with cauda equina syndrome.

Diagnosis

Lab findings are normal. X-ray will show joint space narrowing, osteophyte formation, and subchondral cysts.

Treatment

- NSAIDs for symptomatic relief
- Intra-articular injection of lidocaine provides temporary relief
- Joint replacement as necessary
- Strengthen periarticular muscles

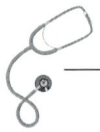

Rheumatoid arthritis: Women are more commonly affected than men.

Connective Tissue Disorders

▶ RHEUMATOID ARTHRITIS (RA)

Definition

A systemic inflammatory disease primarily affecting the synovial membranes. Pannus (granulation tissue) develop in the joint spaces and erode into the articular cartilage and bone.

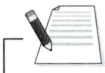

Common deformities in RA:
- **Ulnar deviation** of the digits
- **Boutonniere's deformity:** Hyperextension of the DIP and flexion of the PIP (Figure 2.8-3A)
- **Swan neck:** Flexion of the DIP and extension of the PIP (Figure 2.8-3B)

Signs and Symptoms

- Early symptoms are nonspecific: Malaise, anorexia, fatigue, vague musculoskeletal complaints
- Hypertrophy of synovial tissue
- Prolonged morning stiffness
- Joint pain—most common joints affected: Proximal interphalangeal (PIP), metacarpophalangeal (MCP), wrist, knees, ankles
- Subcutaneous painless rheumatic nodules
- Instability of cervical spine due to bone erosion
- Extra-articular involvement also occurs. Common manifestations include: Vasculitis, pleuritis, pulmonary nodules, and secondary amyloidosis

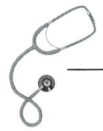

The presence of RF generally signifies more significant disease.

Diagnosis

At least four out of the following seven criteria must be present to diagnose rheumatoid arthritis; criteria 1 through 4 must have been present for ≥ 6 weeks:

1. Morning stiffness for ≥ 1 hour
2. Arthritis of three or more joint areas

TABLE 2.8-2. Common Serology of Rheumatologic Conditions

	ANTIBODY	HLA
SLE	Anti-DS (60–70%) (indicates disease activity) Anti-SM (Smith) (25%) Anticardiolipin Lupus anticoagulant	DR2, DR3
DIL (drug-induced lupus)	Antihistone (sensitive, use to rule out DIL)	DR3
Sjögren's	Anti-SSA(Ro) Anti-SSB(La)	
Ankylosing spondylitis		B27
Reiter's		B27
MCTD		Anti-U_1RNP
Poly/dermatomyositis	Anti-Jo (polymyositis) Anti-Mi2 (dermatomyositis) Anti-PM1	DR3
Systemic sclerosis	Anti-topoisomerase-1 (SCL-70) Antinucleolar	
CREST	Anticentromere	
RA	Rheumatoid factor	DR4 (associated with severe disease)
Behçet's		B5

3. Arthritis of hand joints (see Figure 2.8-3)
4. Symmetric arthritis
5. Rheumatoid nodules
6. Positive serum rheumatoid factor (see Table 2.8-2 for common serology of rheumatologic conditions)
7. Radiographic changes

LABORATORY

- Rheumatoid factor (RF)—positive in 80% of patients with RA
- Anemia of chronic disease
- Elevated ESR

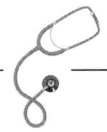

If the WBC count is low in an RA patient, think of *Felty's syndrome:*
- **Rheumatoid arthritis**
- **Splenomegaly**
- **Leukopenia**

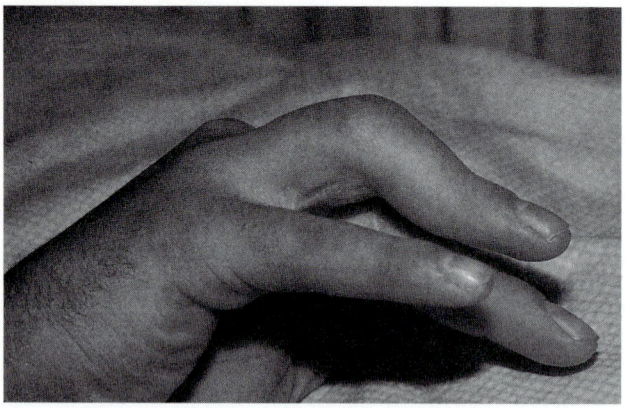

A

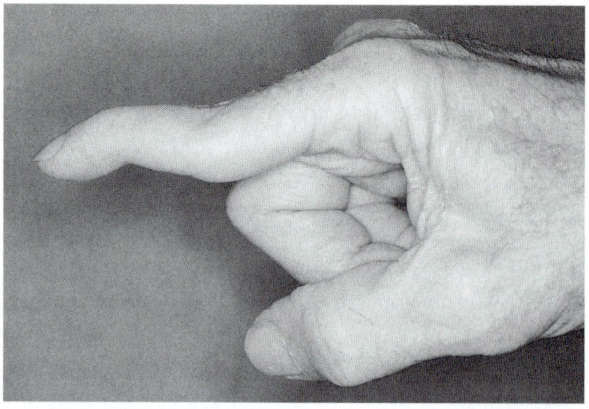

B

FIGURE 2.8-3. Boutonniere (A) and Swan neck (B) deformities of rheumatoid arthritis.

(Reproduced, with permission, from Knoop KJ, Stack LB, Storrow AB. *Atlas of Emergency Medicine.* New York: McGraw-Hill, 1997:291.)

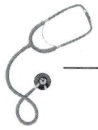

Most arthritis patients (regardless of the type of arthritis) have taken NSAIDs for long periods of time. This places them at high risk for ulcers.

Rheumatoid arthritis: Pain improves with use. **Osteoarthritis:** Pain worsens with use.

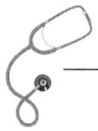

OA is also called "wear-and-tear disease" and "degenerative joint disease" (DJD).

TREATMENT

- Consider NSAIDs, glucocorticoid injections, and/or low-dose steroids for symptomatic relief.
- Physical therapy to maintain strength and range of motion
- Disease-modifying antirheumatic drugs (DMARDs) have been shown to slow or even reverse joint damage. DMARDs should be begun within 3 months of diagnosis and include:
  - Methotrexate
  - Leflunomide
  - Minocycline
  - Gold compounds
  - Hydroxychloroquine
  - Sulfasalazine
  - Cyclosporine
  - Azathioprine

▶ SYSTEMIC LUPUS ERYTHEMATOSUS (SLE)

DEFINITION

- A chronic inflammatory disease that can affect virtually every organ system, including kidney, skin, joints, lungs, CNS
- Classified as an autoimmune disorder with elaboration of characteristic autoantibodies
- Can present with overlapping rheumatologic syndromes (though 90% have skin and joint involvement)
- Associated with HLA-DR2 and HLA-DR3

Epidemiology

- Women > men
- Blacks > whites.
- Though more common in American blacks, SLE is virtually nonexistent in African blacks.

Signs and Symptoms

- Fever, fatigue, weight loss
- Anemia (often Coombs' positive)
- Alopecia
- Arthralgias (symmetric)
- Photosensitive rash
- Raynaud's phenomenon
- Serositis
- Nephritis/nephrotic syndrome
- Recurrent abortions
- Purpura

Diagnosis

American College of Rheumatology (ACR) criteria : ≥ 4 of the following at any given time (sensitivity and specificity ~96%):

1. Malar rash: "Butterfly" distribution; spares nasolabial folds
2. Discoid rash: Raised erythematous patches; scaling; may scar
3. Photosensitivity
4. Oral ulcers: Usually painless
5. Symmetric arthritis: ≥ 2 joints
6. Serositis: Pleuritis/pericarditis
7. Renal disorder: Multiple types
8. Neurologic disorder: Seizures, psychosis, "lupus cerebritis"
9. Hematologic disorder: Any cell line can be affected.
10. Immunologic disorder: Autoantibodies, false-positive syphilis tests (RPR, VDRL)
11. Antinuclear antibody (ANA)

Labs

Autoantibodies:

- **ANA**—present in about 95%
- **Anti-Smith (Sm)**—specific for SLE
- **Anti-dsDNA**—specific; associated with renal disease if high
- **Anticardiolipin** and **lupus anticoagulant**—associated with recurrent fetal loss, thrombocytopenia, heart disease; congenital heart block in the fetus (*Note:* Lupus anticoagulant is a misnomer—it is a prothrombotic state, though it paradoxically causes an elevated PTT.)

Flares can be associated with transaminitis, anemia, elevated ESR, proteinuria, hematuria, and granular casts in urine.

Treatment

- Avoid stress or medical procedure/surgery during flare (exacerbates SLE)
- NSAIDs

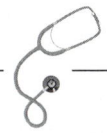

Note that in drug-induced SLE there is no kidney or CNS involvement.

OA can cause morning stiffness but is it usually short-lived (in contrast to RA).
OA affects the **O**uter joints on the hand—the DIPs.
RA affects the inner joints—MCPs and PIPs.

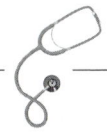

OA is not a systemic inflammatory disease; therefore, lab studies should be normal.

Typical scenario:
A 27-year-old black female presents with general malaise, arthralgias, oral ulcers, and a photosensitive rash. *Think: Systemic lupus erythematosus.*

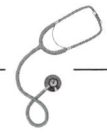

UV light causes flare-ups, so many SLE patients are sensitive to sunlight.

Typical scenario:
A 24-year-old woman presents with a history of multiple miscarriages. She has no known medical history. Which antibodies would you test for? *Lupus anticoagulant and anticardiolipin.* Diagnosis: Antiphospholipid syndrome.

- Antimalarials (chloroquines): Improves skin rash and arthritis
- Glucocorticoids with severe disease/end-organ damage
- Steroid-sparing threapy: Cyclophosphamide/azathioprine reserved for severe disease
- Avoid drugs known to cause SLE-like syndrome.

Prognosis

Poorer prognosis:
- Hypocomplementemia
- + Anti-dsDNA
- Nephritis/nephrotic syndrome
- Hypoalbuminemia
- Cr > 1.5

Better prognosis:
- + AntiU_1RNP

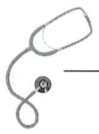

SLE can cause a drop in the RBCs, WBCs, or platelets.

▶ DRUG-INDUCED LUPUS (DIL)

Definition

A distinct entity from SLE—idiopathic reaction to certain drugs. It is distinguished by:
- Complete resolution of disease once offending drug is discontinued
- Presence of serum antihistone antibodies (very sensitive)
- Lack of renal or CNS involvement

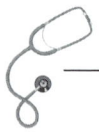

SLE mean survival rate (from diagnosis):
85% at 5 years
80% at 10 years
75% at 20 years

Etiology

- Procainamide: Most common offender—used in the treatment of atrial fibrillation in patients with WPW
- Hydralazine: Second most common offender—used to treat preeclampsia.
- Isoniazid: Used to treat tuberculosis (TB)
- Quinidine: Used to treat malaria and leg cramps
- Methyldopa: Old antihypertensive drug, still used in obstetrics
- Chlorpromazine: Antiemetic also associated with dystonic reactions
- Penicillamine: Used to treat Wilson's disease
- Alpha-interferon: Experimental, used to treat multiple sclerosis (MS) and other autoimmune and viral conditions

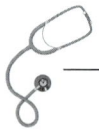

Drugs associated with DIL:
H&P, IQ CAMP
Take H&P. If you're smart (in the high IQ CAMP), you'll discontinue these drugs in patients with a malar rash.

Treatment

Discontinue the offending drug; supportive therapy.

▶ SCLERODERMA (AKA SYSTEMIC SCLEROSIS)

Definition

An autoimmune disorder characterized by widespread small vessel fibrosis secondary to overproduction of collagen and other extracellular matrix proteins.

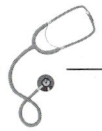

The skin changes in scleroderma at first may actually cause the patient to appear more youthful. The skin becomes tight and wrinkles disappear.

Signs and Symptoms

- Raynaud's phenomenon (vasospasm of arteries in hands in response to cold or emotional stress, resulting in discoloration of hands)
- Thickened, tight skin
- Nailfold capillaries—giant loops formed by abnormal capillaries at nailfold
- Dysphagia due to esophageal fibrosis
- Renal artery fibrosis
- Pulmonary hypertension
- Telangiectasias
- Cardiac conduction disease/pericardial effusion

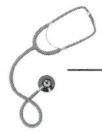

Renal artery fibrosis leads to malignant HTN, the leading cause of death.

In the limited form of the disease symptoms are generally limited to the **CREST syndrome:**

Calcinosis (calcium deposition forming nodules)
Raynaud's phenomenon
Esophageal dysmotility
Sclerodactyly (stiffness of skin of fingers)
Telangiectasias

Laboratory

- ANA positive in 95%
- Anti SCl-70 (topoisomerase antibody)
- Antibody to centromere—specific to CREST variant
- Antibody to nucleolar Ag
- Normochromic, normocytic anemia
- Elevated ESR
- Decreased vital capacity on pulmonary function tests (restrictive lung disease)

Treatment

- Penicillamine—may inhibit collagen cross-linking
- Captopril—helps control the renal hypertension
- Calcium channel blockers—diminish the Raynaud's phenomenon
- Steroids—rarely effective in altering the disease course

▶ SARCOIDOSIS

Definition

- A systemic illness with no known cause, primarily affecting the lungs
- Characterized by noncaseating granulomas
- More common among blacks and women

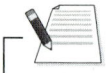

Typical scenario:
A 40-year-old black woman presents with dyspnea, malaise, visual disturbances, and a rash. Chest x-ray shows bilateral hilar adenopathy.
Think: Sarcoidosis.

Signs and Symptoms

Almost any part of the body can be affected. Some typical extrapulmonary findings are:

Skin—erythema nodosum (erythematous nodes on extensor surfaces of lower extremities, also seen in other conditions)
Kidney—hypercalciuria (macrophages increase metabolism of vitamin D to 1,25-dihydroxyvitamin D)
Eyes—uveitis (inflammation of uveal tract, iris, ciliary body, choroid)
Cardiac—conduction defects
Nervous—Bell's palsy (self-limited 7th nerve palsy of unknown etiology)
Lofgren's syndrome—triad of erythema nodosa, arthritis, and bilateral hilar lymphadenopathy (good prognosis)

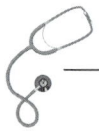

In sarcoidosis, remember, when you go from stage II to stage III, you actually lose the hilar adenopathy.

Staging

I. Bilateral hilar adenopathy
II. Hilar adenopathy plus lung parenchymal involvement
III. Lung parenchymal involvement alone
IV. Pulmonary fibrosis

Diagnosis

Requires transbronchial biopsy to prove existence of noncaseating granulomas, but not sufficient on its own to make diagnosis; requires clinical, laboratory, and radiographic adjuncts

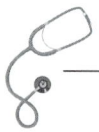

Since early HIV can mimic sarcoidosis in all aspects, patients should have HIV testing as part of their workup.

Laboratory

Diagnosis cannot be made or excluded on the basis of laboratory findings alone. Common laboratory findings include:

- Lymphocytosis on bronchoalveolar lavage
- Eosinophilia
- False positive RF and ANA
- Elevated angiotensin-converting enzyme (ACE)
- Skin anergy to common antigens
- Elevated 24-hour urine calcium
- Chest x-ray shows **bilateral hilar adenopathy** and perihilar calcifications (see Figure 2.8-4)
- Elevated ESR

Treatment

Corticosteroids

Prognosis

Most patients have resolution of their disease within 2 years. Death from pulmonary failure occurs in a minority of patients.

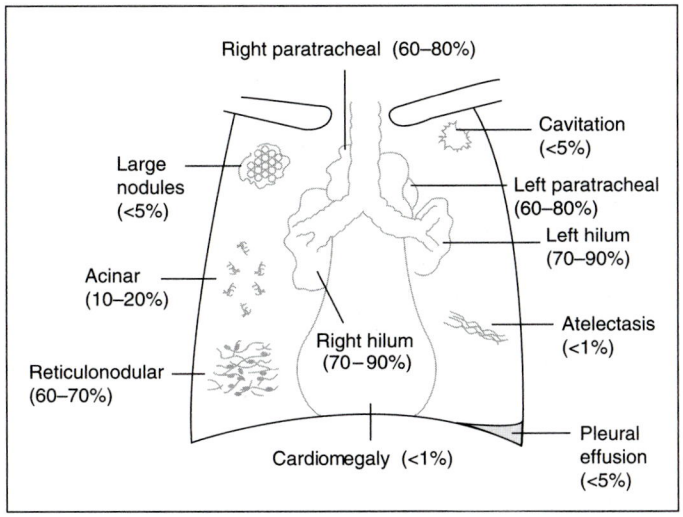

FIGURE 2.8-4. Abnormal CXR findings in sarcoidosis.

(Reproduced, with permission, from Fauci AS et al [eds]. *Harrison's Principles of Internal Medicine*, 14th ed. New York: McGraw-Hill, 1998:1925.)

▶ SJÖGREN'S SYNDROME

Definition

A lymphocytic infiltrate in salivary and lacrimal glands causing decreased secretions from these glands

Etiology

- Autoimmune
- Found in many with coexisting connective tissue diseases (any)

Signs and Symptoms

- Dry mouth, dry eyes
- Can have any symptoms associated with other CTDs

Labs

- + RF in 90%
- + ANA in 70%
- + La (SS_B) in 40 to 50%
- DR3 association

Diagnosis

- Lip biopsy of minor salivary glands
- By symptoms

Treatment

- Treat symptoms
- Corticosteroids

Both polymyositis and dermatomyositis are more common in women.

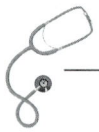

Polymyositis and dermatomyositis can be distinguished from myasthenia gravis by the lack of ocular involvement (ptosis).

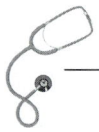

The rash of dermatomyositis involves the upper eyelids; the rash of SLE does not.

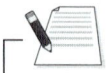

Typical scenario:
A 57-year-old woman complains of difficulty getting out of a chair and difficulty combing her hair. *Think: Polymyositis.*

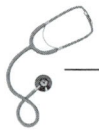

Note both azathioprine and methotrexate suppress the bone marrow. Azathioprine is also hepatotoxic.

Prognosis

> 40% risk of lymphoma

► POLYMYOSITIS AND DERMATOMYOSITIS

Definitions

- Connective tissue disease causing proximal muscle weakness.
- Associated with HLA-DR3
- Dermatomyositis has similar manifestations to polymyositis plus skin involvement.

Etiology

Unknown; many viruses implicated (coxsackie, influenza)

Signs and Symptoms

- Weakness first occurring in legs
- Difficulty with squatting, kneeling, rising from chair, climbing stairs
- Dysphagia
- Abnormal ECG (with advanced disease)
- With dermatomyositis: Purple-red papular/scaly photosensitive rash on face, neck ("V sign," "shawl sign"); erythema, scaling on extensor surfaces of joints (Gottron's papules; very specific); periorbital edema, heliotropic rash

Diagnosis

Four criteria:

1. Muscle weakness
2. Increased creatine phosphokinase (CPK)/aldolase
3. Muscle biopsy showing T-cell infiltrate with myonecrosis
4. EMG shows myopathy: Decreased amplitude, increased spike amplitude

Labs

- Positive antinuclear antibody (ANA)
- Elevated CPK, LDH, AST, aldolase
- ESR is elevated in only ~50% of cases.
- One-third have myositis-specific antibodies (see below).
- CXR may show interstitial pulmonary disease.

Myositis-Specific Antibodies

- **Anti-Jo:** One third with pure myositis
- **Anti-Mi2:** Dermatomyositis specific
- **Anti-PM1**

Treatment

- Glucocorticoids (for poly or dermato): 80% respond within 6 weeks
- If poor response to glucocorticoids, high suspicion of malignancy
- Methotrexate, azathioprine if steroid resistant

Prognosis

- Approximately 15% have malignancy, especially with dermatomyositis.
- Insidious, progressive disease

Seronegative Arthritides

Include ankylosing spondylitis, psoriatic arthritis, ulcerative colitis, and Reiter's syndrome. Many (not all) associated with HLA-B27 genotype. Unlike SLE, rheumatoid arthritis, and scleroderma, these have *asymmetric* arthritis and often have spinal involvement (sacroiliitis, spondylitis).

▶ ANKYLOSING SPONDYLITIS

Definition

Chronic systemic inflammatory disorder affecting primarily the axial skeleton, but can affect multiple organs.

Signs and Symptoms

- Peak onset of symptoms between ages 20 and 30
- Affects men to women 3:1
- Low back pain with reduced range of motion most common presenting symptom
- Worse at night, better with exercise/worse with inactivity
- Spinal ankylosis is a late manifestation of the disease.
- Highly variable disease course (may be self-limiting weith spontaneous remission)
- Extra-articular involvement: Uveitis, neurologic symptoms, pulmonary, renal, genitourinary abnormalities, gastrointestinal, cardiac

Typical scenario:
A young man with stiffness in the lower back that improves with exercise.
Think: Ankylosing spondylitis.

Diagnosis

- Pelvic radiograph: Sacroiliitis is the hallmark of ankylosing spondylitis.
- Osteitis and bone erosions at sites of osseous attachment of ligaments and tendons (enthesopathy)
- Spine radiograph: Syndesmophytes—vertical bridging between vertebrae and ossification of spinal ligaments seen in late disease ("bamboo spine"; see Figure 2.8-5)
- Elevated ESR, CRP
- HLA-B27

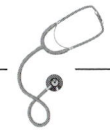

The brittle spine of ankylosing spondylitis is prone to fracture even with minimal trauma. Patients should be restricted from high-risk activities such as skydiving, bungee jumping, and contact sports.

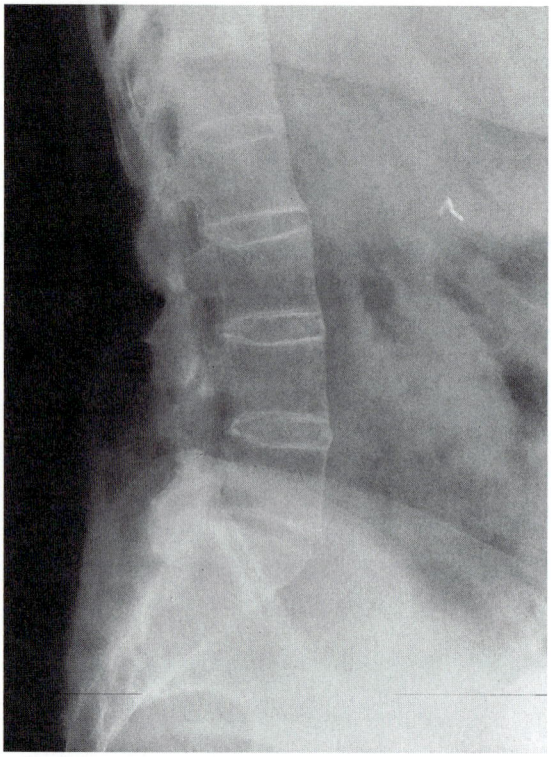

FIGURE 2.8-5. Bamboo spine of ankylosing spondylitis. Note the bridging syndesmophytes.

(Reproduced, with permission, from Wilson FC, Lin PP. *General Orthopedics.* New York: McGraw-Hill, 1997:454.)

TREATMENT

- Exercise/physical therapy
- Smoking cessation: Ankylosing spondylitis patients may develop costochondritis with restrictive pulmonary problems, worsened by development of COPD
- Avoid falls (high risk of vertebral fracture and cauda equina syndrome)
- NSAIDs
- For advanced disease, sulfasalazine, DMARDs, and newer drugs such as anti-TNF therapy are being utilized.

▶ REITER'S SYNDROME AND REACTIVE ARTHRITIS

Reiter's syndrome: "Can't see, can't pee, can't climb a tree"

DEFINITION

An HLA-B27 associated syndrome involving the musculoskeletal, GU, and ocular systems. Occurs in two forms:

1. Sexually transmitted (1 to 2 weeks after exposure); more common in men
2. Postdysentery (most commonly due to *Salmonella, Shigella, Yersinia,* and *Campylobacter*) form more common in women and children

Signs and Symptoms

- Conjunctivitis
- Urethritis/cervicitis
- Arthritis: Asymmetric, lower extremities
- Oral ulcerations
- Balanitis

Laboratory

- Elevated ESR
- Urethral culture may reveal *C. trachomatis*.

Treatment

- NSAIDs for arthritis
- Doxycycline for urethritis/cervicitis

▶ BEHÇET'S SYNDROME

Definition

Autoimmune disease associated with HLA-B5

Signs and Symptoms

- Aphthous (oral) ulcers
- Genital ulcers
- Deep vein thrombophlebitis
- Arthritis (nondeforming)
- Uveitis
- Colitis
- Psychiatric disturbances

Diagnosis

Must have recurrent oral ulcers plus two of the following:

- Recurrent genital ulcers
- Eye lesions
- Skin lesions
- Positive pathergy test

Laboratory

- Elevated ESR
- Hypergammaglobulinemia
- Cryoglobulinemia

Treatment

- Colchicine or interferon-α for arthritis
- Aspirin or antiplatelet agents for thrombophlebitis
- Steroids for uveitis and CNS manifestations

Behçet's syndrome: "Though I enjoyed the experience, I was afterward *beset* with oral and genital ulcers."

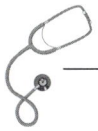

Behçet's ulcers pain the male but spare the female (painless in women).

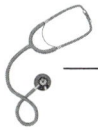

Pathergy test: Inflammatory reaction of skin to any scratches.

▶ GONOCOCCAL SEPTIC ARTHRITIS

Definition

A disseminated gonococcal infection; more common in women than men

Etiology

- *Neisseria gonorrhoeae*
- More likely during pregnancy and menstruation

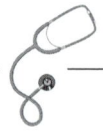

Upper extremities favored in gonococcal arthritis.

Signs and Symptoms

After 1 to 4 days of a **migratory polyarthritis,** 60% of patients develop a tenosynovitis and 40% a purulent monarthritis. Patients will sometimes have fever but, surprisingly, urethritis is rarely seen. Most patients develop a characteristic skin lesion—**small necrotic pustules**—over their extremities, usually the fingers and toes.

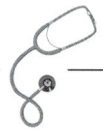

If there is no response to antibiotics for presumed gonococcal arthritis, consider Reiter's syndrome.

Diagnosis

- Synovial fluid shows elevated WBCs.
- Gram stain and blood culture are positive in < 50% of cases.
- Joint cultures are usually negative.

Treatment

- Very sensitive to antibiotic therapy (e.g., ceftriaxone)
- Surgical drainage is not usually necessary.

Vasculitis

▶ POLYARTERITIS NODOSA (PAN)

Definition

Systemic necrotizing vasculitis of small and medium-sized muscular arteries

Signs and Symptoms

- Nonspecific symptoms predominate: Fever, weight loss, malaise
- Specific symptoms depend on organ involved. Most common ones are:
  - Glomerulonephritis, arthritis, mononeuritis multiplex
  - Other systems that may be involved are GI, skin, cardiac, GU, and CNS. Note conspicuous absence of pulmonary involvement.

Laboratory

- Red cell casts in urine
- One third of patients have hepatitis B antigenemia.
- Diagnosis is made by tissue biopsy of affected organ.

Treatment

- Prednisone
- Cyclophosphamide

▶ CHURG-STRAUSS DISEASE

Definition

Medium vessel arteritis, also known as allergic angiitis and granulomatosis; it is very similar to PAN except that the pulmonary findings predominate.

Signs and Symptoms

- Bronchospasm (asthma)
- Eosinophilia
- Fever
- Erythematous maculopapular rashes, palpable purpura, and cutaneous nodules
- Red casts in urine

PAN—spares the lungs
Churg–Strauss—Lung symptoms predominate

Treatment

Steroids; if steroids fail, consider azathioprine and cyclophosphamide.

▶ WEGENER'S GRANULOMATOSIS

Chronically relapsing small artery vasculitis of upper and lower respiratory tracts and glomerulonephritis

Signs and Symptoms

- Kidney: Glomerulonephritis
- Lungs: Hemoptysis, pulmonary infiltrates
- Nasopharynx: Sinusitis, otitis
- Arthralgias/arthritis
- Fever
- Weight loss

Goodpasture's is the other disease that involves both lungs and kidney. Its triad is:
- **Glomerulonephritis,**
- **Pulmonary hemorrhage**
- **Anti-GBM Ab**

Diagnosis

- Granulomatous vasculitis on lung biopsy
- Postive c-ANCA titer
- Exclusion of Goodpasture's syndrome, tumors, and infectious disease

Treatment

Steroids, cyclophosphamide

▶ TAKAYASU'S ARTERITIS

Definition

An arteritis of unknown (possibly autoimmune) etiology that is seen commonly in young people of Asian descent; usually affects medium and large-sized arteries. More common in women.

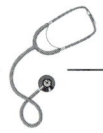

Takayasu's is also called "pulseless disease" and "aortic arch syndrome."

Signs and Symptoms

- Loss of pulses in arms and carotids bilaterally
- Raynaud's phenomenon
- Signs of transient brain ischemia such as blindness and hemiplegia
- Abdominal pain, atypical chest pain

Diagnosis

- Arteriography shows narrowing of aorta +/– aneurysm.
- MRA is helpful if arteriography is not available.

Treatment

- Steroids
- Methotrexate

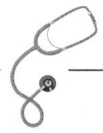

Temporal arteritis is also called giant cell arteritis.

▶ TEMPORAL ARTERITIS

Inflammation of medium and large-sized arteries, commonly the temporal artery. See the neurology chapter.

Joint Disorders

▶ GOUT

Definition

Inflammation and severe joint pain (arthralgia) secondary to urate crystal deposition. Caused by either overproduction or underexcretion of uric acid.

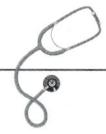

Hyperuricemia is caused by:
- Increased urate production
- Decreased urate excretion

Epidemiology

- Men > women
- Typical age of onset: 45
- For serum urate > 9–10 mg/dL, incidence of attack 5%/year

Etiology

1. Increased production: Idiopathic, leukemia/tumor lysis syndrome, hemolytic anemia, strenuous exercise; excessive fructose ingestion, G6PD, Lesch–Nyhan, high-protein diet, nicotinic acid
2. Decreased excretion: Chronic renal disease, lead nephropathy, EtOH ingestion, DKA, thiazide diuretics

Signs and Symptoms

- Rapid onset of extreme joint pain and swelling
- Fifty percent of first attacks are in the great toe (podagra; see Figure 2.8-6).
- **Tophi:** Aggregates of urate crystals and giant cells, which may cause tissue erosion

Fifty percent of first gout attacks involve first metatarsophalangeal joint.

Diagnosis

Aspirate

- Negatively birefringent urate crystals in joint aspirate
- Large number of PMNs (5,000–7,000)
- Decreased viscosity of joint fluid (low hyaluronate)

Labs

- Increased WBC count, proteinuria, elevated ESR, elevated uric acid, isosthenuria
- 24-hour urinary uric acid level: > 750 mg indicates overproducer

Gout:
Small joints
Negative birefringence
Pseudogout:
Large joints (e.g., knee)
Positive birefringence

Treatment

Acute Attack

- Colchicine: May be poorly tolerated secondary to GI effects, cytopenias
- NSAIDs, particularly indomethacin

Chronic

- Initiate allopurinol and/or probenecid treatment only after acute attack is resolved; otherwise, may prolong or worsen attack.
  - Allopurinol: Use in overproducers and those with renal insufficiency.
  - Probenecid, sulfinpyrazine, uricosurics: Increase excretion of uric acid. Do not use in patients with chronic renal insufficiency.

A man comes in with swollen, painful joint. What is the first step?
Joint fluid aspiration and analysis

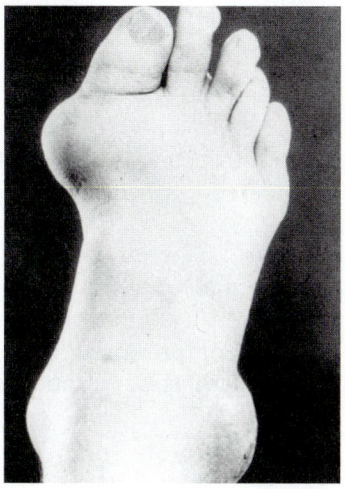

FIGURE 2.8-6. Podagra.

(Reproduced, with permission, from Fauci AS et al [eds]. *Harrison's Principles of Internal Medicine*, 14th ed. New York: McGraw-Hill, 1998:2162.)

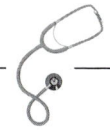

What is isosthenuria? The inability of the kidney to concentrate or dilute urine, resulting in urine of the same concentration as that of protein-free plasma.

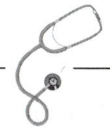

Aspirin is *contraindicated* in acute gout because it decreases urate excretion.

▶ PSEUDOGOUT

Definition

Deposition of calcium pyrophosphate dihydrate (CPPD) crystals in joint spaces causing chondrocalcinosis

Etiology

- Acute inflammatory reaction to the deposition of CPPD in joint spaces
- Changes related to age that make the synovial fluid environment more hospitable to CPPD growth
- Associated with hemochromatosis, hypothyroidism, hyperparathyroidism

Signs and Symptoms/Diagnosis

Similar to gout, the affected joints are painful and red. Unlike gout:

- Large joints are affected (knees, wrists, shoulder).
- The crystals are rhomboid (gouty crystals are needle shaped).
- Radiographs demonstrate calcification in the articular cartilage.
- There is **positive birefringence** of crystals.

Treatment

- NSAIDs can alleviate symptoms.
- Aspirating synovial fluid shortens the duration of the attacks.
- No therapy is available to remove CPPD crystals.

▶ NONGONOCOCCAL SEPTIC ARTHRITIS

Definition

Nongonococcal septic arthritis is seen when there is previous joint damage or bacteremia. It is monarticular and affects the large joints (knee, hip, shoulder, and wrist).

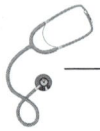

Nongonococcal septic arthritis: Patients will often describe previous trauma to the joint.

Etiology

Young Adults

- *S. aureus*, beta-hemolytic strep, and gram-negative bacilli
- Lyme must also be considered.

Sickle Cell Anemia Patients

- *Salmonella* and *S. aureus* (equal)

IV Drug Users and Immunocompromised

- Gram-negative organisms such as *E. coli* and *Pseudomonas aeruginosa*, as well as *S. aureus*

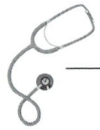

IV drug abuser with septic joint: Must do echo to rule out endocarditis

Risk Factors

- Rheumatoid arthritis
- Prosthetic joints
- Immunodeficiency
- Age
- IV drug abuse

Signs and Symptoms

- Pain, swelling, and warmth over the joint
- Limited range of motion
- Fever

Diagnosis

- Blood cultures are positive in 50% of cases.
- ESR and CRP will be elevated.
- Gram stain can pick up 75% of *S. aureus* infections.

Arthrocentesis is both diagnostic and therapeutic. Joint fluid will reveal an elevated white count (need > 1,000,000 cells/mm^3), predominantly polymorphonucleocytes and a low glucose level. The arthrocentesis releases fluid thereby lowering pressure within the joint capsule and alleviating pain. Arthrocentesis should be avoided if the overlying skin is infected or if there is bacteremia because the procedure introduces a portal of entry for bacteria into the joint.

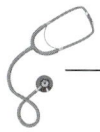

Arthrocentesis should never be attempted in hemophiliacs until the clotting disorder is corrected with the appropriate blood product.

Treatment

- Systemic antibiotics
- Serial arthrocentesis may be necessary if synovial fluid rapidly accumulates
- Surgical drainage is needed for septic hip, and for septic joints that do not improve with intravenous antibiotics within 72 hours.

► AVASCULAR NECROSIS (AVN) OF THE HIP

Definition

The limited blood supply to the head of the femur makes this site particularly vulnerable to AVN.

AVN of the hip in children is called Legg–Calvé–Perthes disease.

Etiology

Seen with a variety of conditions such as trauma, long-term steroid therapy, excessive radiation, alcoholism, sickle cell disease, and Gaucher's disease

Signs and Symptoms

Pain, often referred to the **knee,** exacerbated by internal rotation of the hip

Diagnosis

MRI or bone scan is needed for early detection of the disease. Plain radiographs will be positive only in the late stage.

Treatment

Total hip replacement

▶ COSTOCHONDRITIS

Definition

Painful swelling of the costochondral articulations at the anterior chest wall. Chest pain often confused with PE or MI.

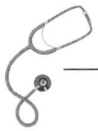

In patients with risk factors for MI, be sure to obtain ECG.

Etiology

Associated with:

- Recent upper respiratory tract infection
- Trauma
- Overuse

Signs and Symptoms

- Typically affects the second through fifth costochondral joints
- Pain is sharp, worse with deep breathing and movement; may radiate to the shoulders and arms.
- Pain is reproducible with palpation.

Diagnosis

Diagnosis is clinical. Can do a chest x-ray to look for metastatic lesions to the sternal bone marrow, which can produce similar symptoms; however, chest x-ray is usually normal.

Treatment

NSAIDs; avoid overuse of muscles.

▶ CARPAL TUNNEL SYNDROME

Definition

Painful compression of the median nerve as it passes through the carpal tunnel; more common in women (see Figure 2.8-7).

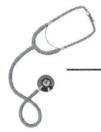

Patients who work extensively with their hands and pregnant women (due to edema) are at increased risk for carpal tunnel syndrome.

Etiology

Anything that increases pressure within the carpal tunnel can cause it. Most common causes are trauma to carpal bones and flexor tenosynovitis. Can be secondary to systemic illnesses such as RA, sarcoidosis, acromegaly, hypothyroidism, diabetes.

Signs and Symptoms

- Muscle weakness and atrophy—mostly in the thenar eminence
- **Phalen's sign:** Presence of paraesthesias along median nerve distribution after holding wrist flexed at 90° for 30 sec
- **Tinel's sign:** Pain radiating down the fingers following percussion over the carpal tunnel

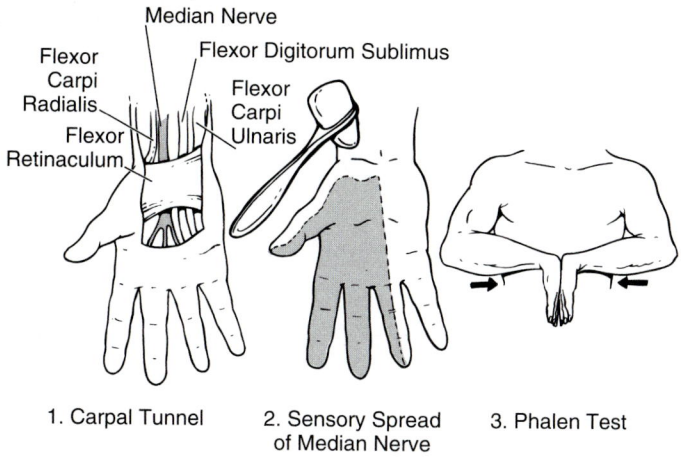

FIGURE 2.8-7. Carpal tunnel syndrome.

1. The flexor retinaculum in the wrist compresses the median nerve to produce hypoesthesia in the radial 3½ digits. 2. Percussion on the radial side of the palmaris longus tendon produces tingling in the 3½ digital region (Tinel sign). 3. Phalen test. Hyperflexion of the wrist for 60 seconds may produce pain in the median nerve distribution; this is relieved by extension of the wrist. (Reproduced, with permission, from DeGowin DL, Brown DD. *DeGowin's Diagnostic Examination,* 7th ed. New York: McGraw-Hill, 2000:720.)

TREATMENT

- Rest with wrist splint worn as much as possible and elevation of the hand to reduce inflammation
- Steroids injected into carpal tunnel are suitable for temporary situations.
- Surgical division of the flexor retinaculum

NOTES

HIGH-YIELD FACTS IN

Neurology

Stroke 306

Brain Herniation 312

CNS Infections 312

- Rabies 312
- Bacterial Meningitis 313
- Viral Meningitis 314
- Botulism 315

Seizure Disorders 316

Brain Neoplasms 316

Neuropathies 318

- Myasthenia Gravis 318
- Guillain–Barré Syndrome 319

Headache 320

- Migraine Headache 320
- Tension Headache 321
- Cluster Headache 322
- Headache of Temporal (Giant Cell) Arteritis 322
- Acute Vision Loss 323

Neurological Disorders 324

- Dementia 324
- Alzheimer's Disease 324
- Parkinson's Disease 325
- Normal Pressure Hydrocephalus (NPH) 326
- Features of Brain Death 327

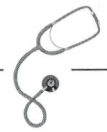

Ischemic penumbra: The tissue surrounding an infarcted zone that is dysfunctional but not infarcted and that may recover full functionality if the hypoxic state resolves. The volume of the ischemic penumbra is often greater than that of the infarcted core, and thus its salvage can dramatically reduce the degree of permanent deficit.

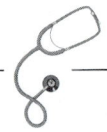

TIAs used to be defined as any stroke whose symptoms resolved completely within 24 hours. With the advent of MRI and the ability to detect "silent" infarctions, the definition has narrowed toward including only those cases with no detectable infarcts.

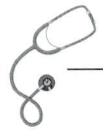

In the United States, someone has a stroke every 45 seconds; someone dies from a stroke every 3.1 minutes.

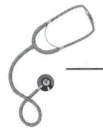

Risk of stroke after TIA:
- First month: 4–8%
- First year: 12–14%
- At 5 years: 24–29%

STROKE

DEFINITIONS

Abrupt onset of new neurologic deficits (see Table 2.9-1) caused by cerebrovascular disease, which can be ischemic or hemorrhagic in nature.

Types of Stroke

- *Stroke:* Cerebral vascular event resulting in infarcted cerebral tissue, regardless of the presence or absence of neurologic deficits
- *Stroke in evolution:* Neurologic deficits continue to fluctuate or increase over time.
- *Completed stroke:* Neurologic deficits have remained stable for 24 to 72 hours.
- *Transient ischemic attack (TIA):* Neurologic deficit resolving completely in 24 hours (usually within 30 minutes) and resulting in no apparent infarcted tissue on magnetic resonance imaging (MRI)
- *Crescendo TIAs:* Two or more TIAs within 24 hours—highly predictive of impending stroke, constitutes a medical emergency

Common Stroke Sequelae

Anosognosia: The inability to identify body dysfunction—patients are unaware of their neurological deficits.
Aphasia: A defect in comprehension or expression of spoken or written language
Broca's aphasia: A deficit in speech and written expression
Wernicke's aphasia: Patients tend to articulate a fluent nonsense with natural rhythm, and comprehension is impaired.
Apraxia: Disturbance in the ability to perform learned motor tasks
Dysarthria: Disturbance in the articulation of speech
Dysphagia: Difficulty swallowing

EPIDEMIOLOGY (SOURCE: WORLD HEALTH ORGANIZATION & AMERICAN STROKE ASSOCIATION)

Worldwide

- There were over 20.5 million strokes in 2001; 5.5 million of these were fatal.
- High blood pressure contributes to over 12.7 million strokes.

In the United States

- Stroke is the third leading cause of death, behind heart disease and cancer. It is the number one cause of long-term disability.
- Each year, about 700,000 people suffer a stroke. About 500,000 of these are first attacks, and 200,000 are recurrent attacks.
- At all ages, more women than men have a stroke.
- Twenty-eight percent of people who suffer a stroke in a given year are under age 65.
- African Americans have a two- to threefold greater risk of ischemic stroke and are more likely to die of stroke.
- About 47% of stroke deaths occur out of hospital.
- Eight percent of men and 11% of women will have a stroke within 6 years after a heart attack.
- 7.6% of ischemic strokes and 37.5% of hemorrhagic strokes result in death within 30 days.

TABLE 2.9-1. Neurological Deficits in Stroke

Artery Occlusion	Deficit	Other
Middle cerebral	■ Contralateral hemiparesis (face and hand more affected) ■ Contralateral hemisensory deficit ■ Homonymous hemianopsia (blindness affecting the right or the left half of the visual fields of both eyes) opposite to occluded artery ■ If dominant MCA affected (left side in 92–94% of people), patient will be aphasic ■ If nondominant MCA affected, confusion, constructional apraxia, contralateral body neglect	
Anterior cerebral (see Figure 2.9-1)	■ Contralateral weakness of leg or foot ■ Broca's aphasia ■ Incontinence ■ Abulia (lack of motivation)	
Internal carotid	■ Presentation similar to MCA occlusion	
Posterior cerebral (see Figure 2.9-2)	■ Homonymous hemianopsia of contralateral visual field (occipital cortex) ■ Other visual field defects including vertical gaze and oculomotor nerve palsy ■ If dominant hemisphere affected, anomia (difficulty naming objects) or alexia (inability to read) may occur	Pupillary reflexes spared
Posterior inferior cerebellar	Clinical: Sudden onset of: ■ Nausea/vomiting ■ Vertigo ■ Hoarseness ■ Ataxia ■ Ipsilateral palate and tongue weakness ■ Contralateral disturbance of pain and temperature sensation ■ Dysphagia, dysarthria, and hiccup ■ Ipsilateral Horner's syndrome (ptosis, miosis, hemianhidrosis, and apparent enophthalmos)	1. Motor system typically spared 2. Lateral medullary (Wallenberg's) syndrome Horner's syndrome: **HORNE** **H**—hemianhidrosis (loss of sweating) **O**—one eye (usually unilateral) **R**—relaxed eyelid (ptosis) **N**—narrow pupil (miosis) **E**—enophthalmos (sunken eyes)
Anterior inferior cerebellar	Definition: Infarction of lateral portion of pons Clinical: ■ Ipsilateral facial weakness ■ Gaze palsy ■ Deafness ■ Tinnitus	No Horner's syndrome, dysphagia, or dysarthria

(continued)

TABLE 2.9-1. Neurological Deficits in Stroke *(continued)*

Artery Occlusion	Deficit	Other
Lacunar	Lenticulostriate branches of the middle cerebral artery (midbrain) become occluded as a result of chronic hypertension. ▪ Symptoms may present gradually over several days. ▪ CT or MRI may not detect stroke. Presentations: ▪ Pure motor hemiparesis: Affecting face, arm, leg without other disturbances ▪ Pure sensory stroke: Hemisensory loss ▪ Ataxic hemiparesis: Pure motor hemiparesis combined with ataxia ▪ Clumsy hand dysarthria: Dysarthria, dysphagia, facial weakness, and weakness/clumsiness of contralateral hand	

- Twenty-two percent of men and 25% of women who have an initial stroke die within a year.

The strongest risk factor is **hypertension,** with **smoking** as a close second.

Risk Factors

Ischemic

- Hypertension
- Smoking
- Diabetes mellitus
- Dyslipidemia
- Atrial fibrillation
- Hypercoagulable state
- Recent MI

Hemorrhagic

- Hypertension
- Arteriovenous malformation (AVM)
- Trauma
- Ruptured aneurysm
- Bleeding diathesis/anticoagulation

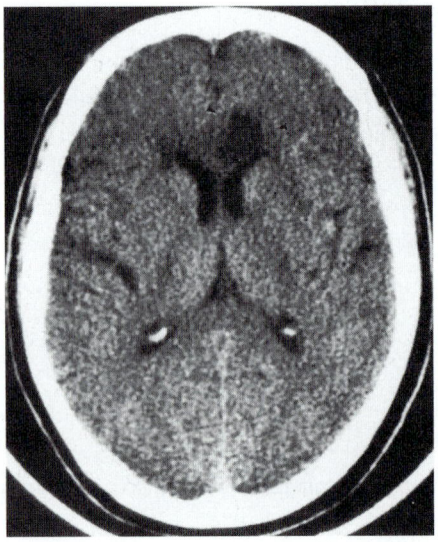

FIGURE 2.9-1. CT of ischemic stroke of the anterior cerebral artery (ACA). Note that the lesion is hypodense.

(Reproduced, with permission, from Johnson MH. CT evaluation of the earliest signs of stroke. *The Radiologist* 1(4):189–199, 1994.)

Classification and Etiology

Ischemic Stroke

- **Thrombotic:**
  - Large-vessel disease—atherosclerosis usually located at bifurcation of carotid, vertebrobasilar system, or middle cerebral artery
  - Small-vessel disease—microatheroma or lipohyalinosis usually due to HTN or DM, causing lacunar infarcts in subcortical tissues
- **Embolic:** Usually of cardiac origin (60%), source often unknown, sometimes carotid (artery-to-artery embolus)
- **Hypoperfusion:** Shock, etc.; most affect *watershed* areas (most commonly parasagittal strips of cortex)

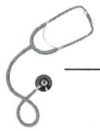

Watershed injury describes ischemic injury to brain tissue located at distal end of cerebrovascular tree, usually due to a low-flow state.

Hemorrhagic Stroke

- **Subarachnoid:** Head trauma most common, aneurysms, AV malformations
- **Intracerebral:** Hypertension, amyloid, bleeding disorders, trauma, tumors

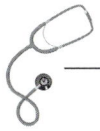

There is < 5% risk of stroke per year in patients with atrial fibrillation.

Metabolic Stroke

- Not necessarily related to vasculature/territories.
- Usually secondary to cerebral energy failure.
- Often resolves without deficits.

Venous Stroke

- Usually from thrombosis of cerebral veins/dural sinus.
- Does not obey territories
- Often hemorrhagic

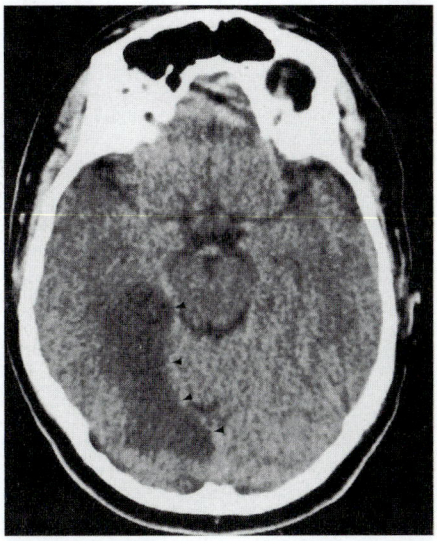

FIGURE 2.9-2. Low attenuation area within the cerebellum posteriorly on the right (arrow) suggestive of infarct in right PICA distribution.

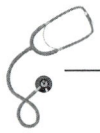

The initial CT should be done *without* contrast as fresh blood is radiolucent relative to old blood and normal cerebral tissue. Contrast-enhanced CT or MRI is useful subsequently to reveal regions of infarct.

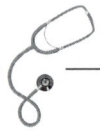

TIAs preceding thrombotic strokes tend to present with similar symptoms because the transient ischemia is locked to the distribution of the stenotic artery. Conversely, TIAs preceding embolic strokes tend to have more variable presentation.

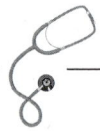

Thrombolytic therapy is not indicated for extremely mild or severe strokes. Other contraindications are the same as for MI.

Pathophysiology

Ischemic Stroke

- Occlusion of artery feeding brain causes oxygen depletion and damage to neurons.
- The ensuing ischemia results in release of inflammatory cytokines, which decreases flow by increasing viscosity. These cytokines further damage neuronal function.
- With reperfusion of ischemic area, oxygen free radicals are produced, which also damage neurons.

Hemorrhagic Stroke (see Figure 2.9-3)

- The extravasation of blood into the central nervous system (CNS) resulting from subarachnoid hemorrhage, hypertension, or bleeding into a prior ischemic stroke

Signs and Symptoms

- Thrombotic strokes often show relatively slow progressive onset, often during sleep.
- Embolic strokes present suddenly, often in discrete steps ("stuttering onset"), most often during waking hours.
- Hemorrhagic strokes evolve over minutes, invariably during waking hours.
- Twenty percent of stroke patients have a history of at least one TIA.

Diagnosis/Workup

- A noncontrast CT scan is useful for quick diagnosis and localization. It can also be helpful to exclude hemorrhagic infarcts.
- MRI/MRA for further study and follow-up
- Carotid ultrasound to screen for carotid stenosis

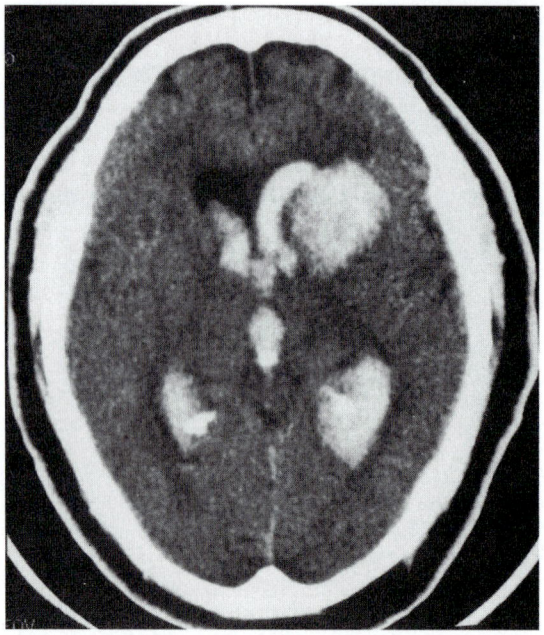

FIGURE 2.9-3. Head CT demonstrating hemorrhagic infarct.

- Cardiac echocardiography may be used to screen for embolic source. Transesophageal echo (TEE) is most sensitive. A bubble study may be performed to evaluate for a patent foramen ovale. Also need to look for atrial/aortic thrombus or dilated atria.
- ECG to look for atrial fibrillation

Treatment

TIA

- Main "treatment" involves assessment of risk factors, and diagnostic studies to see if there is a correctable cause for brain ischemia (e.g., critical carotid stenosis).
- Beyond that, patients should be started on a daily aspirin or alternative antiplatelet agent.

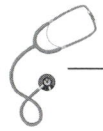

There has been no advantage shown of alternative antiplatelet agents such as clopidogrel or ticlopidine over ASA. Use of these alternative agents should be reserved for those who have a true allergy to aspirin, or those who have had their stroke while on aspirin.

General Measures for Stroke

- Correct hypoxemia (supplemental oxygen), hypoglycemia (D50), hypotension (IVF), and hyperthermia (acetaminophen).
- Deep venous thrombosis (DVT) prophylaxis (compression stockings, low-molecular-weight subcutaneous injections)
- Regular turning of comatose patients to prevent decubitus ulcers
- NPO initially, then parenteral feeding for those without intact gag reflex to avoid risk of aspiration

Ischemic Stroke

- Monitor BP. Do not treat acutely unless other acute conditions such as concurrent myocardial infarction (MI), aortic dissection, hypertensive encephalopathy, congestive heart failure (CHF), or acute renal failure (ARF) are present.
- Treat sBP > 220, dBP > 110, or mean arterial pressure (MAP) > 130. Start with labetalol 10 mg IV. Do not decrease the MAP more than 20%.
- For patients who present within 3 hours of symptom onset, IV t-PA is an FDA-approved option, currently considered standard of care. Patients must have a moderate-sized stroke and have no contraindications to thrombolytic therapy.
- Investigational therapies include intra-arterial t-PA and mechanical clot retrieval via coil introduced through the groin.
- Anticoagulation is not indicated acutely; there is little evidence to support its use in any given case, although you will still see it being used. Often reserved for refractory cases and piosterior circulation stroke.
- Aspirin or other antiplatelet agent both acutely and once daily following hospital discharge

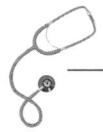

Remember, decreasing the systemic perfusion pressure (BP) causes a corresponding decrease in cerebral perfusion pressure in ischemic stroke and can be detrimental, as it can extend the area of infarct. Be **very** careful when lowering BP in stroke.

Hemorrhagic Stroke

- Elevate head of the bed 30 degrees.
- Provide a quiet environment, analgesia, and sedation as needed.
- Treat elevated intracranial pressure with hyperventilation, hyperosmolar agents (mannitol, glycerol), and steroids as needed.
- Prevent straining (Valsalva) with antitussives and stool softeners as needed.
- Nimodipine 60 mg for subarachnoid hemorrhage (to reduce vasospasm)
- BP control (more important in hemorrhagic than ischemic stroke)

Brain Herniation

Definition

The movement of brain tissue into a space that it does not normally occupy, which can lead to coma and death. It is usually caused by a mass/lesion; can be caused by a bleed.

Classification

Transtentorial herniation: The upper thalamic region herniates downward through the tentorium.

- *Uncal herniation* is a common type of transtentorial herniation in which the gyrus moves through the anterior section of the tentorial opening.
- The third nerve is often affected by the brain tissue that is displaced.
- Patients often present with an enlarged pupil on the ipsilateral side of the herniation as well as a contralateral hemiparesis.
- This is often followed by coma.

Subfalcine herniation: The cingulate gyrus herniates across the midline.

- Clinically, this may compromise blood flow through the anterior cerebral artery and can present as a headache.
- Anterior cerebral artery infarction is a complication of this type of herniation.

Central herniation: The entire cerebral hemisphere herniates across the tentorium as a result of increased intracranial pressure.

Tonsillar herniation: This is a result of increased pressure in the posterior fossa, causing parts of the cerebellum to herniate through the foramen magnum.

- This type of herniation results in compression of the lower brain stem.

CNS Infections

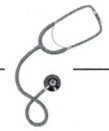

A patient with encephalitis, hydrophobia, and aerophobia should have rabies virus workup.

RABIES

Respiratory failure
Aerophobia,
  Apprehension,
  Aversion to water
Bad pains
Irritability
Excitation
Seizures

▶ RABIES

Definition

A rapidly progressing viral infection affecting the human nervous system; usually from raccoons or bats

Epidemiology

- Fewer than 10 cases per year in United States
- 50% of cases from raccoon bites
- Other cases transmitted by dogs, skunks, foxes, coyotes, bats, and bobcats
- Rare cases from tissue transplantation (cornea)

Signs and Symptoms

- Two phases:
  - *Prodromal phase:* Pain, paresthesias, GI/respiratory symptoms, irri-

tability, apprehension, **hydrophobia** (aversion to swallowing water because of pain), aerophobia (fear of fresh air)
  - *Excitation phase:* Hyperventilation, hyperactivity, disorientation, and seizures
- Patient becomes increasingly lethargic. Further involvement of cardiac and respiratory nerves leads to death.

Diagnosis

- Fluorescent antibody staining, polymerase chain reaction
- Presence of Negri bodies on nuchal biopsy

Treatment

- Wash affected area thoroughly with soap and water.
- No antiviral therapy available
- Supportive treatment:
  - Rabies immunoglobulin (passive immunization)
  - Human diploid cell rabies vaccine (active immunization: Because of long incubation period, early injections provide sufficient time for protective immunity.
  - Active and passive immunization are administered in different parts of body so that immunoglobulin (passive) does not neutralize the vaccine (active).
- Isolation of patient
- Preexposure prevention with vaccine should be used for high-risk individuals like zookeepers and veterinarians.

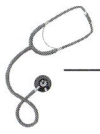

Rabies is universally fatal unless vaccine is given prior to the onset of symptoms. Immunize for:
- **Raccoon bites**
- **Skunk bites**
- **Bat exposure (bite may be too small to see)**
- **Fox bites**
- **Bite from feral dog or cat**

▶ BACTERIAL MENINGITIS

Definition

Acute infection of the subarachnoid space and leptomeninges

Causes
- *Streptococcus pneumoniae* (40 to 60%)
- *Neisseria meningitidis* (young adults)
- *Listeria monocytogenes* (immunocompromised hosts and very young or old)
- Gram-negative bacilli
- *Haemophilus influenzae* (unimmunized adults)
- Group B strep (neonates)

Kernig's sign: Extending the knee with the thigh at right angles causes pain in back and hamstring.
Brudzinski's sign: Forced neck flexion results in flexion at the knee and hip.

Pathophysiology

- Bacteria commonly colonize the nasopharynx, which can then enter the bloodstream.
- Via the blood, the bacteria make their way into the CSF through the choroid plexus.
- Most signs and symptoms are secondary to the body's own inflammatory response.
- Bacteremia, sinusitis, otitis, and direct trauma could predispose to meningitis.

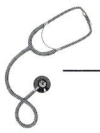

Herniation from LP occurs 1% of time and is more likely to occur in those with focal neurological findings.

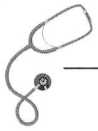

Low glucose is caused by bacterial inhibition of glucose transport into the CSF, not bacterial consumption. The value should be compared to a concurrently determined blood glucose level.

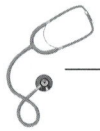

When meningitis is suspected on clinical grounds, do not wait for results of lab tests or imaging studies: Treat empirically!

Signs and Symptoms

- Triad of headache, stiff neck, and fever (95%)
- Mental changes such as confusion, lethargy, or coma in 80%
- Seizures occur in 10 to 30%.
- Nausea, vomiting, and photophobia are common complaints.
- Look for classic maculopapular rash of meningococcemia.

Diagnosis

- Blood culture positive in 50 to 60%
- Lumbar puncture (see Table 2.9-2):
  - Neutrophil count, protein, and opening pressure increased
  - Monocytes may predominate in cases of *Listeria*.
  - Glucose decreased
  - Check Gram stain for presence of microorganisms.
  - Cerebrospinal fluid (CSF) culture positive in 80%
- CT before LP to rule out abscess as source of meningeal irritation/infection and mass effect. These pose risk of herniation during LP.

Treatment

- Good empiric coverage includes third-generation cephalosporin and vancomycin.
- Empiric treatment with antibiotics based on age. This is adjusted once when the Gram stain or sensitivity results are completed.
- *Streptococcus pneumoniae:* Vancomycin + cefotaxime or ceftriaxone
- *N. meningitidis:* Penicillin G or ceftriaxone
- If patient is at risk for *Listeria* (old, young, or immunocompromised), you must add ampicillin.
- Add steroids before antibiotics if *S. pneumoniae* is the cause (decreases neurologic sequelae).

▶ VIRAL MENINGITIS

- Increased incidence in summer, early fall
- Most commonly caused by enterovirus
- Also called aseptic meningitis

TABLE 2.9-2. CSF Findings in Meningitis and Abscess

	WBCs	Diff.	Protein	Glucose	Opening Pressure
Bacterial meningitis	Very high	Polys	High	Low	High
Viral meningitis	High	Lymphs/monos	Norm	Norm	Norm/high
TB/fungal meningitis	High	Lymphs/monos	High	Low	High
Brain abscess	Norm/high	Polys	High	Low	Very high

- More common than bacterial
- Course is more benign.
- Signs and symptoms are similar to bacterial, but less pronounced (patient does not appear toxic).
- CSF shows normal to low protein, normal to high glucose, and lymphocytosis. Cultures and PCR can usually identify the cause.
- Treatment is supportive except in cases of varicella or herpes, in which antiviral therapy might be useful.

▶ BOTULISM

Definition

A paralytic disease caused by the toxin of *Clostridium botulinum*, resulting in presynaptic destruction of neuromuscular junction

Etiology

- Ingestion of improperly prepared home processed foods, canned foods
- Wound contamination

Pathophysiology

- Toxin blocks the release of acetylcholine at the peripheral nerve endings.
- Usual incubation period is 18 to 36 hours.
- A descending paralysis ensues, leading to respiratory failure and death.

Signs and Symptoms

- *Neurologic:* Dry mouth, diplopia, dysphagia, dysarthria, descending weakness of the extremities and muscles of ventilation
- *GI:* Nausea, vomiting, diarrhea, abdominal cramps
- Patient will generally be afebrile.

Diagnosis

Detection of neurotoxin by serology, only in specialized labs

Treatment

Ingestion
- Antitoxin
- Vomiting and cathartics can be used to decrease absorption.

Wound Contamination
- Drainage of lesion, antitoxin, and penicillin

For Both
- Intubation with ventilatory support

Prevention

The toxin can be inactivated after 10 minutes in boiling water. The spores, however, can withstand boiling temperatures for several hours.

Botulinum spores in honey can replicate in the gut of a newborn (who does not have normal bacterial flora yet) and cause botulism.

Signs of botulism
"5 Ds"
- **D**ry mouth
- **D**iplopia
- **D**ysphagia
- **D**ysarthria
- **D**escending weakness

Due to the great potency of the toxin, botulinum has been considered a potential biological weapon.

Seizure Disorders

Status epilepticus is a long continuous seizure lasting 30 minutes or two or more seizures in a row without a lucid interval.

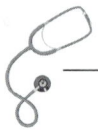

Remember: Status epilepticus is a true emergency, and the ABCs of CPR must be initiated.

3-Hz spike and wave is the pathognomonic EEG pattern of absence seizures.

Loss of bowel or bladder function and tongue biting are important clues in the diagnosis of a seizure.

INH causes seizures refractory to anticonvulsant therapy. They are treated with pyridoxine (B_6).

Definition

- Seizure: Abnormal and excessive neuronal discharge causing a transient disturbance of cerebral function
- Epilepsy: Two or more unprovoked seizures
- One percent of population has disease.
- A range of effects can be seen, from the asymptomatic to overt convulsions.

Classification

- Partial: Focal, only part of cortex involved:
  - Simple: No loss of consciousness (LOC), no postictal state
  - Complex: Postictal state present, LOC may or may not be present
- Generalized: Always associated with LOC, whole cortex is involved:
  - Absence (petit mal): Brief episode of nonresponsiveness to external or internal stimuli; motor tone is preserved
  - Tonic–clonic (grand mal): Generalized convulsion—brief tonic phase (stiffening) followed by clonic phase (rhythmic jerking)

Etiology

- Fever
- Idiopathic
- Head trauma
- Stroke
- Mass lesions
- Meningitis/encephalitis (infectious)
- Metabolic: Hypoglycemia, hyponatremia, hyperosmolarity, hypocalcemia, uremia, hepatic encephalopathy, porphyria, drugs, eclampsia, hyperthermia
- Brain malformation/dysplastic cortex

Diagnosis

- Electroencephalogram (EEG)
- CT or MRI to rule out any lesions
- Routine blood tests and toxicology screen to rule out metabolic or drug-induced seizures

Treatment

- Address underlying cause if appropriate.
- Anticonvulsant therapy:
  - Benzodiazepines to break ongoing seizure
  - Phenytoin, carbamazepine, and valproic acid are common preventive medications for seizure.

Brain Neoplasms

See Table 2.9-3 for individual types.

TABLE 2.9-3. CNS Tumors

Tumor	Description
Astrocytoma	▪ Most common neuroectodermal tumor ▪ Those occurring in adults are usually high grade—poor prognosis. ▪ *Glioblastoma multiforme* (GBM) is an aggressive anaplastic type.
Central nervous system lymphomas	▪ Originate from B cells that have entered the CNS ▪ Commonly affects eyes, spinal cord, or leptomeninges ▪ Presents with headache, vision problems, and behavioral/personality changes ▪ Diagnose by identifying malignant lymphocytes. ▪ Treatment with chemotherapy, radiation, and steroids
Oligodendrogliomas	▪ Tend to calcify ▪ More benign and better prognosis than astrocytoma ▪ Epileptogenic
Ependymoma	▪ In adults, characteristically found in spinal canal ▪ In children, most common location in 4th ventricle ▪ With excision, 5-year survival rate is 80%.
Meningiomas	▪ Most common mesodermal tumor ▪ Usually benign and slow growing, but usually discovered at large size ▪ Clinically, may present as a cranial nerve palsy
Schwannomas	▪ Most common cranial nerve tumor ▪ Vestibular (acoustic) neuromas are 8th cranial nerve tumors. Anyone with unilateral deafness should have this ruled out. ▪ Associated with neurofibromatosis type 1 > type 2
Pituitary tumors	See endocrinology chapter.
Metastatic tumors to CNS	▪ 80,000 per year ▪ More common than primary tumors ▪ Metastases common from lung, breast, and malignant melanoma

Etiology

- Exposure to ionizing radiation
- Hereditary syndromes (i.e., neureofibromatosis, tuberous sclerosis)
- HIV (lymphoma is typically of the B-cell subtype)

Astrocytomas are the most common primary intracranial neoplasms.

Epidemiology

- Kills > 13,000 per year
- Most common solid tumor of childhood
- Originates from brain, spinal cord, or meninges
- Most common:

- Glial origin (50 to 60%)
- Meningiomas (25%)
- Schwannomas (8%)

In migraines, prolonged headache may be followed several hours later by vomiting. In brain tumors, acute headache is followed immediately by vomiting.

Signs and Symptoms

- Headache (40%); usually the result of increased intracranial pressure:
  - Present upon awakening and disappears within 1 hour (but can take any form)
  - Can wake patient from sleep
  - Worse while lying supine
  - New headache in middle-aged or older person
  - Change in headache character in person with chronic headaches
- Nausea or vomiting especially on awakening
- Irritability, apathy
- Sometimes vision loss, weakness of extremities
- Seizures, focal neurologic deficits
- Lethargy, weight loss more common with metastatic disease

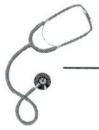

A spinal tap can induce brain herniation in patients. Be careful with mass effect. Remember: CT before LP.

Diagnosis/Workup

- MRI/CT for detection of mass and preliminary diagnosis
- Biopsy for histology and definitive diagnosis
- PET scans and EEG occasionally have some diagnostic role.

Treatment

- Corticosteroids to decrease edema and intracranial pressure
- Surgical resection, if possible
- Radiation and perhaps chemotherapy for high-grade tumors

Neuropathies

▶ Myasthenia Gravis

Forty to 50% of patients with ocular myasthenia gravis go on to develop generalized myasthenia gravis.

Pathophysiology

Autoimmune disease in which antibodies against the postsynaptic nicotinic acetylcholine receptor prevent acetylcholine from binding. Therefore, an end-plate potential is decreased at the neuromuscular junction.

Epidemiology

- Two peaks of incidence:
  - Women in 2nd to 3rd decade
  - Men older than 60
- Twenty percent have thyroid disease.
- 10% thymoma, 70% thymic hyperplasia

Symptoms worsen as day progresses. (This is the opposite of rheumatoid arthritis.)

Signs and Symptoms

- Muscular weakness and fatigue
- Ptosis and diplopia (by affecting muscles of eye)

- Proximal muscle weakness
- Intact reflexes
- Nasal speech, dysphagia
- Myasthenic crisis: Severe, life-threatening exacerbation, usually compromising respiratory status, and often requiring ventilatory support

Diagnosis

- Myasthenia antibodies on serology
- Edrophonium (Tensilon™) test: Edrophonium, which inhibits acetylcholinesterase, is given to the patient and a set of muscle groups is observed. In order for the test to be positive, the patient's muscle strength must improve, which is due to the increased availability of acetylcholine at the postsynaptic receptor (typically this test is used in acute setting).
- *Repetitive nerve stimulation* will display a quick reduction in the amplitude of the action potentials in myasthenic patients.
- CT of chest for thymoma/thymic hyperplasia

Labs and Tests

- Antibody presence against acetylcholine receptor (AChR)
- Chest MRI to evaluate any thymus abnormalities

Treatment

- Most patients are able to have normal lives.
- If mild, anticholinesterase drug
- Thymectomy when indicated (most patients experience long-term improvement)
- Prednisone as first line therapy
- Cyclosporine or azathioprine if prednisone not effective
- Plasmapheresis and immunoglobulin therapy can also be useful.
- Patients in crisis should get steroids, PFTs, ICU admission, but not acetylcholinesterase inhibitors until crisis is under control.

In myasthenia gravis, repetitive muscle use quickly induces fatigue, whereas in Eaton–Lambert syndrome, repetitive muscle use improves muscle strength.

Aminoglycosides can precipitate myasthenic crisis.

▶ GUILLAIN-BARRÉ SYNDROME

Definition

Syndrome of transient immune-mediated ascending paralysis usually following a viral upper respiratory tract infection

Etiology

- Most cases are preceded by a respiratory or GI infection.
- *Campylobacter jejuni*, HSV, CMV, EBV, and *Mycoplasma* have all been identified as potential causes.
- Vaccines have been implicated as a potential cause in the past (i.e., influenza, rabies vaccines).

Pathophysiology

An immune-mediated demyelination of axons/axonopathy can also occur.

Signs and Symptoms

- Initial symptoms include paresthesias in the feet (or arms) and leg weakness, which progresses as an ascending motor paralysis, usually over several days.
- Distal muscle weakness is common soon afterward—may last a few weeks.
- Deep aching pain in back and legs
- Areflexia
- Tachypnea
- Quadriparesis and respiratory muscle paralysis occur in 30% of patients, and one-third of patients will need mechanical ventilation.
- Respiratory muscle paralysis can be fatal.
- Cranial nerves can be involved.

Diagnosis

- CSF shows increased protein, but no WBCs.
- EMG shows signs of demyelination with marked decrease in action potential conduction velocities.
- The diagnosis is usually made clinically since CSF and EMG testing are often normal in the early course of this syndrome.

Treatment

- Most patients will have to be hospitalized.
- Mechanical ventilation for respiratory muscle paralysis
- Plasma exchange and IV immunoglobulin in selected patients
- Reassurance. Most patients make a full recovery, although < 5% of patients die from respiratory failure.
- Most cases resolve spontaneously over the course of several weeks to months.

Headache

Top 10 Causes of Headache

- Chronic headache syndromes (migraine, cluster, tension headaches)
- Subarachnoid hemorrhage
- Meningitis
- Hypertension
- Mass lesion
- Temporal arteritis
- Trigeminal neuralgia
- Brain abscess
- Pseudotumor cerebri
- Subdural hematoma

▶ MIGRAINE HEADACHE

Pathophysiology

According to the vasogenic theory, cerebral vasoconstriction is followed by vasodilation. It is thought that there are genetic and hormonal components to migraines.

Epidemiology

- 60% have family history.
- 12% in United States affected
- Females > males

Signs and Symptoms

1. *Migraine with aura (classic):* Patient suffers from aura approximately 1 hour before onset. The focal neurological dysfunction can include photophobia, sonophobia, nausea, vomiting, vertigo, dysarthria, tinnitus, diploplia, weakness, and ataxia. Patient may also complain of scintillating scotoma or homonymous hemianopsia.
2. *Migraine without aura (common):* Photophobia and sonophobia are again noted, along with anorexia, nausea, vomiting, and general malaise. Specific visual findings are usually not involved.

Both types have prodromal symptoms 1 to 2 days before attack. These include lethargy, craving of food, depression, and fluid retention.

Headache phase of migraine may last several hours. It is characterized by a unilateral, throbbing head pain.

Treatment

- Nonpharmacologic: Avoidance of triggers, stress reduction, dark quiet environment
- Acute treatment:
  - Nonsteroidal anti-inflammatory drugs (NSAIDs)
  - Ergotamine derivatives
  - 5-HT receptor agonists (sumatriptan)
  - Antiemetics (metoclopramide IV)
- Valproic acid, tricyclics, gabapentin

Prophylaxis: Calcium channel blockers, beta blockers, tricyclics, and serotonergic drugs

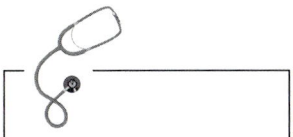

Triggers of migraines include: red wine, chocolate, MSG, lack of sleep, menses, stress.

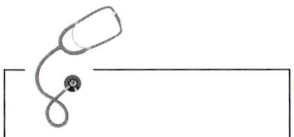

5-HT receptor agonists can cause coronary vasospasm.

▶ TENSION HEADACHE

Signs and Symptoms

- Muscular contractions causing bandlike pain located in head and neck
- Neck stiffness
- Usually bilateral
- No prodrome
- Worsens as the day progresses

Treatment

- Aspirin or acetaminophen
- Narcotics if severe
- Prophylaxis with tricyclics such as amitriptyline
- Relaxation

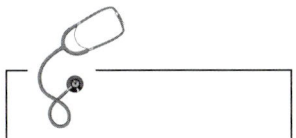

Tension headache may benefit from head and neck massage.

A 38-year-old man presents with drooling and right facial nerve paralysis. On exam, he has vesicular lesions or erythematous bases in the ear canal. *Think: Ramsay Hunt syndrome.*

Causes of painful vision loss:
- Optic neuritis
- Giant cell arteritis
- Acute angle-closure glaucoma

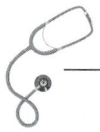

More than 50% of patients with temporal arteritis have polymyalgia rheumatica.

Typical scenario:
A 62-year-old woman presents with headache, pain when she chews, and scalp tenderness. *Think: Temporal arteritis.* Treat with steroids. This can save vision.

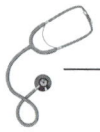

Refer to ophthalmologist when suspecting temporal arteritis to aid in prevention of vision loss.

▶ CLUSTER HEADACHE

Definition

A severe vascular headache that clusters in the same area of the head and time of day, usually lasting for several weeks

Epidemiology

- Increased incidence in males than females
- Increased incidence after alcohol, nitrates, or stress

Signs and Symptoms

- Unrelenting unilateral facial pain, which tends to occur in clusters
- Pain so severe it can lead to suicide
- Headaches are often seasonal.
- Accompanied by ipsilateral autonomic signs, including conjunctival injection, lacrimation, rhinorrhea, nasal congestion, ptosis, miosis, eyelid edema, and facial sweating

Treatment

Acute Episodes
- High-flow oxygen
- Intranasal lidocaine
- Ergotamine, sumatriptan, and antiemetics if the above fail

Prophylaxis
- Verapamil, methysergide, high-dose prednisone followed by rapid taper, lithium, or indomethacin

▶ HEADACHE OF TEMPORAL (GIANT CELL) ARTERITIS

Definition

Idiopathic inflammation of medium and large arteries, usually the temporal artery, histologically characterized by giant multinucleated cells

Etiology

Thought to be part of a systemic vasculitis that has gone undetected except for the temporal and ophthalmic artery involvement

Epidemiology

More common in women and persons older than 60

Signs and Symptoms

- Unilateral headache in distribution of temporal artery
- Thickened, tender temporal arteries
- Ipsilateral visual loss (ophthalmic artery)

- Claudication of the masseter, temporalis, and tongue muscles
- Scalp tenderness
- Pulsating temporal artery, also sometimes nodular

Diagnosis

- High erythrocyte sedimentation rate (ESR), C-reactive protein
- Definitive diagnosis by temporal artery biopsy
- Anemia is frequently seen.

Treatment

- Corticosteroids as soon as suspected; can lead to blindness if treatment is delayed
- NSAIDs for pain relief

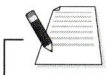

The most common cause of blindness in the United States is macular degeneration.

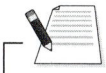

Causes of painless vision loss:

- Central retinal artery occlusion (pallor and cherry red spot)
- Central retinal vein occlusion (thunderstorm)
- Retinal detachment (curtain)

▶ ACUTE VISION LOSS

See Table 2.9-4 for differential diagnosis.

TABLE 2.9-4. Differential Diagnosis for Acute Vision Loss

Differential Diagnosis	Description	Treatment
Central retinal artery occlusion	▪ Typically painless loss of vision ▪ Causes ischemic stroke of retina ▪ Cherry red spot on fovea	Dissolve or dislodge embolus
Retinal detachment	▪ Symptoms include flashes of light. ▪ Floaters ▪ Vision loss	Surgery or laser treatment
Vitreous hemorrhage	▪ Caused by bleeding into vitreous humor ▪ Common causes are diabetic retinopathy and retinal tears. ▪ Symptoms initially include floaters, which progress to vision loss.	Photocoagulation or vitrectomy
Optic neuritis	▪ Painful, unilateral vision loss with partial resolution ▪ Inflammation of optic nerve or absence of clinical findings ▪ Caused by demyelination ▪ Visual acuity at its worst in 1 week ▪ Other symptoms include headache and eye pain with movement. ▪ Many patients have progression to multiple sclerosis.	Steroids
Temporal (giant cell) arteritis	▪ See description under Headaches	

NEUROLOGICAL DISORDERS

▶ DEMENTIA

Causes of dementia:
Vincent Van Gogh was demented.
Vitamin deficiency
Infection
NPH
CVA
Epilepsy
Neurodegeneration
Trauma, tumors, toxins

DEFINITION

Loss of cognitive function with normal sensorium

ETIOLOGY

- Stroke
- Infection (particularly syphilis, AIDS, Creutzfeldt–Jakob)
- Epilepsy
- Vitamin deficiency (folate, B_{12}, thiamine, niacin)
- Normal pressure hydrocephalus (NPH)
- Neurodegenerative disorders (Alzheimer's, Parkinson's, Huntington's, amyotrophic lateral sclerosis)
- Trauma
- Toxins
- Tumors

DIAGNOSIS/WORKUP

Dementia workup should include CBC, electrolyte panel, B_{12}, folate, rapid plasma reagin (RPR), and head CT.

TREATMENT

- Treat underlying disorder.
- Optimize sensory function (vision aids, hearing aids).
- Simplify activities of daily living (simplify floor plans, stairs).
- Ensure physical safety (bedrails, companions).

▶ ALZHEIMER'S DISEASE

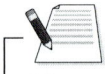

Alzheimer's is the most common cause of dementia.

DEFINITION

- Slowly progressive dementia characterized by amyloid plaques and neurofibrillary tangles in the neurons of the cerebral cortex (mostly temporal lobe)

EPIDEMIOLOGY

- Older people
- Family history (apolipoprotein E genotype)
- Higher incidence in patients with Down syndrome

SIGNS AND SYMPTOMS

- Usually present with subtle onset of memory deficits accompanied by a progressive dementia

- The earliest signs may include the inability to pay bills, go shopping, or other routine daily activities.
- Later on, patients will display aphasia, apraxia, confusion, and hallucinations.
- Patients may become incontinent, mute, and require constant assistance with most tasks.

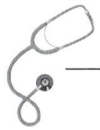

Alzheimer's disease is definitively diagnosed by tissue examination on autopsy.

Diagnosis

- Diagnosis is mainly clinical; other causes of dementia need to be ruled out.
- Cortical atrophy on CT or MRI (see Figure 2.9-4)
- EEG slowing later in disease

Treatment

- Donepezil, tacrine, and selegiline may slow cognitive decline.
- Memantine, vitamin E, exercise, and mental activity may be protective.
- Behavioral symptoms can be treated with neuroleptics, anxiolytics, and antidepressants.

▶ PARKINSON'S DISEASE

Definition

Complex progressive disorder involving movement and higher cognitive function

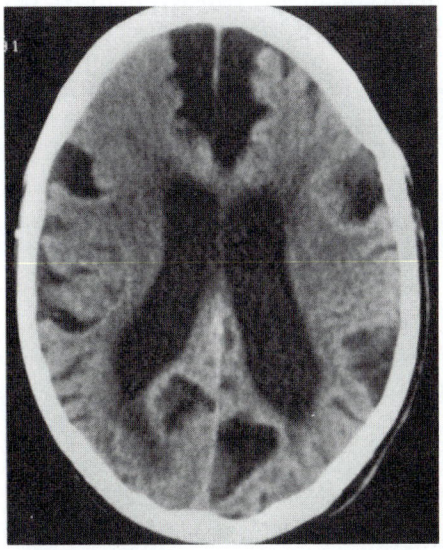

FIGURE 2.9-4. Alzheimer's disease. Note the severe frontal atrophy.

(Reproduced, with permission, from Lee SH, Rao K, Zimmerman RA [eds]. *Cranial MRI and CT.* New York: McGraw-Hill, 1999:194.)

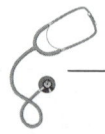

Remember: Parkinson's is marked by a resting tremor, and essential tremor occurs with movement.

Etiology

- Degeneration of neurons in the substantia nigra
- May be secondary to toxins (manganese, carbon monoxide, designer drugs) and encephalitis

Epidemiology

Mean age is 55; more common in men (3:2).

Signs and Symptoms

Signs and symptoms fluctuate:

- **Pill-rolling resting tremor** (thumb rubs fingers)
- **Cogwheel rigidity** (actually a tremor)
- **Bradykinesia**
- Shuffling gait, festinating gait
- Mask facies
- Depression, hallucinations
- Impaired autonomic dysfunction (gastroparesis, orthostatic hypotension)

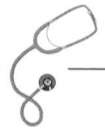

Cognitive decline is a late feature of Parkinson's.

Diagnosis

- Clinical presentation
- Response to levodopa–carbidopa

Treatment

The pathophysiologic opposite of Parkinson's disease (dopamine paucity) is schizophrenia (dopamine excess).

- Amantadine may improve tremor and bradykinesia in early disease by blocking reuptake of dopamine into presynaptic neurons.
- Levodopa: Converted to dopamine in substantia nigra; co-administer with carbidopa (does not cross BBB) to block metabolism of levodopa in peripheral tissues.
- Anticholinergics: Block cholinergic inhibition of dopaminergic neurons in substantia nigra; commonly trihexyphenidyl, benztropine mesylate
- Selegiline: Selective MAO-B inhibitor, blocks central metabolism of dopamine
- Dopamine receptor agonists such as bromocriptine, pergolide, pramipexole

▶ NORMAL PRESSURE HYDROCEPHALUS (NPH)

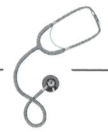

NPH is one of the few reversible causes of dementia.

Definition

A distinct clinical syndrome in the setting of hydrocephalus without increased intracranial pressure

Etiology

Most patients have no clear cause for the NPH; however, it can sometimes be seen after a CNS event (SAH, meningitis, trauma, tumor).

Signs and Symptoms

Classic Triad

- Gait disorder (most responsive to treatment)
- Urinary incontinence
- Dementia (most refractory to treatment)

Diagnosis

- Normal pressure on lumbar puncture (LP)
- Enlarged ventricles on CT or MRI
- Clinical improvement after LP and removal of a volume of CSF

Treatment

- CSF ventricular shunt
- Choroid plexectomy in some cases

A 58-year-old man went to a movie theater and experienced acute nausea, headache, and blurred vision. Exam shows dilated pupils with shallow anterior chamber. *Think: Acute angle-closure glaucoma.*

FEATURES OF BRAIN DEATH

- Preserved cardiac function
- No spontaneous respiratory function
- No cranial nerve reflexes (especially pupils)
- No posturing (decerebrate or decorticate)
- No evidence of hypothermia
- No known reversibility of state (drugs)

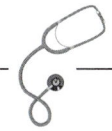

Brain death is death.

NOTES

HIGH-YIELD FACTS IN

Dermatology

Overview 331

- Top Causes of Rash with Fever 331
- Important Questions to Ask in Any Skin Condition 333

Immune-Mediated Diseases Associated with Skin Findings 333

- Immediate Type I Hypersensitivity Reactions (IgE Mediated) 333
- Hypersensitivity (Leukocytoclastic) Vasculitis 334

Eczema/Dermatitis 336

- Atopic Dermatitis/Eczema 336
- Allergic Contact Dermatitis 337
- Irritant Contact Dermatitis 337

Miscellaneous Inflammatory Conditions 338

- Pityriasis Rosea 338
- Psoriasis 339
- Erythema Nodosum 340
- Erythema Multiforme 341
- Stevens–Johnson Syndrome 343
- Toxic Epidermal Necrolysis 343
- Decubitus Ulcers 344

Skin Diseases Due to Microbial Agents 346

- Erysipelas 346
- Cellulitis 348
- Toxic Shock Syndrome (TSS) 349
- Meningococcemia 350
- Bacterial Endocarditis 351
- Rocky Mountain Spotted Fever (RMSF) 351
- Herpes Zoster 353
- Cutaneous Fungal Infections 355
- Lyme Borreliosis (Lyme Disease) 356
- Acne Vulgaris 357

Skin Cancers 358
Basal Cell Carcinoma 358
Squamous Cell Carcinoma 359
Malignant Melanoma 359

OVERVIEW

▶ TOP CAUSES OF RASH WITH FEVER

- Rubella
- Measles
- Staphylococcal scalded syndrome
- **Toxic shock syndrome**
- Scarlet fever
- **Meningococcemia**
- **Disseminated gonococcal infection**
- **Bacterial endocarditis**
- **Rocky Mountain spotted fever (RMSF)**
- Kawasaki's disease
- **Erythema nodosum**
- **Hypersensitivity vasculitis**

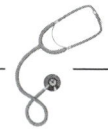

Rashes that can be seen on palms and soles: ***Mrs. E***

- **M**eningococcemia
- **R**MSF
- **S**yphilis
- **E**rythema multiforme

TABLE 2.10-1. Definitions of Primary Skin Lesions

Macule	A flat, nonpalpable area of skin discoloration (vitiligo, café au lait spot)
Papule	An elevated, palpable solid area of skin < 0.5 cm diameter (acne, lichen planus)
Plaque	An elevated area of skin > 2 cm diameter that has a larger surface area compared to its elevation above the skin (psoriasis, seborrheic keratosis)
Wheal	An elevated, rounded or flat topped area of dermal edema that disappears within hours (urticaria)
Vesicle	A circumscribed, elevated fluid-containing lesion of < 0.5 cm diameter (varicella zoster)
Bullae	A circumscribed, elevated fluid-containing lesion of > 0.5 cm diameter (pemphigus vulgaris)
Pustule	A circumscribed, elevated pus-containing lesion (acne, disseminated gonococcal infection)
Nodule	An elevated, palpable solid lesion > 0.5 cm diameter (nodulocystic acne, erythema nodosum)
Petechiae	A red-purple nonblanching macule < 0.5 cm diameter, usually pinpoint in size (meningococcemia)
Purpura	A red-purple nonblanching macule > 0.5 cm diameter (Henoch–Schönlein purpura)
Telangiectasia	A blanchable dilated blood vessel (rosacea, cirrhosis, Osler–Weber–Rendu)

TABLE 2.10-2. Definitions of Secondary Skin Lesions

Scale	An accumulation of dead, exfoliating epidermal cells
Crust	Dried serum, blood, or purulent exudate that accumulates on the skin surface (scab)
Erosion	A superficial loss of epidermis, leaving a denuded, moist surface; heals without scarring because doesn't penetrate through dermal–epidermal junction
Excoriation	A linear erosion produced by scratching
Ulcer	A loss of epidermis extending into dermis; heals with scarring because it penetrates into dermis
Scar	Replacement of normal skin with fibrous tissue as a result of healing
Atrophy	Thinning of skin
Lichenification	Thickening of epidermis with accentuation of normal skin markings

TABLE 2.10-3. Diagnostic Procedures Used in Dermatology

Diascopy	Pressing of a glass slide firmly against a red lesion will determine if it is due to capillary dilatation (blanchable) or to extravasation of blood (nonblanchable).
KOH preparation	Used to identify fungus and yeast. Scrape scales from skin, hair, or nails and treat with a 10% KOH solution to dissolve tissue material. Septated hyphae are revealed in fungal infections, and pseudohyphae and budding spores are revealed in yeast infections.
Tzanck preparation	Used to identify vesicular viral eruptions. Scrape the base of a vesicle and smear cells on a glass slide. Multinucleated giant cells will be identified in herpes simplex, herpes zoster, and varicella infections.
Scabies preparation	Scrape skin of a burrow between fingers, side of hands, axilla, or groin. Mites, eggs, or feces will be identified in scabies infection.
Use of Wood's lamp	Certain conditions will fluoresce when examined under a long-wave UV light ("black" lamp). Tinea capitis will fluoresce green or yellow on hair shaft.
Patch testing	Detects type IV delayed hypersensitivity reactions (allergic contact dermatitis). Nonirritating concentrations of suspected allergen are applied under occlusion to the back. Development of erythema, edema, and vesicles at site of contact 48 hours later indicates an allergy to offending agent.
Biopsy	Type of biopsy performed depends on the site of lesion, the type of tissue removed, and the desired cosmetic result. Shave biopsy is used for superficial lesions. Punch biopsy (3–5 mm diameter) can remove all or part of a lesion and provides tissue sample for pathology. Elliptical excisions provide more tissue than a punch biopsy and are used for deeper lesions or when the entire lesion needs to be sent to pathology.
Therapeutic modalities	Cryosurgery, curettage and electrodesiccation, phototherapy

► IMPORTANT QUESTIONS TO ASK IN ANY SKIN CONDITION

1. When did it start?
2. Where did it start?
3. Does it hurt? Itch? Other symptoms?
4. How has it spread?
5. How has each lesion changed over time?
6. What makes it worse? (sun, heat, pregnancy, cold, medications, exposures)
7. Previous treatments?

Immune-Mediated Diseases Associated with Skin Findings

► IMMEDIATE TYPE I HYPERSENSITIVITY REACTIONS (IgE MEDIATED)

- Immunologic reaction mediated by immunoglobulin E (IgE) and mast cells, characterized by vasodilation and transudation of fluid
- As the antigen binds to IgE on the mast cell surface, the mast cell degranulates and releases histamine, serotonin, heparin, leukotrienes, and prostaglandins.
- These inflammatory mediators cause vasodilation, increased capillary permeability, and smooth muscle contraction.
- Leakage of plasma into the dermis causes a swelling, characterized by a wheal.

Urticaria (Hives)

- Characterized by **wheals:** An abrupt development of transient edematous pink papules and plaques that may be localized or generalized and are usually pruritic
- Wheals may develop after exposure to circulating antigens (drugs, food, insect venom, animal dander, pollen), hot and cold temperatures, exercise, and pressure or rubbing (dermographism).
- Wheals usually last < 24 hours and may recur on future exposure to the antigen.

Angioedema

- Describes a deeper involvement of subcutaneous tissues with less demarcated swelling, usually characterized by swelling of the eyelids, lips, and tongue (see Figure 2.10-1).
- A hereditary form also exists, characterized by recurrent attacks of abdominal pain, vomiting, and edema of soft tissue, caused by a deficiency of C1 esterase.

Urticaria, angioedema, anaphylaxis, and atopic dermatitis are examples of type I hypersensitivity reactions occurring in the skin.

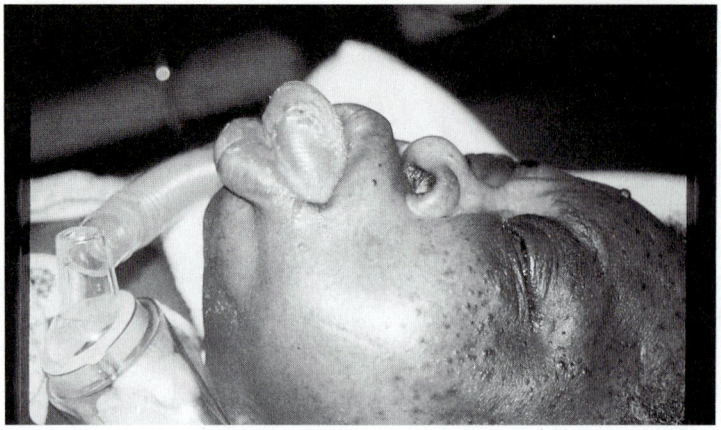

FIGURE 2.10-1. Angioedema.

(Reproduced, with permission, from Knoop KJ, Stack LB, Storrow AB. *Atlas of Emergency Medicine.* New York: McGraw-Hill, 1997:127.)

Anaphylaxis

The most severe systemic form of type I hypersensitivity reaction, is characterized by bronchoconstriction and hypotension.

Treatment of Type I Hypersensitivity Reactions

- Airway protection
- Antihistamines
- Corticosteroids
- Epinephrine (for anaphylaxis)

▶ HYPERSENSITIVITY (LEUKOCYTOCLASTIC) VASCULITIS

Henoch–Schönlein purpura:
- Associated with strep infection + penicillin
- Small-vessel vasculitis
- Purpura of lower extremities and buttocks
- Abdominal pain
- IgA deposits in glomeruli
- More common in children

Definition

- A group of vasculitides in which immune complexes lodge in small blood vessels, resulting in inflammation, fibrinoid necrosis, and painful, palpable purpura
- Patients have a hypersensitivity to antigens in the immune complex: Drugs, infectious agents, or other sources.
- Henoch–Schönlein is a classic example.

Signs and Symptoms

- Pruritus and pain, associated with fever and malaise
- **"Palpable purpura"**—multiple, scattered nonblanchable red papules distributed over lower extremities, arms, and buttocks (see Figure 2.10-2)
- May be crusted due to necrosis of tissue overlying the blood vessel

Epidemiology

All ages, equal in males and females

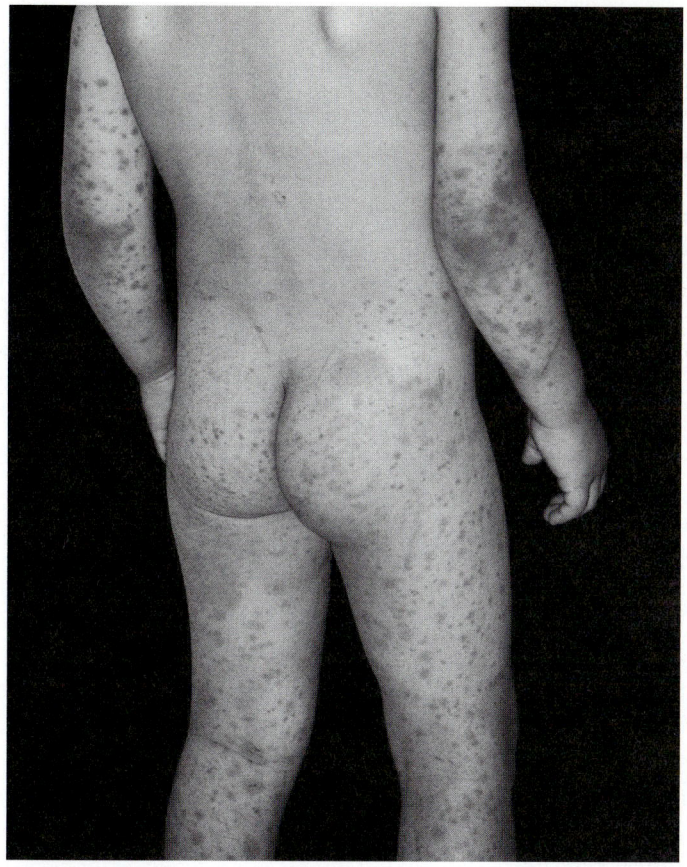

FIGURE 2.10-2. Henoch–Schönlein purpura.

(Reproduced, with permission, from Knoop KJ, Stack LB, Storrow AB. *Atlas of Emergency Medicine*. New York: McGraw-Hill, 1997:345.)

Etiology

Idiopathic in 50% of cases; infectious diseases (hepatitis B and C, *Staphylococcus aureus*); sulfonamides and penicillin; neoplasms (lymphoproliferative disorders, renal cell carcinoma); connective tissue disorders (SLE, Sjögren's syndrome, rheumatoid arthritis)

Diagnosis

American College of Rheumatology criteria for diagnosis includes at least three of the following:

1. Age > 16 at disease onset (development of symptoms)
2. Medication taken at disease onset
3. Palpable purpura
4. Maculopapular rash
5. Biopsy demonstrating eosinophilic material (fibrinoid) deposited in venule walls and necrotic vessel walls

Complications

Renal insufficiency, bowel ischemia, central nervous system (CNS) involvement

Treatment

- Eliminate and/or treat causative agent
- Systemic corticosteroids
- Immunosuppressive agents (cyclophosphamide or azathioprine)

Eczema/Dermatitis

▶ ATOPIC DERMATITIS/ECZEMA

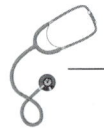

Allergic triad:
- **A**topic dermatitis
- **A**llergic rhinitis
- **A**sthma

Definition

An acute or chronic relapsing pruritic type I (IgE) immediate hypersensitivity inflammatory reaction where scratching and rubbing lead to further lichenification of skin

Risk Factors

- Family history of atopy: Asthma, allergic rhinitis, hay fever, eczema, and increased IgE
- Exacerbating factors: Scratching, stress, infection, wool, skin dehydration, pregnancy, menstruation, and foods (milk, eggs); symptoms are usually worse in winter

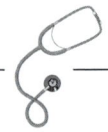

Atopic dermatitis is also called "the itch that rashes."

Epidemiology

- Affects all ages but onset is in first 6 months of life. Two thirds of patients outgrow the dermatitis by age 10.
- Familial predisposition

Signs and Symptoms

- Pruritus
- Lesions vary with patient's age:
  - Infantile eczema: Red, exudative, crusty, and oozy lesions primarily affecting the face and extensor surfaces; spares diaper area; may clear by 2 years of age
  - Juvenile and adult eczema: Dry, lichenified pruritic plaques distributed over flexural areas (antecubital, popliteal, neck)

Atopic dermatitis:
Affected areas: **FACE**
Flexor surfaces get **A**dults
Children get **E**xtensor surfaces

Diagnosis

Supported by a personal or family history of atopy or eczema

Complications

Secondary bacterial and viral infections with *Staphylococcus*, herpes simplex virus, and molluscum contagiosum.

Treatment

- Avoid scratching (will provoke the rash).
- Lubricate dry skin.
- Avoid wool and fragrances.
- Use mild cleansers and detergents.
- Oral antihistamines
- Oral antibiotics only if clinical signs of secondary infection (don't culture skin; 90% of atopic patients are carriers of *S. aureus*)
- Topical corticosteroids (mainstay of therapy)
- Avoid oral corticosteroids (associated with an excellent response, but patients become steroid dependent or rebound when steroids are discontinued).

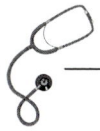

Most children have progressive improvement with increasing age, but some may evolve into adult eczema.

▶ ALLERGIC CONTACT DERMATITIS

Definition

Dermatitis resulting from skin contact with a substance causing a delayed (type IV) hypersensitivity immune response

Triggers

Poison ivy, oak, sumac; nickel (jewelry); formaldehyde; rubber; chemicals in shoes

Signs and Symptoms

Intensely pruritic rash with linear, papular, erythematous lesions with indistinct margins in the distribution of the exposure

Diagnosis

History and physical exam is most reliable.

Treatment

- Avoid exposure
- Mild/moderate: Topical corticosteroids, soothing lotions
- Severe: Systemic steroids and antihistamines

▶ IRRITANT CONTACT DERMATITIS

Definition

Dermatitis resulting from exposure to substances that cause physical, mechanical, or chemical irritation to the skin

Triggers

Common exposures after daily repetitive use of soapy water, cleansers, rubbing alcohol

Signs and Symptoms

Erythematous pruritic chapped skin, dryness, fissuring; most commonly affects hands

Diagnosis

History and physical, but patch testing may be necessary to differentiate from allergic contact dermatitis

Treatment

Goal is to restore normal epithelial barrier and then protect.

- Decrease exposure to soap and water
- Emollients
- Severe cases: Topical corticosteroids

Miscellaneous Inflammatory Conditions

► PITYRIASIS ROSEA

Definition

A common self-limiting eruption of a **single herald patch** (see followed by a generalized secondary eruption within 2 weeks.

Etiology

Herpes simplex virus type 7 is suspected.

Typical scenario:
A young person presents with a pruritic, spotted rash on the trunk that began as one solitary larger patch.
Think: Pityriasis rosea.

Epidemiology

Affects children and young adults, primarily ages 10 to 35. Clusters of cases in spring and fall.

Signs and Symptoms (See Figure 2.10-3)

- Mild pruritus
- 2- to 10-cm solitary, oval erythematous **"herald plaque"** with a collarette of scale precedes the generalized eruption in 80% of patients
- Within days, multiple smaller pink oval scaly patches appear over trunk and upper extremities.
- Secondary eruption occurs in a Christmas tree distribution, oriented parallel to the ribs.

Treatment

Symptomatic. No treatment shortens disease course:

- Cool baths
- Calamine lotion
- Topical corticosteroids
- Oral antihistamines
- UVB phototherapy or sunlight

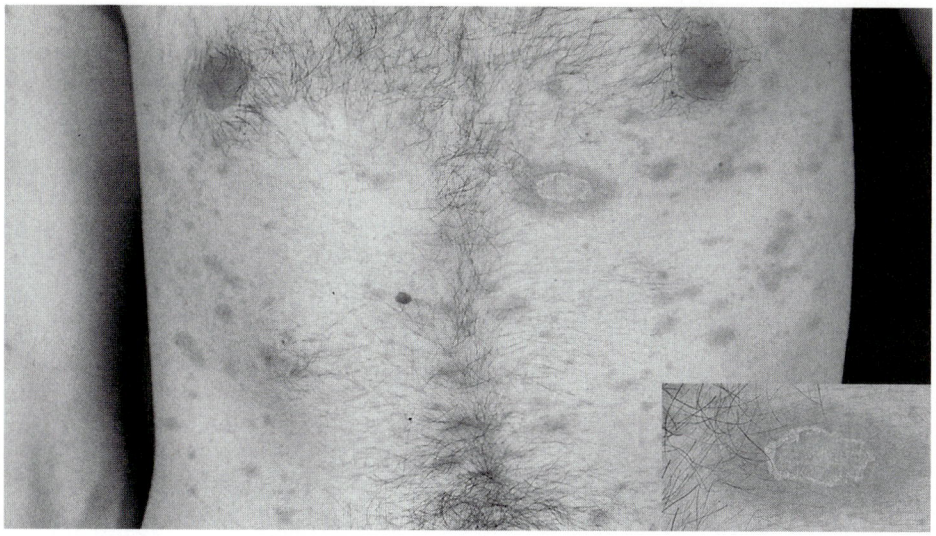

FIGURE 2.10-3. Pityriasis rosea.

Papules and small erythematous plaques; note herald patch, an erythematous plaque with scale in central portion of lesion and collarette on border. (Reproduced, with permission, from Wolff K, Johnson RA, Suurmond D. *Fitzpatrick's Color Atlas & Synopsis of Clinical Dermatology*, 5th ed. New York: McGraw-Hill, 2005:119.)

▶ PSORIASIS

Definition

- A chronic, noninfectious hyperproliferative inflammatory disorder characterized by thick adherent scales (see Table 2.10-2 for definitions of secondary skin lesions)
- Presents with multiple exacerbations and remissions

Pathophysiology

Increased epidermal cell proliferation due to a shortened epithelial cell cycle results in keratinization defects, forming thick adherent scales.

Epidemiology

Affects 1 to 3% of the population. Common among ages 15 to 40. Rare under the age of 10. Forty percent have a positive family history.

Psoriasis is worse in winter.

Risk Factors

Trauma, infection, emotional stress, and drugs (lithium, beta blockers, iodine, and antimalarials)

Signs and Symptoms

- Mild pruritus
- Well-demarcated, thick, "salmon-pink" **plaques** with an adherent silver-white scale
- Distributed bilaterally over **extensor surface** of extremities, often on elbows and knees, and trunk and scalp

Typical scenario:
A 35-year-old has salmon-colored papules covered with silvery white scale on his scalp, elbows, and knees. *Think: Psoriasis.*

- Nails are commonly involved: Pitting of nails, oil spots (yellow-brown spots under nail plate), onycholysis (separation of distal nail plate from nail bed), subungual hyperkeratosis (thickening of epidermis under nail plate)
- Can occur at site of injury (Koebner phenomenon)
- Pinpoint capillary bleeding occurs if scale is removed (Auspitz sign).

Complications

Psoriatic arthritis, a destructive arthritis of the distal interphalangeal joints of hands and feet **(rheumatoid factor negative)**

Treatment

For mild psoriasis, the following can be applied to plaques:

- Topical coal tar or anthralin (inhibit DNA synthesis)
- Topical corticosteroids
- Calcipotriene (Dovonex is a synthetic vitamin D analog that decreases cellular proliferation)
- Combination therapy

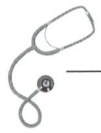

Psoriasis is a chronic disease and complete remission is often not achieved. Goal is to decrease scale and achieve a better cosmetic result.

If the plaques fail to improve, or if psoriasis is extensive and affects > 20% of body surface area, systemic treatment should be implemented:

- UVB phototherapy
- PUVA (psoralen + UVA; psoralen is taken orally 1 to 2 hours prior to UV exposure and is photoactivated in the skin by UV radiation)
- Retinoids (etretinate, tazarotene, acitretin)
- Methotrexate (inhibits DNA synthesis)
- Combination therapy of retinoids or methotrexate with PUVA
- Cyclosporine

▶ ERYTHEMA NODOSUM

Definition

- An inflammatory disorder of subcutaneous fat (panniculitis) characterized by painful erythematous nodules on lower legs
- Thought to be an immunological reaction precipitated by multiple etiologies

A 23-year-old woman has a cough and a CXR showing mediastinal lymphadenopathy. She has painful skin nodules on the skin of the tibia. *Think: Erythema nodosum* as a manifestation of sarcoidosis.

Epidemiology

Occurs more often in women, age 15 to 30

Etiology

- Forty percent of cases are idiopathic.
- Drugs: Sulfonamides, oral contraceptives
- Infectious: Streptococci, tuberculosis, leprosy, histoplasmosis, coccidioidomycosis, blastomycosis, *Chlamydia*, *Yersinia*
- Autoimmune: **Sarcoidosis,** inflammatory bowel disease, Behçet's disease

Signs and Symptoms

- Fever, malaise, and arthralgias
- Painful, deep-seated, indurated erythematous nodules scattered over lower legs, bilaterally but not symmetrically (see Figure 2.10-4)
- May also occur on forearms, thighs, or any other area with fat

Diagnosis

Confirmed by a careful history and laboratory evaluation including a complete blood count (CBC), throat culture, antistreptolysin-O titer, and chest x-ray

Treatment

- Removal and/or treatment of causative agent
- Bed rest and elevation of legs
- Anti-inflammatory medication for pain
- Systemic corticosteroids (only if etiology is known)

▶ ERYTHEMA MULTIFORME

Note: Erythema multiforme, Stevens–Johnson syndrome, and toxic epidermal necrolysis are considered by many to be part of the same spectrum of disease.

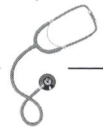

Fifty percent of erythema multiforme cases are idiopathic.

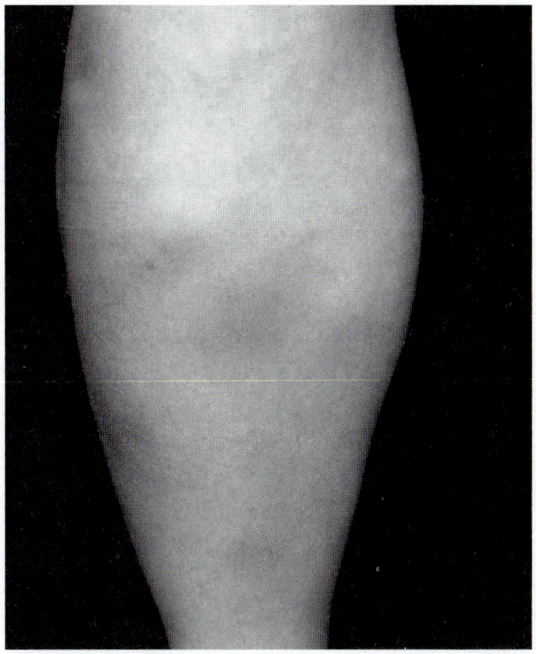

FIGURE 2.10-4. Erythema nodosum.

(Reproduced, with permission, from Wolff K, Johnson RA, Suurmond D. *Fitzpatrick's Color Atlas & Synopsis of Clinical Dermatology,* 5th ed. New York: McGraw-Hill, 2005:149.)

Definition

A general name used to describe an immune complex–mediated hypersensitivity reaction to different causative agents

Causes

- **Drugs** (penicillins, sulfonamides, barbiturates, NSAIDs, thiazides, phenytoin)
- **Viruses** (usually herpes simplex virus, but also hepatitis A and B)
- **Bacteria** (*Streptococcus, Mycoplasma*)
- Fungi
- Malignancy
- Radiotherapy
- Pregnancy

Epidemiology

Older children and adults

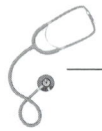

Herpes simplex virus accounts for most cases of recurrent erythema multiforme.

Signs and Symptoms

Although characterized by **target lesions,** multiforme refers to the wide variety of lesions that may be present, including papules, vesicles, and bullae (see Figure 2.10-5). Affected sites include dorsa of hands, palms and soles, penis (50%), feet, and face.

Treatment

- Discontinue offending agent.
- Treat any underlying infections (e.g., oral acyclovir to prevent herpes outbreak).

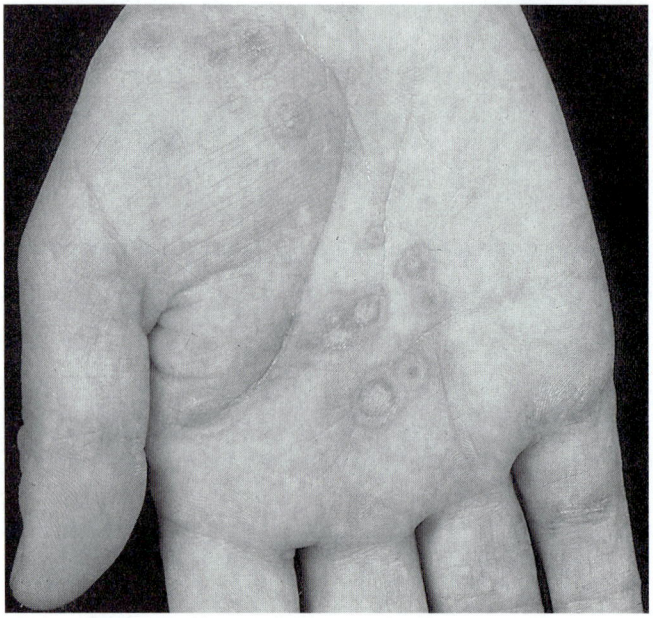

FIGURE 2.10-5. Erythema multiforme.

(Reproduced, with permission, from Wolff K, Johnson RA, Suurmond D. *Fitzpatrick's Color Atlas & Synopsis of Clinical Dermatology*, 5th ed. New York: McGraw-Hill, 2005:141.)

▶ STEVENS–JOHNSON SYNDROME

- Erythema multiforme with systemic illness (fever, malaise) and multiple mucous membrane involvement (oral, vaginal, conjunctival) (see Figure 2.10-6).
- Extensive targetlike lesions and mucosal erosion covering < 10% body surface area
- Ocular involvement may result in scarring, corneal ulcers, or uveitis; 5% mortality.
- May evolve to toxic epidermal necrolysis

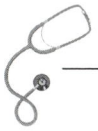

Stevens–Johnson syndrome and toxic epidermal necrolysis are severe variants of erythema multiforme that are potentially life threatening.

▶ TOXIC EPIDERMAL NECROLYSIS

Definition

Widespread full-thickness necrosis of skin covering > 30% body surface area

Signs and Symptoms

- Prodrome of fever and influenza-like symptoms.
- Pruritus, pain, tenderness, and burning
- Classic targetlike lesions symmetrically distributed on dorsum of hand, palms, soles, face, and knees

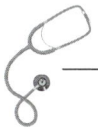

Nikolsky's sign is sloughing off of the epidermis with gentle manual pressure.

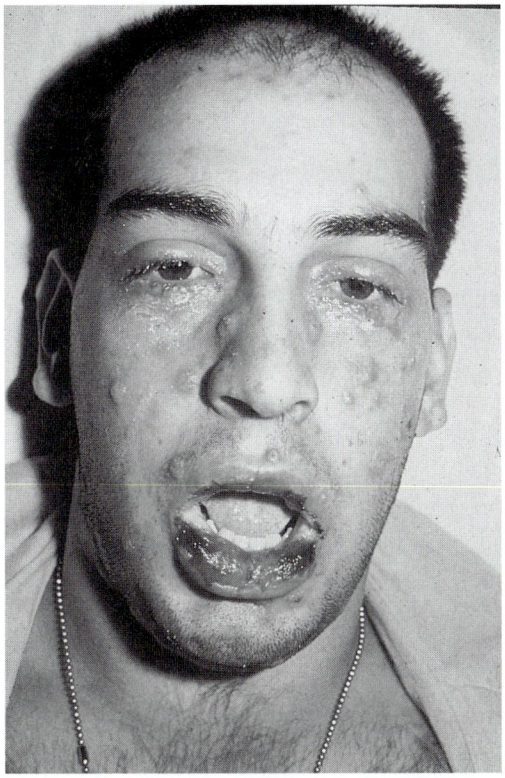

FIGURE 2.10-6. Stevens–Johnson syndrome.

(Reproduced, with permission, from Knoop KJ, Stack LB, Storrow AB. *Atlas of Emergency Medicine.* New York: McGraw-Hill, 1997:343.)

- Initial **target lesions** can become confluent, erythematous, and tender, with bullous formation and subsequent loss of epidermis.
- Epidermal sloughing may be generalized, resembling a second-degree burn, and is more pronounced over pressure points.
- Positive Nikolsky's sign
- Ninety percent of cases have mucosal lesions—painful, erythematous erosions on lips, buccal mucosa, conjunctiva, and anogenital region.

Diagnosis

Confirmed by biopsy

Complications

- Secondary skin infections
- Fluid and electrolyte abnormalities
- Prerenal azotemia
- Increased risk of death (denudation of skin results in fluid loss and infections)
- 30% mortality rate

Treatment

- Removal and/or treatment of causative agent (suppressive therapy with acyclovir to prevent recurrences of herpes simplex virus)
- Hospitalization for severe disease
- Fluid and electrolyte replacement
- Systemic corticosteroids

▶ DECUBITUS ULCERS

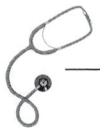

Decubitus ulcers are also called bedsores and pressure ulcers.

Definition

- Any pressure-induced ulcer that occurs secondary to external compression of the skin, resulting in ischemic tissue necrosis
- May extend to underlying subcutaneous tissue, muscle, joints, or bones
- Fifty percent of ulcers are hospital-acquired and usually develop within the first 2 weeks of hospitalization.

Etiology

Pressure induces ischemia and tissue necrosis.

Risk Factors

- Immobility, fracture
- Malnutrition
- Age > 70
- Hypoalbuminemia
- Spinal cord injury
- Fecal incontinence
- Diabetes mellitus (DM)
- Inadequate nursing care
- Decreased level of consciousness

Signs and Symptoms

- Appearance depends on extent of damage.
- Localized, blanchable erythema develops prior to ulcer formation.
- Early ulcers have irregular, ragged borders, but chronic ulcers have smooth, well-demarcated borders.
- Eschar represents devitalized tissue at the base. Purulent exudate surrounding the ulcer suggests an infection.

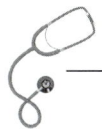

Decubitus ulcers develop over bony prominences: sacrum, ischial tuberosities, iliac crests, greater trochanters, heels, elbows, knees, occiput. Can develop at any site that can be compressed against a hard surface.

Stages

I—nonblanching erythema of intact skin
II—partial-thickness skin loss involving epidermis and/or dermis (superficial ulcer)
III—full-thickness skin loss involving epidermis and dermis (deep, crateriform ulcer). May involve damage to subcutaneous tissue, extending down to but not through fascia.
IV—full-thickness skin loss with extensive damage to muscle, bone, or other supporting structures

Diagnosis

- Elevated WBC and erythrocyte sedimentation rate (ESR) suggest an underlying infection (osteomyelitis, bacteremia).
- Wound culture can be used to differentiate infection from colonization.
- Culture of base detects only surface bacteria; therefore, recommend deep punch biopsy for optimal culture.
- Infection is usually polymicrobial: *S. aureus*, *Streptococcus*, *Pseudomonas*, *Enterococcus*, *Proteus*, *Clostridia*, and *Bacteroides*.

Complications

Osteomyelitis, bacteremia, sepsis

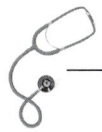

With proper treatment, stage I and II ulcers heal within 1 to 2 weeks. Stage III and IV ulcers heal within 6 to 12 weeks.

Treatment

Prophylaxis

- Mobilizing patients as soon as possible
- Repositioning patients every 2 hours
- Pressure-reducing devices (foam, air, or liquid mattresses)
- Correction of nutritional status.

Local Wound Care

- Proper cleansing with mild agents
- Moisturizing to maintain hydration and promote healing
- Polyurethane, hydrocolloid, or absorptive dressings, and topical antibiotics for wound
- Necrotic tissue may require surgical debridement, flaps, and skin grafts.
- Appropriate antibiotic therapy for infected ulcer

Skin Diseases Due to Microbial Agents

For commonly tested infectious causes of rash see Table 2.10-4.

▶ ERYSIPELAS

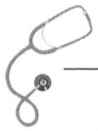

Erysipelas: High morbidity rate if untreated.

Definition

An acute onset of superficial spreading cellulitis, arising in inconspicuous breaks in skin (see Figure 2.10-7)

Etiology

Group A beta-hemolytic *Streptococcus pyogenes*

Epidemiology

Increased incidence in young children and older adults

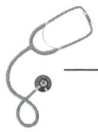

Erysipelas, erysipeloid, and necrotizing fasciitis are variants of cellulitis.

Signs and Symptoms

- Local pain and tenderness
- An erythematous, shiny area of warm and tender skin with a well demarcated and indurated advancing border
- Less edematous than cellulitis, but margins are more sharply demarcated and elevated

TABLE 2.10-4. Fever and Rash—Commonly Tested Infectious Causes

Disease	Etiology	Skin Finding(s)	Rash Characteristics	Other Clinical Findings
Measles	Paramyxovirus	Blanching erythematous maculopapular rash that becomes confluent	Rash starts at hairline and behind ears → centrifugally to face → neck/trunk, extremities	Koplik's spots Fever Cough, coryza Conjunctivitis
Rubella	Rubella virus	Similar to measles but patient doesn't look as "sick"	By second day, facial exanthem fades	Prominent postauricular, posterior cervical lymph nodes
Varicella (chickenpox)	Varicella-zoster virus	Pruritic vesicular lesions in successive crops; vesicles evolve to pustules and crust over time	First lesions begin on face/scalp → trunk/back	Herpes zoster (shingles): Painful vesicular lesions; does **not** cross midline

TABLE 2.10-4. Fever and Rash—Commonly Tested Infectious Causes (continued)

Disease	Etiology	Skin Finding(s)	Rash Characteristics	Other Clinical Findings
Erythema infectiosum (fifth disease)	Parvovirus B19	Erythematous macules and papules giving lacy "reticulated" appearance	"Slapped cheek" in children	
Roseola infantum ("exanthem subitum")	HHV-6, HHV-7	Multiple blanchable macules and papules trunk → extremities (after high fever prodrome)	Rash spares face	Primarily in infants High fever 3–4 days prior to appearance of rash
Infectious mononucleosis	Epstein–Barr virus	Generalized maculopapular rash in 100% of patients with administration of ampicillin/amoxicillin		Splenomegaly
Scarlet fever	Group A streptococcus	Course, erythematous blanching rash, circumoral pallor, strawberry tongue, linear petechiae in skin folds (Pastia's lines)	Rash fades in several days → desquamation of skin	Rash appears 1–3 days after strep pharyngitis
Acute rheumatic fever	Group A streptococcus	Erythema marginatum (transient macular rash with central clearing found on proximal extremities)	Subcutaneous nodules on bony prominences	

- Face is most commonly involved, but can affect any area, especially sites of chronic edema.

Diagnosis

Gram stain reveals gram-positive cocci in chains.

Treatment

Penicillin: If allergic, use a cephalosporin, macrolide, or vancomycin.

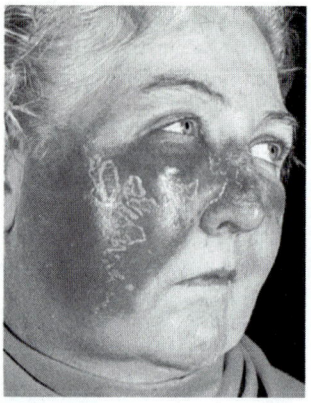

FIGURE 2.10-7. Erysipelas.

(Reproduced, with permission, from Fauci AS et al [eds]. *Harrison's Principles of Internal Medicine,* 14th ed. New York: McGraw-Hill, 1998:10–34.)

▶ CELLULITIS

Typical scenario:
A 54-year-old insulin-dependent diabetic male presents with a warm, erythematous, slightly tender rash with poorly demarcated borders that began on his calf yesterday and has now spread up his leg. *Think: Cellulitis.*

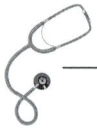

A detailed history is particularly important to reveal the portal of entry in cellulitis.

Definition

An acute deep infection of dermis and subcutaneous tissue characterized by erythema, tenderness, and warmth of involved area.

Etiology

- *Staphylococcus aureus*
- Group A beta-hemolytic *Streptococcus pyogenes*
- *Hemophilus influenzae*

Risk Factors

- Injury to affected area such as abrasions, burns, surgical wounds, lymphadenectomy, mucosal infections, bites, tattoos, nail cutting, acupuncture, etc.
- Underlying dermatosis
- Drug and alcohol abuse
- Immunocompromised states

Signs and Symptoms

- Warmth and tenderness of infected site
- Erythematous, edematous, **shiny area of warm and tender skin** with poorly demarcated, **nonelevated** borders
- Usually overlying site of wound or trauma
- Lower leg is more frequently involved due to interdigital tinea.

Diagnosis

Confirmed by Gram stain demonstrating gram-positive cocci in clusters or chains. Culture of lesion or blood will be positive only 25% of the time.

Treatment

Penicillin: If penicillin allergic or methicillin-resistant *S. aureus* (MRSA), use vancomycin or cephalosporins. For *H. influenzae*, use cefotaxime or ceftriaxone.

▶ TOXIC SHOCK SYNDROME (TSS)

Definition

A toxin-mediated disease characterized by acute onset of fever, hypotension, diarrhea, and generalized skin and mucous erythema, followed by failure of multiple organ systems.

Epidemiology

- Ages 20 to 30
- Increased incidence in women using high-absorbency tampons, and in patients with burns, ulcers, surgical wounds, and nasal packs

Etiology

- *Staphylococcus aureus* producing TSS toxin-1 (TSST-1)
- Group A beta-hemolytic streptococci (rare)

Signs and Symptoms

- Acute onset of fever, hypotension, tingling sensation in hands and feet, myalgia, headache, confusion, disorientation, and diarrhea.
- A generalized erythematous macular eruption occurs most intensely at affected site followed by desquamation of palms and soles 1 to 2 weeks after onset of illness with edema of face, hands, and feet.
- Erythema of oral mucosa, bulbar conjunctiva, vagina, and tympanic membrane

Diagnosis

Centers for Disease Control and Prevention (CDC) Criteria for Diagnosis

- Fever > 102°F
- Hypotension (systolic blood pressure < 90 mm Hg for adults or an orthostatic decrease in blood pressure > 15 mm Hg)
- Involvement of three or more of the following organ systems:
  1. Gastrointestinal: Vomiting or diarrhea at onset of illness
  2. Muscular: Myalgia or creatine phosphokinase (CPK) > 2 times upper limit of normal
  3. Mucous membrane: Vaginal, oropharyngeal, and conjunctival hyperemia
  4. Renal: Blood urea nitrogen (BUN) or creatinine > 2 times upper limit of normal, or 5 WBC/HPF
  5. Hepatic: Total bilirubin, SGOT, SGPT > 2 times upper limit of normal
  6. Hematologic: Platelets < 100,000/μL
  7. Central nervous system (CNS): disorientation or alteration in consciousness
- Gram stain reveals gram positive cocci in clusters.
- Culture grows TSST-1–producing staphylococcus.

Treatment

- Admission to intensive care unit
- Removal of potential foreign bodies
- IV anti-staphylococcus antibiotics
- Management of organ system failure

▶ MENINGOCOCCEMIA

Definition

A potentially fatal disease resulting from meningococcal bacteremia

Epidemiology

- Highest incidence in 6 months to 1-year-old children
- Increased incidence in alcoholics, asplenic, and complement-deficient patients

Etiology

Neisseria meningitidis

Signs and Symptoms

- Prodrome of spiking fever, cough, headache, sore throat, nausea, and vomiting followed by chills, arthralgias, myalgias, and hypotension
- Patients appear **acutely ill** and **listless.**
- Seventy-five percent of patients have discrete **pink macules, papules,** and **petechiae,** which can be distributed over trunk, extremities, and palate (see Figure 2.10-8) (see Table 2.10-1 for definitions of primary skin lesions).
- With fulminant disease, patients have **purpura,** ecchymosis, and confluent area of gray-black necrosis.
- Signs of meningeal irritation

Diagnosis

- Blood cultures reveal meningococci 100% of the time.
- Cerebrospinal fluid (CSF) culture is usually positive.
- Skin biopsy cultures are positive 85% of the time.
- Gram stain reveals gram-negative diplococci.

Meningococcemia is fatal if untreated. Treat empirically prior to completion of tests if suspected on clinical grounds.

Complications

- Meningitis (50 to 90%)
- Waterhouse–Friderichsen syndrome (fulminant meningococcemia with adrenal hemorrhage)

Treatment

- Admission to intensive care unit
- Vancomycin and ceftriaxone IV at first clinical suspicion of meningococcemia.

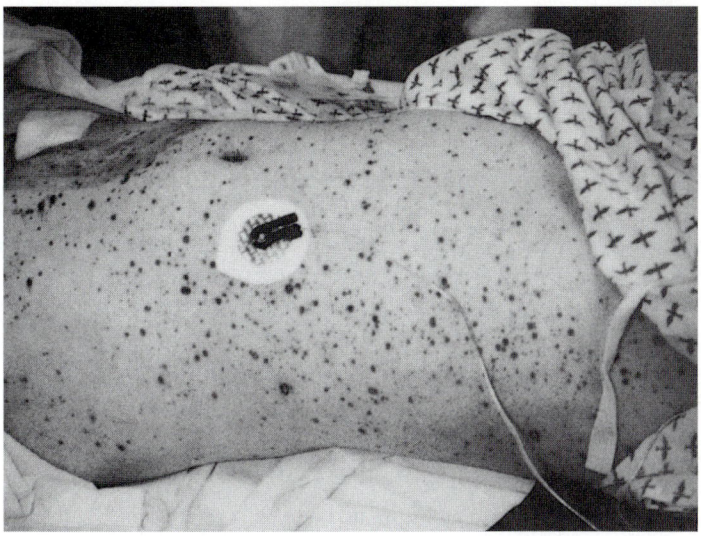

FIGURE 2.10-8. Meningococcemia.

(Reproduced, with permission, from Knoop KJ, Stack LB, Storrow AB. *Atlas of Emergency Medicine*. New York: McGraw-Hill, 1997:404.)

▶ BACTERIAL ENDOCARDITIS

Covered in the cardiovascular chapter

▶ ROCKY MOUNTAIN SPOTTED FEVER (RMSF)

Definition

- A potentially life-threatening disease due to a tick bite
- The infected tick adheres to vascular endothelium, resulting in vascular necrosis and extravasation of blood.

Epidemiology

- Highest incidence in children aged 5 to 10 years old.
- Ninety-five percent of cases occur from April through September.
- Occurs only in the Western hemisphere, primarily in southeastern states and most often in Oklahoma, North and South Carolina, and Tennessee
- Rarely occurs in the Rocky Mountains
- Only 60% of patients report a history of a tick bite.

Etiology

Rickettsia rickettsii, transmitted via female *Dermacentor* tick

Signs and Symptoms

- Sudden onset of high **fever,** myalgia, severe headache, rigors, nausea, and photophobia within first 2 days of tick bite.

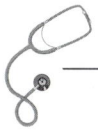

RMSF rash spreads from extremities to trunk.

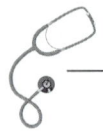

In real time, RMSF is a clinical diagnosis (because current diagnostic tests aren't back fast enough). It is important not to delay treatment.

- Fifty percent develop rash within 3 days. Another 30% develop the rash within 6 days.
- Rash consists of 2- to 6-mm pink **blanchable macules** that first appear peripherally on wrists, forearms, ankles, **palms,** and **soles** (see Figure 2.10-9).
- Within 6 to 18 hours the exanthem spreads centrally to trunk, proximal extremities, and face.
- Within 1 to 3 days the macules evolve to deep red papules, and within 2 to 4 days the exanthem is hemorrhagic and no longer blanchable.
- Up to 15% have no rash.
- Many patients have exquisite tenderness of the gastrocnemius muscle.

Diagnosis

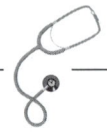

A delay in treatment of RMSF is associated with increased morbidity and mortality. Increased risk of death with delayed diagnosis and older age of patient.

- Indirect fluorescent antibody (IFA) assay:
  - Titer > 1:64 is diagnostic.
  - Most sensitive and specific test
- Other, less sensitive tests include:
  - Indirect hemagglutinin, Weil–Felix, complement fixation, and latex agglutination tests
- Biopsy would demonstrate necrotizing vasculitis.

Complications

Some patients develop long-term sequelae lasting > 1 year, including paraparesis, hearing loss, peripheral neuropathy, bladder/bowel incontinence, and cerebellar, vestibular, and motor dysfunction.

Treatment

- Most patients, except those with very mild disease, require intravenous antibiotics.
- Doxycycline considered drug of choice

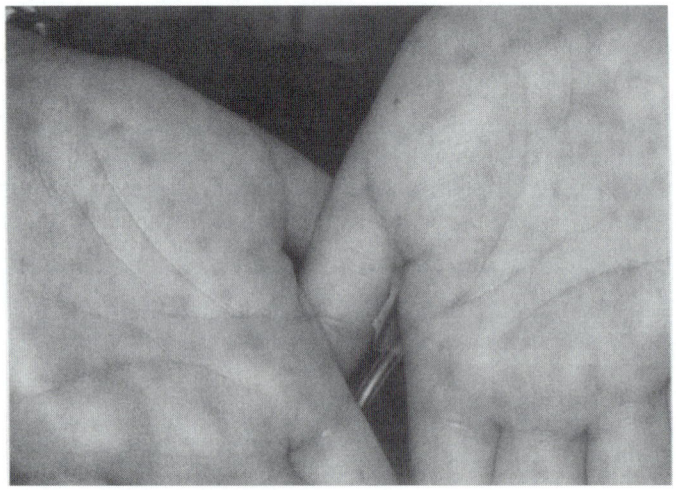

FIGURE 2.10-9. Rocky Mountain spotted fever.

(Reproduced, with permission, from Fauci AS et al [eds]. *Harrison's Principles of Internal Medicine,* 14th ed. New York: McGraw-Hill, 1998:10–48.)

- Chloramphenicol for pregnant patients, children younger than 8 years (due to concern of staining the teeth), and severe disease
- Treatment is continued until patient is afebrile for 48 hours.

▶ HERPES ZOSTER

Definition

- An acute dermatomal viral infection caused by reactivation of latent varicella-zoster virus that has remained dormant in a sensory root ganglion
- The virus travels down the sensory nerve, resulting initially in dermatomal pain, followed by skin lesions.

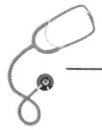

Patients with zoster can infect nonimmune contacts with chickenpox. Exposed nonimmune contacts should be treated with varicella-zoster immune globulin (VZIG).

Etiology

Varicella-zoster virus

Epidemiology

Age > 50

Risk Factors

Age, malignancy, immunosuppression, and radiation

Signs and Symptoms (See Figure 2.10-10)

- **Prodrome of pain,** burning, itching, and paresthesia in affected dermatome precedes eruption by 3 to 5 days; accompanied by fever, headache, and malaise and heightened sensitivity to stimuli (allodynia).

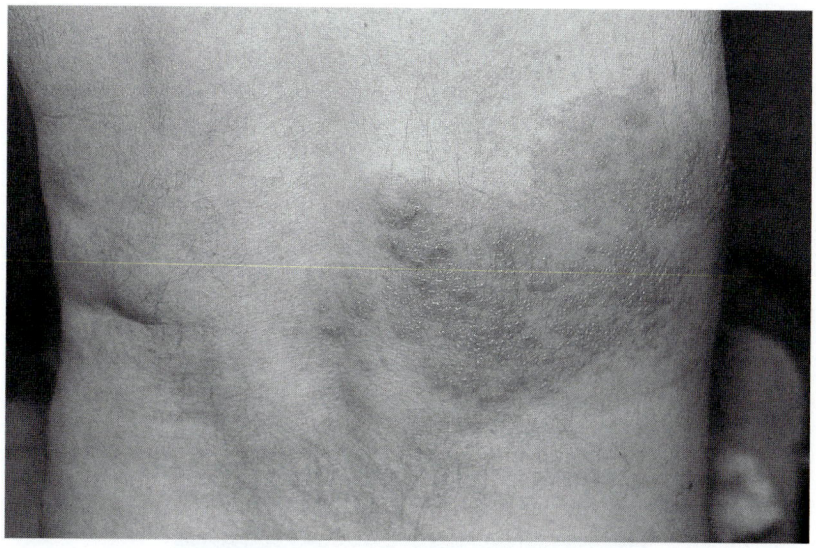

FIGURE 2.10-10. Varicella-zoster virus infection: herpes zoster in T8 to T10 dermatome. Note typical dermatomal distribution of rash.

(Reproduced, with permission, from Wolff K, Johnson RA, Suurmond D. *Fitzpatrick's Color Atlas & Synopsis of Clinical Dermatology*, 5th ed. New York: McGraw-Hill, 2005:823.)

A 24-year-old medical student working in the ICU held a patient's endotracheal tube with his ungloved hand to keep it from falling out. Two weeks later he has a vesicular lesion on an erythematous base that is extremely painful. *Think: Herpetic whitlow.*

- **Grouped vesicles** on an erythematous base distributed unilaterally along a dermatome
- Crust formation within 5 to 10 days
- **Some vesicles may occur outside of involved dermatome.**
- Thoracic nerves are the most commonly involved.

Diagnosis

Confirmed by **Tzanck preparation** revealing multinucleated giant cells, and culture of lesions.

Complications

- Secondary bacterial superinfection
- **Postherpetic neuralgia** (more common in the elderly and may persist for weeks to years after infection)
- Herpes zoster ophthalmicus: Lesions on nasal tip or eye indicate zoster involvement of nasociliary branch of ophthalmic nerve, resulting in uveitis, conjunctivitis, retinitis, optic neuritis, or glaucoma. An ophthalmic consult is necessary.
- Ramsay Hunt syndrome: Lesions on external surface of ear or auditory canal indicate zoster involvement of facial and auditory nerve, resulting in facial paralysis, hearing loss, ear pain, and vertigo.
- Herpetic whitlow is HSV of fingers (see Figure 2.10-11). Occurs in medical personnel exposed to patient's secretions (even without clinical herpes; virus may be shed in saliva). Treat with wet-to-dry dressing. Do not open vesicles or infection will spread.

Treatment

- Moist and cool compresses to affected dermatome
- Oral acyclovir, valacyclovir, or famciclovir (accelerate healing of lesions

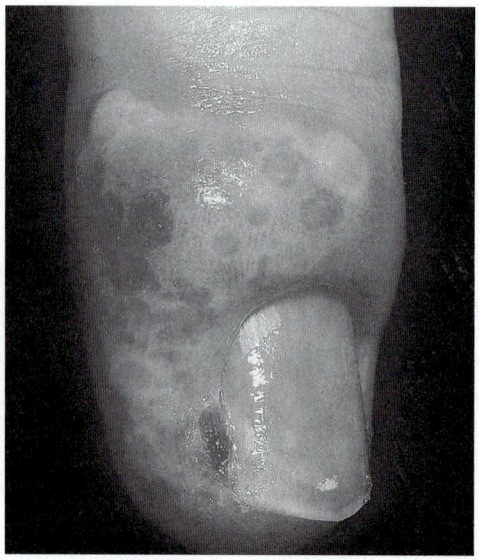

FIGURE 2.10-11. Herpes simplex virus infection: herpetic whitlow.

(Reproduced, with permission, from Wolff K, Johnson RA, Suurmond D. *Fitzpatrick's Color Atlas & Synopsis of Clinical Dermatology*, 5th ed. New York: McGraw-Hill, 2005:805.)

and decrease duration of pain if started within 3 days of infection) for immunocompetent patients
- IV acyclovir for severe infections and immunocompromised individuals
- Adequate analgesia
- Epinephrine (for anaphylaxis)

▶ CUTANEOUS FUNGAL INFECTIONS

See Table 2.10-5.

TABLE 2.10-5. Cutaneous Fungal Infections

	DERMATOPHYTES	CANDIDIASIS	PITYRIASIS (TINEA) VERSICOLOR
Definition	Group of noninvasive fungi that infect keratinized tissue of epidermis, nails, and hair resulting in tinea infection	Superficial yeast infection found on mucosal surfaces typically in moist occluded areas	Chronic asymptomatic scaling condition characterized by well-demarcated patches with variable pigmentation usually on the trunk
Etiology	*Trichophyton, Microsporum,* and *Epidermophyton*	*Candida albicans* (most often) **Predisposing factors:** Diabetes, obesity, heat, maceration, steroid use (systemic and topical); invasive disseminated candidiasis in immunocompromised hosts	*Plasmodium ovale* (aka *Malassezia furfur*)
Types	Tinea pedis (athlete's foot) Tinea cruris (jock itch) Tinea corporis (ringworm) Onychomycosis (nail infection)	Genital (balanitis, vulvovaginitis) Diaper dermatitis Oropharynx (thrush) Nail (chronic paronychia) Intertrigo	
Diagnosis	**KOH → multiple septated hyphae** **Wood's lamp** → bright green fluorescence in hair shaft (tinea capitis)	**KOH → pseudohyphae** (elongated yeast without true septations)	KOH → round yeast and elongated pseudohyphae **("spaghetti and meatballs")**
Treatment	Prevention (well-ventilated, cotton clothing); topical antifungals (not for hair or nails); systemic antifungals (if no response to topicals)	Keep areas dry, topical antifungals (nystatin, azole, imidazole creams), oral antifungals for recurrent infections	Topical agents (selenium sulfide shampoo, azole creams)

▶ LYME BORRELIOSIS (LYME DISEASE)

Definition

- A multisystem disease transmitted by the bite of an *Ixodes* genus deer tick infected with a spirochete
- Characterized by three stages of disease: localized, disseminated, and chronic
- Patients are often unaware of tick bite.

Etiology

Borrelia burgdorferi

Epidemiology

- More frequent in late May through early fall
- Increased prevalence in Northeast and North Central regions, primarily Connecticut, Rhode Island, New York, New Jersey, Delaware, and Pennsylvania

Signs and Symptoms

History—acute onset of fever, chills, myalgia, weakness, headache, and photophobia
Symptoms—local burning, itching, or pain
Physical exam:

- **Erythema chronicum migrans** (ECM) develops at site of tick bite in 75% of patients within 1 month (an expanding erythematous annular plaque with a central clearing) (see Figure 2.10-12).
- Usually affects the trunk, proximal extremities, axilla, and inguinal area
- May have multiple ECM lesions if multiple tick bites present
- Fifteen percent of patients develop secondary annular lesions that resemble ECM but are smaller and migrate less.

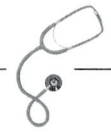

Lyme disease: If untreated, lesions fade within 28 days. If treated adequately, lesions fade within days and the late manifestations of the disease are prevented. If delayed diagnosis, may have permanent neurologic or joint disabilities.

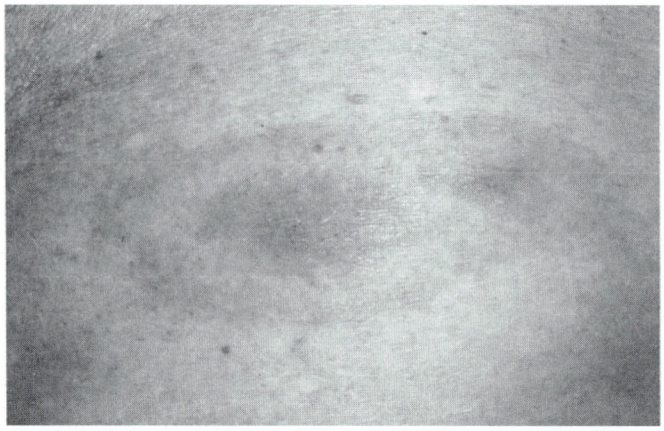

FIGURE 2.10-12. Erythema chronicum migrans rash of Lyme disease.

(Reproduced, with permission, from Fauci AS et al [eds]. *Harrison's Principles of Internal Medicine*, 14th ed. New York: McGraw-Hill, 1998:10–47.)

Diagnosis

- Clinical, confirmed by serology
- IgM titers are elevated in acute disease and peak 3 to 6 weeks after exposure.
- IgG levels peak when arthritis develops.
- An elevated IgG titer in absence of an elevated IgM indicates prior exposure as opposed to recent infection.
- May have false-negative results in first 2 to 4 weeks and false-positive results with other spirochetal infection and in patients with some autoimmune disorders (systemic lupus erythematosus, rheumatoid arthritis).
- PCR can detect spirochete DNA in CSF and synovial fluid. Forty percent of skin biopsies reveal spirochetes.

Complications

- Sixty percent of untreated cases with disseminated infection develop arthritis (mediated by immune complex formation) 4 to 6 weeks following tick bite.
- May also develop neurologic (meningitis, encephalitis, or Bell's palsy) and cardiac involvement (carditis, atrioventricular block)

Treatment

Amoxicillin or doxycycline

ACNE VULGARIS

Definition

Inflammation of pilosebaceous units of certain areas of the body including face, trunk, upper arms, and upper back

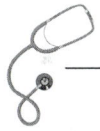

Acne vulgaris can be distinguished from acne rosacea by the presence of comedones and absence of telangiectasias.

Pathogenesis

1. Hyperkeratotic "plug" (increased proliferation and decreased desquamation of keratin)
2. Increased sebum production
3. Propionibacterium acnes within the follicle
4. Inflammation

Epidemiology

Puberty (10–17-year-old females, 14–19-year-old males); may appear at > 25 years

Etiology

- *Propionibacterium acnes*
- Drug related (lithium, steroids, androgens)

Signs and Symptoms

Comedones—open (blackheads) and closed (whiteheads), nodules or cysts in more severe cases

Treatment

Goal is to remove plugging and treat infection (combination treatment is best)

- Mild: Topical antibiotics (clindamycin, erythromycin), benzoyl peroxide, topical retinoids
- Moderate: Consider adding oral antibiotic (e.g., minocycline) or oral contraceptives in females
- Severe: Isotretinoin (Accutane)

Skin Cancers

▶ BASAL CELL CARCINOMA

Definition

- The **most common** type of skin cancer due to a malignancy of the epidermal basal cells
- Basal cells invade locally but almost never metastasize.

Epidemiology

> 40 years of age. Occurs mainly in white males.

Risk Factors

- Fair-skinned people with poor tanning capacity
- Chronic sun exposure
- Radiation therapy

Signs and Symptoms

Physical exam is variable, depending on type of basal cell cancer:

- Nodular type: A single translucent, **"pearly,"** waxy nodule or papule with telangiectasias and a rolled border, distributed on face and neck. May develop central necrosis with adherent crust (rodent ulcer).
- Superficial spreading type: Multiple erythematous scaly plaques with a well-defined border distributed primarily on trunk, with no relation to sun exposure
- Sclerosing type: Yellowish white sclerotic waxy plaques with poorly defined borders, resembling scar tissue or morphea
- Pigmented type: May have any of the above characteristics with pigmentation and is easily confused with malignant melanoma

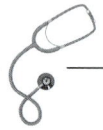

Typical scenario:
A 47-year-old white male presents with pearly, painless, ulcerated nodules with overlying telangiectasias.
Think: Basal cell carcinoma.

Diagnosis

Clinical, confirmed by biopsy that reveals a palisading pattern of cells at the tumor's periphery

Treatment

Depends on type and location:

- Curettage and desiccation
- Surgical excision

- Radiation therapy (if surgery is contraindicated)
- Regular follow-up to detect recurrences

▶ SQUAMOUS CELL CARCINOMA

Definition

- A tumor of malignant keratinocytes accounting for the second most frequent type of skin cancer
- Growth may arise de novo, from an actinic keratosis, or from an underlying skin lesion.
- Lesions arising from an actinic keratosis have the least potential of metastasizing.

Actinic keratosis is a premalignant precursor to squamous cell carcinoma.

Epidemiology

> 55 years of age, commonly occurs in men, people with sun exposure, and outdoor workers

Risk Factors

- Sun and x-ray exposure
- Radiation therapy
- Tar, pitch, mineral oil, or arsenic exposure
- Immunosuppression
- Topical nitrogen mustard
- Human papillomavirus (HPV) infection
- Xeroderma pigmentosum.

Signs and Symptoms

- An erythematous scaling plaque that may be eroded or ulcerated with crust
- Hyperkeratotic center
- Distributed primarily on sun exposed skin of lips, cheeks, helix of ears, scalp, and dorsum of hand

Diagnosis

Clinical, confirmed by biopsy demonstrating malignant keratinocytes invading the dermis with keratin pearls

Treatment

- Surgical excision
- Radiotherapy (if surgery is contraindicated)

▶ MALIGNANT MELANOMA

Definition

- A malignant proliferation of melanocytes (pigment cells), accounting for 3% of all cancers
- May arise from normal-appearing skin (70%) or from a preexisting melanocytic nevi (mole) or skin lesion (30%)

Dysplastic nevus is a premalignant precursor to malignant melanoma.

Pathophysiology

- Characterized by two different growth phases: horizontal and vertical
- During the horizontal growth phase there is lateral extension within the epidermis and dermis, without metastasizing.
- When the tumor enters the vertical phase, it penetrates downward into the dermis, with a high risk of metastasis.
- Prognosis is based on the thickness of the primary tumor, measured histologically according to the depth of invasion from the surface to the deepest part of the tumor (Breslow's classification) or according to the depth of penetration in relation to the different layers of the dermis (Clark's classification).

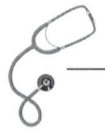

Melanomas can be brown, black, white, or blue.

Epidemiology

Incidence has been increasing worldwide, possibly related to increased exposure to sunlight.

Risk Factors

- Sunlight exposure
- Fair skin
- Positive family history (5%)

Signs and Symptoms

Commonly recognized clinical variants of melanoma include:

1. *Superficial spreading melanoma*—accounts for 70% of melanomas and is characterized by a prolonged horizontal growth phase. May develop as a new mole or as a change in a preexisting mole. During its horizontal growth phase, it appears as an elevated plaque with irregular borders and variegated colors, but it evolves into a nodule with bleeding and ulceration during its vertical phase.
2. *Nodular melanoma*—accounts for 15% of melanomas and is characterized only by a vertical growth phase. Develops as a blue, gray, or black papule or nodule that may ulcerate or bleed. Associated with a poor prognosis because metastasizes early.
3. *Lentigo maligna melanoma*—accounts for 10% of melanomas and occurs on sun exposed areas of the skin in elderly patients. During its vertical growth phase it develops as a slow growing macule that gradually forms irregular borders, indistinct edges, or variable shades of color. May be present for years as a macule (lentigo maligna) before development of melanoma.
4. *Acral lentiginous melanoma*—accounts for < 5% of melanomas, and is common in black and Asian people. Develops as a flat, variably pigmented macule on the palms, soles, and nail beds that enlarges peripherally during its horizontal growth phase, and becomes nodular during its vertical growth phase.

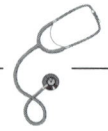

Suspicious features of malignant melanoma include the ABCDEE's:

- **A**symmetry
- **B**order (irregular)
- **C**olor (variegated and mottled)
- **D**iameter (> 0.6 cm)
- **E**levation
- **E**nlargement

Diagnosis

Clinical, based on change in size and color or development of bleeding and ulceration

Treatment

- Surgical excision with margins of at least 1 cm, depending on depth of lesion
- Follow-up

Prognosis

Bad Prognostic Factors

- Tumors with a prolonged vertical growth phase
- Proximal tumors
- Palpable nodes

Good Prognostic Factors

- Tumors with < 0.76 mm in depth have almost a 100% cure rate.
- Women have a better prognosis than men.

NOTES

HIGH-YIELD FACTS IN

Health Maintenance and Evidence-Based Medicine

General Preventive Care 365

- Leading Causes of Death in the United States 365
- Annual Exams 365
- Adult Vaccinations 366

Health Promotion in Women 367

- Hormone Replacement Therapy (HRT) 367
- Domestic Violence 367
- Depression 368

Substance Abuse 369

- Alcohol Abuse 369
- Tobacco Use 370
- Opioid Use 371
- Sympathomimetics 371

Injury Prevention 372

- Motor Vehicle Injuries 372
- Falls 372

Nutritional Disorders 373

- Malnutrition 373
- Obesity 373
- Vitaminoses 374

Environmental Exposures 375

- Heat Exhaustion 375
- Heatstroke 375

Cold-Related Illness 375

Frostbite 375
Hypothermia 376
Principles of Medical Ethics 376
Principles of Evidence-Based Medicine 376
Statistical Concepts 378

General Preventive Care

► LEADING CAUSES OF DEATH IN THE UNITED STATES

1. Heart disease (29.0%)
2. Cancer (23.2%)
3. Stroke (6.8%)
4. Chronic obstructive pulmonary disease (COPD)
5. Unintentional injury (4.1%)
6. Diabetes mellitus (3.1%)
7. Influenza and pneumonia (2.7%)
8. Alzheimer's disease (2.5%)
9. Nephritis (1.7%)
10. Septicemia (1.4%)

Note: Suicide replaces Alzheimer's disease in persons < 65 years old.

► ANNUAL EXAMS

History and Counseling

Health Maintenance
- Nutrition
- Exercise (recommend 30 minutes of aerobic exercise 3×/wk)
- Weight gain/loss

Accident Prevention
- Safety belt/helmet use
- Smoke detectors
- Firearm safety

Toxic Habits
- Alcohol consumption (CAGE criteria; see Alcohol section)
- Tobacco use
- Illicit drug use

Sexuality
- Contraception
- Sexually transmitted disease (STD) prevention

Domestic Violence
- Elder abuse
- Spousal abuse

Tests and Exams

Gynecologic Cancer Screening
- Pap smear and pelvic exam (annually, beginning when first sexually active or at 18 yrs)
- Mammogram (40+, q2y; 50+, qy)
- Breast exam (annually, beginning at age 40)

Colon Cancer Screening
- Digital rectal exam
- Guaiac (50+)
- Sigmoidoscopy (50+, q3y)

Prostate Screening (controversial!)
- PSA and digital rectal exam yearly starting at 50
- No screening after age 70

The only cancer screenings that are effective:
- Breast cancer (mammogram)
- Cervical cancer (Pap smear)
- Colon cancer (sigmoidoscopy/colonoscopy)
- Prostate cancer (PSA, controversial)

Cardiovascular
- Lipid profile (m: 35+, f: 45+)
- Blood pressure

Classification of Hypertension in Adults
- Normal: < 120/80 mmHg
- Prehypertension: 120–139/80–89 mmHg
- Stage 1 hypertension: 140–159/90–99 mmHg
- Stage 2 hypertension: > 160/100 mmHg

Age-Related Changes
- Height: Decreases as bone mass is lost with age
- Vision and auditory screening (65+)

▶ ADULT VACCINATIONS

Vaccinations for AIDS patients:
- Influenza
- Hepatitis B
- Hib
- Childhood vaccines, if missed

Tetanus

Who: Everyone
When: DTaP series in childhood, booster q10y (or if > **5**y with a dirty wound)

Hepatitis B

Who: Everyone
When: One series of three injections (each 1 month apart)

Influenza

Who: Health care workers, age > 65, the chronically ill, and household contacts of these people
When: Annually, autumn (new vaccine each year based on prediction of prevalent strains)

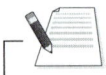

Live vaccines:
- MMR
- Oral polio
- Yellow fever
- BCG
- Typhoid

Do not give to pregnant or immunocompromised patients (except AIDS patients **can** receive MMR).

Pneumococcal

Who: Age > 65, the chronically ill
When: Once every 5 years

Measles, Mumps, Rubella (MMR)

Who: All persons born after 1956 who lack evidence of immunity to measles

When: First one age 12 to 15 months, second one between 4 and 6 years, then a booster during adulthood if not previously received or not immune

Varicella

Who: Healthy adults with no history of varicella infection or previous vaccination

When: Two doses of varicella vaccine delivered 4 to 8 weeks apart are recommended.

Health Promotion in Women

▶ HORMONE REPLACEMENT THERAPY (HRT)

Benefits

Estrogen decreases risks of:

- Osteoporosis by 25%
- Senile dementia
- Urinary incontinence, urinary tract infections (UTIs), and vaginal atrophy (local estrogen also effective)
- Reduces hot flashes

Risks

- Endometrial cancer: Associated with unopposed estrogen use. Can be prevented by using estrogen–progestin combination.
- Breast cancer: Women with estrogen receptor–positive breast cancer worsen with HRT. Increases risk as well.
- Coronary artery disease and stroke: Recent trials (HERS and HERS II) show increased risk.
- Venous thromboembolism

▶ DOMESTIC VIOLENCE

Epidemiology

- Lifetime prevalence 20% for women
- In the United States, approximately 2,000 women die each year as a direct result of injuries.

Signs and Symptoms

- Frequent or unexplained injuries
- Depression/suicide attempts
- Substance abuse

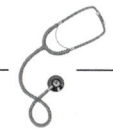

- Estrogen inhibits osteoclast bone resorption.
- Estrogen elevates high-density lipoprotein (HDL), lowers low-density lipoprotein (LDL), but raises triglycerides.

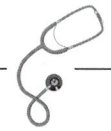

Raloxifene mimics estrogenic effects on osteoclasts but has no effect on breast, endometrium, or lipid profile. Useful for prevention of osteoporosis in women at high risk for breast cancer. Other benefits are lost.

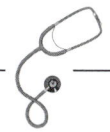

HERS and HERS II trials show increased risk of MI and stroke with hormone replacement therapy.

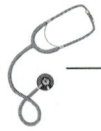

Domestic violence help is more commonly sought during pregnancy.

- Anxiety
- Headaches
- Chronic pain

Screening

- Women should be routinely asked about domestic violence due to its high prevalence.
- Routine screening of women by physicians is thought to yield positive results in about **half** of all cases.

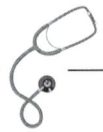

How to ask:
- "Have you ever been hit, hurt, or threatened by your partner?"
- "Have you ever been a victim of domestic violence?"
- "Many of my patients with your symptoms have experienced physical violence. Has this happened to you?"

Treatment

- Treat medical conditions.
- Assess safety of patient's current situation.
- Provide information (shelters, social agencies).
- Reassure patient that no one deserves to be abused.

▶ DEPRESSION

Epidemiology

- Debilitating mood disorder that has a lifetime prevalence of about 15%
- Incidence higher in women
- Mean age is 40 years.

Risk Factors

- Family history of depression, suicide, substance abuse
- Presence of chronic disease
- Personal history of substance abuse
- Lack of support system

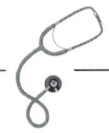

Differential diagnosis of depression:
- Bereavement
- Substance abuse
- Hypothyroidism
- Medication side effect
- Organic brain disease

Signs and Symptoms

Depressed mood with sadness, weight loss, guilt, fatigue, insomnia or hypersomnia, anhedonia, psychomotor agitation or retardation, difficulty concentrating or suicidal ideation, for at least 2 consecutive weeks

Treatment

- All patients should be asked specifically about suicidal intent.
- Patients who are actively suicidal require inpatient evaluation by a psychiatrist.
- Evaluate for antidepressant medication.

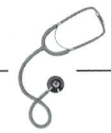

How to ask about depression:
"Have you been feeling overwhelmingly sad lately?"
"Have you lost pleasure in the things you used to enjoy?"

SUBSTANCE ABUSE

▶ ALCOHOL ABUSE

DEFINITION

Alcohol abuse is associated with failure to fulfill work or social obligations, physical danger because of alcohol use, or recurrent legal problems due to alcohol use.

Alcohol dependence is at least three of the following: tolerance, withdrawal, taking more than intended, desire to cut down, time spent obtaining alcohol, aspects of life sacrificed.

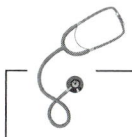

How to ask about suicidal intent:
"Have you ever thought that life was not worth living?"
"Have you ever thought about killing yourself?"
"Have you ever made a plan to kill yourself?"

SCREENING

CAGE Questions

1. Have you ever tried cut down your drinking?
2. Have you ever been angry/annoyed when people ask about your drinking?
3. Have you ever felt guilty about your drinking?
4. Have you ever had an eye-opener (drink on waking up in the morning)?

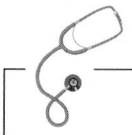

Cancers due to alcohol use:
- Head and neck cancers
- Esophageal and gastric cancers
- Pancreatic cancer
- Liver cancer
- Breast cancer

Systemic Effects

See Table 2.11-1.

TABLE 2.11-1. Systemic Effects of Alcohol Abuse

	ACUTE	CHRONIC
Central nervous system	CNS depression, amnesia, fragmented sleep	Peripheral neuropathy, Wernicke's and Korsakoff's syndromes (thiamine deficiency), cerebellar degeneration, alcoholic dementia
Cardiovascular system	Decreased myocardial contractility, peripheral vasodilation	Hypertension, cardiomyopathy, increased HDL cholesterol
Gastrointestinal system	Esophageal and gastric inflammation, acute pancreatitis	Mallory–Weiss tear, esophageal varices, portal hypertension, chronic pancreatitis
Liver	Impaired gluconeogenesis	Alcohol-induced hepatitis, cirrhosis
Hematopoietic system	Macrocytosis	Thrombocytopenia, hypersplenism, decreased platelet aggregation
Genitourinary system	Erectile dysfunction	Testicular atrophy, amenorrhea, ovarian atrophy, increased risk of spontaneous abortion, fetal alcohol syndrome

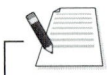

Alcohol and benzodiazepine withdrawal are life threatening. Opioid and cocaine withdrawal are not.

Withdrawal Syndrome

Can range from mild anxiety and tremor to alcohol withdrawal seizures and delirium tremens. Alcohol withdrawal is life threatening. Treat with benzodiazepine taper. Usual onset is 12 to 48 hours after last drink.

Delirium Tremens

- Tachycardia, fever, hallucinations
- 5 to 30% mortality if untreated
- Treatment: Sedation with benzodiazepines and intensive care

▶ TOBACCO USE

DEFINITION

- Single largest cause of preventable death in the United States
- About 450,000 people in the United States die each year from tobacco-related disease:
  - 40% cardiovascular
  - 35% due to cancer
  - 20% respiratory
  - 5% cerebrovascular

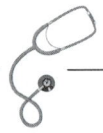

Types of tobacco-related cancer: "CANCER PLUS"
Colon
A
Neck
Cervix
Esophagus
Renal
Pancreas
Lung
Urogenital (bladder)
Stomach

Tobacco-Related Disease

Smoking:

- Promotes atherosclerosis, thrombosis, arrhythmias
- Reduces oxygen carrying capacity of the blood
- Reduces elasticity in the lungs and causes COPD and emphysema
- During pregnancy associated with increased risk of spontaneous abortion, fetal death, and sudden infant death syndrome

Smokeless tobacco products cause oral and head and neck cancers.

Smoking Cessation Counseling

Should be a primary focus of all physician encounters with smokers:

- Identify all smokers and tobacco users by routine questioning during history.
- Instruct all tobacco users to stop, giving personalized advice and support (e.g., "If you stop smoking, your cough will improve").
- Evaluate each patient for readiness and motivation. If the patient is not motivated, reinforce that support for smoking cessation will be available when the patient is ready.
- Formulate a plan with the patient, including a quit date, nicotine replacement or other pharmacologic therapy, and follow-up appointment for support.

The most effective way to extend life expectancy is smoking cessation.

Smoking Cessation Pharmacotherapy

- Nicotine patches are associated with a 40% quit rate.
- Bupropion is associated with a 55% quit rate.
- Combination is associated with a 66% quit rate.
- Ongoing counseling may improve abstinence.

▶ OPIOID USE

Signs and Symptoms

- Depressed mental status
- Respiratory depression
- Pupillary constriction (or dilation with profound respiratory depression)
- Overdose can cause death.

Treatment

- Naloxone is an opioid antagonist that rapidly reverses toxicity, but is short acting (< 30 min).
- Use is both diagnostic and therapeutic.

Opiate Withdrawal Syndrome

Not life threatening, except in very young and very old, but may lead to relapse, using street drugs, and exposure to needle sharing with its attendant risks such as acquisition of HIV and hepatitis C.

Signs and Symptoms

- Nausea
- Vomiting
- Diarrhea
- Mydriasis
- Piloerection
- Diffuse muscle pain
- Desire for more drug

Treatment

- Long-acting opioid (e.g., methadone)
- Symptomatic relief
- Supportive care

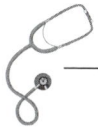

A patient on opioids for true pain control has little risk of developing opiate dependence.

▶ SYMPATHOMIMETICS

Signs and Symptoms

- Syndrome of catecholamine excess
- Agitation
- Tachycardia
- Hypertension
- Hyperthermia

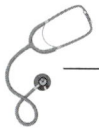

3% of all patients seen in the emergency department and 6% of all patients admitted to the hospital with cocaine chest pain will have biochemical evidence for a myocardial infarction.

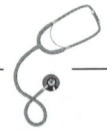

Beta blockers are contraindicated in patients with cocaine use due to the risk of unopposed alpha-adrenergic tone, which may worsen vasoconstriction.

- Psychosis
- Seizures
- Chest pain

TREATMENT

- Benzodiazepines to control excess sympathetic discharge and anxiety
- Cooling measures to control hyperthermia
- Nitroglycerin and heparin to control chest pain

INJURY PREVENTION

▶ MOTOR VEHICLE INJURIES

Statistics

- Cause about 30% of all deaths between ages 15 and 25
- Disproportionately affect the young, so responsible for more years of life lost than any other single cause
- Alcohol is implicated in 44% of all traffic fatalities.

Seatbelt Use

Associated with an 89% reduction in mortality, and concurrent airbag use further reduces mortality

Motorcycle Collisions

Motorcycle use is associated with a fatality rate 20 times greater than that of passenger cars.

Helmet Use

Reduces motorcycle fatalities by 37% and reduces the incidence of head injury by 67%.

Screening

- Ask all patients about seatbelt use, airbag availability, helmet use, child safety seat use, and alcohol use.
- Intervene when patients show behaviors that put others in danger (e.g., adult does not provide toddler with a child safety seat).

▶ FALLS

Most common cause of injuries

RISK FACTORS

- Elderly
- Disability
- Alcohol intoxication

Prevention

- Assess gait of each patient.
- Assess vision of each patient.
- Provide corrective devices or referral for identified impairment.
- Counsel alcohol use cessation.

Nutritional Disorders

▶ MALNUTRITION

Definitions

- Marasmus: Starvation
- Kwashiorkor: Protein deficiency
- Essential fatty acids: Linoleic and linolenic acids

Risk Factors

- Low socioeconomic class
- Nursing home and hospitalized patients

Complications

- Anemia
- Hypoalbuminemia
- Poor wound healing
- Weakness
- Decubitus ulcers
- Infection
- Death

OBESITY

Definition

Body mass index (BMI) > 30 kg/m^2

Complications

- Atherosclerosis
- Type 2 diabetes
- Sleep apnea
- Osteoarthritis
- Gout
- Venous stasis
- Biliary disease
- Endometrial cancer
- Postmenopausal breast cancer

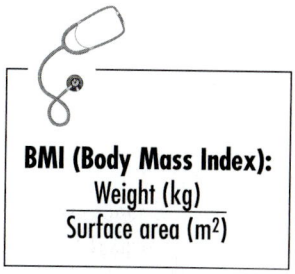

Treatment

- Behavior modification, exercise
- Low-calorie diet with < 25% of calories from fat
- Goal: 10% weight loss over 6 months

If the above fail, consider:

- Pharmacologic therapy
- Bariatric surgery (for BMI > 40 m^2 or > 35 m^2 with comorbid disease)

▶ VITAMINOSES

See Table 2.11-2.

TABLE 2.11-2. Syndromes of Vitamin Deficiency and Excess

Vitamin	Deficiency	Excess
Vitamin A	Early: Night blindness Late: Keratomalacia, blindness	Acute: GI symptoms, headache, papilledema Chronic: Joint pain, hair loss, fissured lips, anorexia, weight loss, hepatomegaly
Vitamin C	Scurvy: Petechial hemorrhage, ecchymoses, gum bleeding, poor wound healing, anemia	Uricosuria, kidney stones
Vitamin E	Areflexia, decreased proprioception, gait abnormality	Potentiates oral anticoagulants
Vitamin K	Prolonged bleeding time	Attenuates oral anticoagulants
Niacin	(aka Pellagra): Chronic wasting, dermatitis, dementia, diarrhea	GI symptoms, flushing, pruritus, hepatotoxicity
Thiamine (vitamin B_1)	Beriberi (dry) Peripheral neuropathy Wernicke's encephalopathy (horizontal nystagmus followed by lateral rectus palsy, fever, ataxia, encephalopathy, death) Korsakoff's syndrome (retrograde amnesia, confabulation)	
Pyridoxine (vitamin B_6)	Seizures Glossitis, cheilosis GI symptoms Weakness Peripheral neuropathy	

Environmental Exposures

▶ HEAT EXHAUSTION

- Normal core temperature, symptoms due to dehydration and salt loss
- Characterized by headache, nausea and vomiting, weakness, irritability, and cramps.
- Treat with oral or IV hydration with salt-containing fluids, and patient should rest in a cool environment.

How to remember the 3 D's of niacin deficiency: Three doctors drank a nice Pellegrino.

▶ HEATSTROKE

- Failure of thermoregulation
- Associated with elevated core temperature and central nervous system (CNS) dysfunction such as altered mental status, focal deficits, hemiplegia, and posturing
- Exertional heatstroke is a result of exercise or physical labor in a high heat-index environment
- Classic or nonexertional heatstroke is usually seen in elderly or nonacclimated patients during summer heat waves.

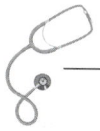

Patients who are dehydrated, disabled, or chronically ill or who are alcohol or drug users are more prone to developing heatstroke.

Treatment of Heatstroke

- Rapid cooling by cooling blanket, evaporation, ice packs to axilla and groin, or gastric or peritoneal lavage is critical to prevent rhabdomyolysis, multiorgan failure, and death.

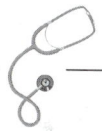

Cooling should be halted when the patient's core temperature reaches 39°C to prevent hypothermia.

Cold-Related Illness

Risk Factors

- Overwhelming cold exposure
- Extremes of age
- Intoxicated patients
- Homelessness
- Concurrent illness
- Iatrogenic

▶ FROSTBITE

- Caused by exposure of the skin to freezing temperatures; usually seen on the extremities, nose, and ears.
- As the body reduces cutaneous blood flow in freezing temperatures to maintain the core body temperature, capillary blood becomes more viscous, and ice crystals form in the extracellular space. This causes direct tissue injury and osmotic pressures that cause intracellular dehydration.

Frostbite is more common in diabetics due to neuropathy.

Treatment

- Rapid rewarming with clean water at 40 to 42°C
- Tetanus prophylaxis
- Debridement of tissues and prophylactic antibiotics remains controversial.

▶ HYPOTHERMIA

Definition

Core (rectal) temperature:
- Mild: 35 to 32°C
- Moderate: 32 to 28°C
- Severe: < 28°C

Signs and Symptoms

- Shivering
- Poor judgment
- Paradoxical undressing
- Cardiac dysrhythmias
- Osborne wave: A convex, upward deflection of the J point on the ECG

Treatment

Rewarming by:
- Warming blanket
- Warm packs to groin and axillae
- Infusion of warmed IV fluid

For severely hypothermic or pulseless patients:
- Warm-fluid lavage of bladder, stomach, peritoneum, and pleural space
- Extracorporeal rewarming techniques (cardiac bypass)

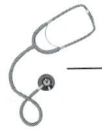

Rewarm patients and continue cardiac resuscitation before declaring death. "You're not dead until you're warm and dead."

▶ PRINCIPLES OF MEDICAL ETHICS

See Table 2.11-3.

▶ PRINCIPLES OF EVIDENCE-BASED MEDICINE

Definition

- Practice of incorporating the best available evidence from the medical literature for a diagnostic test or treatment into daily patient care
- Best evidence obtained from randomized clinical trials

Steps

1. Identify a clinical problem.
2. Formulate a question.
3. Search for the best evidence.

TABLE 2.11-3. Principles of Medical Ethics

Principle	Definition
Autonomy	▪ Ability to function independently and to make decisions about one's care free from the undue influence or bias of others ▪ All patients are considered autonomous if they have the ability to understand the situation as evaluated with competency examination by psychiatrist (capacity) and are not a danger to self or others (suicidal, homicidal, demented, delirious).
Nonmalfeasance	▪ The principle of *primum non nocere,* or first, do no harm
Beneficence	▪ The principle of doing good ▪ The practice of doing whatever is best for the patient without the consideration of the patient's wishes is called *paternalism.*
Distributive justice	▪ The principle of equal and fair allocation of benefit. Patients of different race, gender, and disability should be treated differently only on the basis of medical need and projected benefit.
Advance directives	▪ Oral or written instructions from a patient to family members and health care professionals about health care decisions ▪ May include living wills, designation of a health care proxy, specific instructions about which therapies to accept or decline including intubation, surgery or medical treatments, and Do Not Resuscitate (DNR) orders ▪ A DNR order applies only to advanced cardiac life support (ACLS) resuscitation, and does not include intubation and ventilation unless specifically addressed.

4. Appraise the evidence.
5. Apply the information to the clinical problem.

Sources of Medical Evidence

- **Meta-analysis:** Evaluates the data of many trials that address the same question, and attempts to combine the information. These studies are best used when the clinical problem is infrequent and large randomized trials cannot be done.
- **Randomized controlled clinical trial:** The selected population is randomized to receive either the treatment in question or a placebo, and the outcome is measured. The ideal RCT is triple-blinded, meaning that both the treating physician, the patient, and the investigators, do not know which treatment has been given until the analysis is complete. These studies can establish cause and effect.
- **Cohort study:** The selected population is identified as being exposed or not exposed, and is monitored for subsequent effects. These studies are used when the exposure cannot be assigned for logistical or ethical reasons.
- **Case control study:** Populations with and without a given outcome are selected, and historical (retrospective) data is collected on exposure to a given agent or treatment.

See Tables 2.11-4 and 2.11-5.

TABLE 2.11-4. Statistical Concepts

Concept	Definition
Sensitivity	▪ Measures the ability of a test to accurately detect true-positive results: TP/(TP + FN) (true positive test results/all patients with the disease). ▪ The more sensitive a test, the less likely the test is to fail to detect a positive result. This is sometimes called a true-positive rate (TPR).
Specificity	▪ Measures the ability of a test to accurately detect true-negative results: TN/(FP + TN) (true negative test result/all patients without the disease). ▪ The more specific a test, the less likely the test is to fail to detect a negative result. This is sometimes called a true-negative rate (TNR).
Positive predictive value	▪ Measures the chance that a patient with a positive test result in truth has the disease: TP/(TP + FP) (true positives/test positives). Depends on disease prevalence.
Negative predictive value	▪ Measures the chance that a patient with a negative test result in truth does not have the disease: TN/(TN + FN) (true negatives/test negatives). Depends on disease prevalence.
Likelihood ratio	▪ Measures the fixed relationship between the chance of given test result in a patient with the disorder and the chance of the same test result in a patient without the disorder. ▪ Likelihood ratio for a positive test result is expressed as: sensitivity/(1-specificity) or true-positive rate (TPR)/false-positive rate (FPR). ▪ Likelihood ratio for a negative test result is expressed as: (1-sensitivity)/specificity or false-negative rate (FNR)/true-negative rate (TNR). ▪ A test with known likelihood ratios can help a clinician with decision making; the pretest likelihood that a patient has a disease can be either improved with a high positive likelihood ratio (> 2) or reduced with a low negative likelihood ratio (< 0.5).
Confidence interval	▪ Range around a sample mean that contains the true population mean to any desired degree of probability (frequently 95%).
Number needed to treat	▪ Measures the number of patients with a given disease that a clinician would need to treat with the tested therapy in order to see one beneficial event or prevent one adverse event.
Prevalence	▪ Number of individuals with a given disease in a population at one point in time (number with disease/number in population)
Incidence	▪ Number of new events (new cases of disease) over a specific period of time (number of new events/number in population)

TABLE 2.11-5. Sensitivity and Specificity vs. Positive and Negative Predictive Value

	Disease Present	Disease Absent	
Test Positive	True Positive (TP)	False Positive (FP)	Positive predictive value = TP/(TP+FP)
Test Negative	False Negative (FN)	True Negative (TN)	Negative predictive value = FN/(FN+TN)
	Sensitivity = TP/(TP/FN)	Specificity = FP/(FP+TN)	

NOTES

SECTION 3: CLASSIFIED

Awards and Opportunities for Students Interested in Medicine

- General Awards
- Research Awards
- Summer Externships
- Year-Long Fellowships
- For Minority Students
- Ethnic
- For Women
- Evidence-Based Medicine Links

The Paul & Daisy Soros Fellowships for New Americans

The fellowships are grants for $20,000 for up to 2 years of graduate study in the United States. The recipients are chosen on a national competitive basis. Thirty fellowships will be awarded each year.

A New American is an individual who (1) is a resident alien (i.e., holds a green card) or (2) has been naturalized as a U.S. citizen or (3) is the child of two parents who are both naturalized citizens.

The purpose of The Paul & Daisy Soros Fellowships for New Americans is to provide opportunities for continuing generations of able and accomplished New Americans to achieve leadership in their chosen fields. The program is established in recognition of the contributions New Americans have made to American life and in gratitude for the opportunities the United States has afforded the donors and their family. *Contact:* 400 West 59th Street, New York, NY 10019. Phone: 212-547-6926; Fax: 212-548-4623; *www.pdsoros.org.*

AMERICAN ASSOCIATION FOR THE HISTORY OF MEDICINE OSLER MEDAL

The medal is awarded for the best unpublished essay on a medico-historical subject written by a student in a school of medicine or of osteopathy in the United States or Canada. Essays appropriate for consideration by the committee may pertain either to the historical development of a contemporary medical problem or to a topic within the health sciences of a discrete past period. The essay should demonstrate either original research or an unusual appreciation and understanding of the problem or situation discussed. Winner will receive $500 in travel money to deliver paper at the American Association for the History of Medicine.

Ty Cobb Scholarship Program

For medical students who are legal residents of Georgia. *Contact:* Ty Cobb Foundation, Post Office Box 725, Forest Park, GA 30298, or e-mail *tycobb@mindspring.com.*

Coe Memorial Scholarship

For medical students who are from the Auburn, New York, area. *Contact:* Norstar Trust Company, Coe Memorial Scholarship Fund, 120 Genesee St., Auburn, NY 13021.

COUNTRY DOCTOR SCHOLARSHIP PROGRAM

$10,000 annually, $40,000 aggregate

Georgia residents qualify for funding to obtain primary care medical degrees such as internal medicine, general surgery, OB-GYN, pediatrics, and family practice. In return, the student must practice in a Georgia board-approved town of 15,000 or less population. *Contact:* Joe B. Lawley, Ph.D., State Medical Education Board, 270 Washington St. SW, 7th Floor, Room 7093, Atlanta, GA 30334.

Southern Medical Association Medical Student

$500 to $2,500 awards for students who are SMA members in their first year of medical school, of superior ability with demonstrated financial need.

Olive D. Hoffman Scholarship

$5,000 scholarship for students committed to community service. *Contact:* Olive D. Hoffman Memorial Inc., 1474 North Pointe Village, Center Suite 280, Reston, VA 22094.

ILLINOIS HOSPITAL ASSOCIATION SCHOLARSHIP

$500 award for students who are Illinois residents with demonstrated financial need and academic acheievement. *Contact:* Scholarship, The Illinois Hospital Association, Center for Health Affairs, 1151 East Warrenville Rd., P.O. Box 3015, Naperville, IL 60566.

International Order of the King's Daughters and Sons

$1,000 scholarships for medical students. *Contact:* Health Careers Director, Mrs. Fred Cannon, Box 1310, Brookhaven, MS 39602-1310.

NEW YORK ACADEMY OF MEDICINE: DAVID E. ROGERS FELLOWSHIP PROGRAM

The David E. Rogers Fellowship Program is national fellowship for medical students in support of a project initiated during the summer between the first and second years of medical school. Ten fellowships of $2,500 will be awarded. The fellowship is meant to enrich the educational experiences of medical students through projects that couple medicine with the needs of underserved or disadvantaged patients or populations. For more information, contact the Rogers Fellowship at *rogers@nyam.org* or the New York Academy of Medicine. Contact your school's financial aid office for more info.

DoctorsCare Internationale Foundation Scholarships

DoctorsCare is an independent nonprofit organization created to promote scientific research, education, and medical health programs that contribute toward improving the health of mankind. The foundation has funds for annual grants for needy men and women in the field of medicine. Applications may be obtained by sending a self-addressed, stamped envelope to: Grants Department, Doctors Care Internationale Foundation, P.O. Box 1111, Houston, TX 77251-1111.

Wilderness Society Charles S. Houston Award

Award for a project proposal that is likely to result in a substantive contribution to the field of wilderness or environmental medicine. The applicant will conduct his project during the calendar year and present results at the Annual Meeting of the Society. Award: $1,500.

U.S. DEPARTMENT OF HEALTH AND HUMAN SERVICES INNOVATIONS IN HEALTH AWARD

An annual competition for innovative proposals for health promotion and disease prevention. The proposal must be concerned with disease prevention or health promotion. It could describe a community risk-reduction effort; a project for a whole community or a special population group, such as the aged or children; a health promotion program at the worksite; or a preventive approach for community education, such as primary and secondary school programs. Awards range from $250 to $3,000.

Life and Health Insurance Medical Research Fund Medical Scientist Scholarship

A five-year scholarship program for an MD/PhD student who will have completed 2 years of medical school before July and is usually not already funded. $16,000 per year.

Johnson & Johnson Student Paper

Students are invited to submit papers expressing original ideas in the broad area of engineering in medicine and biology.

American Academy of Medical Ethics William Liley Essay Contest

An essay contest for medical students and residents on a topic designated by the Academy. $250– $2,000 prizes.

PAUL W. MAYER SCHOLARSHIP IN MEDICINE AND BIOLOGY

Sponsored by the Alliance for Engineering, this is a scholarship to encourage student excellence in the field of biomedical engineering. Grant is $200. Contact your school's financial aid office for more info.

Jerry L. Memorial Pettis Scholarship

Sponsored by the American Medical Association Education and Research Foundation, this scholarship will be awarded to a junior or senior medical student with a demonstrated interest in the communication of science. Financial need of nominees will not be a consideration. *Contact:* American Medical Association Education and Research Foundation, 515 North State Street, Chicago, IL 60610. Phone: 312-464-5357; Fax: 312-464-5973; *www.ama-assn.org/med-sci/erf/toc.htm*.

Student Paper Competition in Medical Informatics

Students are invited to submit papers expressing original ideas in the broad areas of medical informatics and computer applications in medical care for the SCAMC (Symposium on Computer Applications in Medical

Care). Awards consist of the Martin N. Epstein Award of $1,000 and two cash prizes of $600 and $400 for second and third place. Contact your school's financial aid office for more info.

AMERICAN COLLEGE OF LEGAL MEDICINE SCHWARTZ AWARD

Each year the ACLM presents the Schwartz Award for the outstanding paper on legal medicine. The award provides a $1,000 honorarium, transportation, accommodations and meals at the ACLM annual meeting. Contact your school's financial aid office for more info.

Medical History Society of New Jersey Stephen Wickes Prize in the History of Medicine

Any currently enrolled undergraduate, graduate, or professional student is eligible to submit an original essay on a historical subject in the medical or allied fields. The topic may be historical aspects of a current problem, or it may deal with a specific subject in a defined period of the past. Prize: $100. Contact your school's financial aid office for more info.

Northeastern Ohio University College of Medicine William Carlos Poetry Competition

The Human Values in Medicine at Northeastern Ohio Universities College of Medicine is sponsoring this annual poetry-writing competition for students attending schools of medicine or osteopathy in the United States. Prize: $100–$300. Contact your school's financial aid office for more info.

New York Academy of Medicine:

The Paul Klemperer Fellowship in the History of Medicine and the Audrey and William H. Helfand Fellowship in the Medical Humanities

Each year the New York Academy of Medicine offers the Paul Klemperer Fellowship and the Audrey and William H. Helfand Fellowship to support work in history and the humanities as they relate to health, medicine, and the biomedical sciences. The Klemperer Fellowship supports research using the Academy Library as a historical resource. It is intended specifically for a scholar in residence in the collections of the Academy Library.

The Helfand Fellowship more broadly supports work in the humanities, including both creative projects dealing with health and the medical enterprise, and scholarly research in a humanistic discipline—other than history of medicine—as applied to medicine and health. Although residence is not obligatory, preference in the selection process will be given applicants whose projects require use of the resources of the Academy Library and who plan to spend time at the Academy. The Helfand Fellowship and the Klemperer Fellowship each provide stipends of up to $5,000 to support travel, lodging, and incidental expenses for a flexible period between June 1, 2001, and May 31, 2002. Besides completing research or a creative project, each Fellow will be expected to make a presentation at the Academy and submit a final report on the project. Applications are accepted from anyone—regardless of citizenship, academic discipline, or academic status—who wishes to use the Academy's collections for historical research or for a scholarly or creative project in the medical humanities. *Contact:* Fellowship Program Coordinator, New York Academy of Medicine, 1216 Fifth Avenue, Room 612, New York, NY 10029. Phone: 212-822-7204; Fax: 212-996-7826.

AGENCY FOR INTERNATIONAL DEVELOPMENT INTERNSHIP

Sponsoring Agency: A.I.D.
Two-week educational program (over Christmas holiday) for graduate students from the Caribbean and South and Central America, which may lead to summer placement in transnational corporations over summer. Program focuses on U.S. foreign policy and Latin American indebtedness. Travel costs to seminar in Baton Rouge paid.

Alpha Omega Alpha Essay Award

The purpose of these $500–$750 awards is to stimulate medical students to address general topics in medicine and to enable the society to recognize in a tangible way excellent and thoughtful presentations. The topic of the essay may be any nontechnical aspect of medicine including, medical education, medical ethics, philosophy as related to medicine, reflections on illness, science, and the culture and history of medicine.

American Bureau for Medical Advancement in China

Open to fourth-year students. Several university teaching hospitals in Taiwan offer clinical clerkships to qualifying students. Electives of 2 months are optimal, although shorter ones will be considered. It is expected that students will be able to provide for their own transportation and room and board, but Warner–Lambert has provided a grant to accommodate several partial scholarships.

AMERICAN COLLEGE OF NUTRITION

Award based on original scientific work in Clinical Nutrition. Award: $500 plus transportation to meeting.

American College of Preventive Medicine

$1,000 award for the best paper on preventive medicine—oriented topics; papers concerned with women's health issues encouraged.

National Council on Aging—Geriatric Fellowship

Sponsored by Travelers Insurance Aging, Inc., this program is designed to increase students' technical knowledge of geriatrics and to help sensitize them to social and personal problems facing older people. A fellowship of $3,000 will be provided.

JOSEPH AND ROSE KENNEDY INSTITUTE OF ETHICS NATIONAL HUMANITIES IN MEDICINE SEMINAR

This seminar was established to achieve three purposes: to provide selected medical students with an intensive experience in research and writing in the history of medicine, or philosophy of medicine, or literature and medicine; to encourage these students to develop programs of research and writing in a discipline of the humanities, which they will carry out during subsequent years of professional education and training and during careers as clinicians and humanists; and to link these students with other humanists in medicine across generational and disciplinary boundaries. Each student will receive a stipend of $1,200 to cover room and board. Students will be reimbursed for round-trip air fares to and from their school or home.

ACP-ASIM Medical Student Abstract Competition

Wanted: Students involved in research projects through their medical schools or community service programs they want to share with others, or who have come across as interesting case during an internal medicine rotation or through an internal medicine preceptorship program. If you are a medical student member of the ACP-ASIM, you are invited to submit an abstract to the annual Medical Student Abstract Competition. Ten winners will be awarded an expense-paid trip to the annual session. Abstracts may be submitted electronically using our online form at *www.acp.org*.

Medical Student Membership in the American College of Physicians–American Society of Internal Medicine

ACP-ASIM membership entitles you to special discounts on various college products, free attendance at ACP-ASIM annual session (the annual scientific meeting) and local chapter meetings, and a subscription to IMpact, the medical student newsletter.

AMA POLITICAL ACTION COMMITTEE (AMPAC)

AMPAC is a bipartisan group that serves to advance the interest of medicine within Congress, specifically by supporting candidates for office that are friendly to medicine. They also provide numerous programs to educate physicians, medical students, and their families on political activism. The board directs the programs and activities of this extremely important political action committee. Adding medical students to the leadership of this group will provide for better medical student representation within the group, as well as greater student involvement in this important process. Terms are for 2 years. Contact the American Medical Association for more information.

AMA Foundation Leadership Award Program

This award is an exciting opportunity to advance your leadership skills within organized medicine. Medical students who have demonstrated strong nonclinical leadership skills in medicine or community affairs and have an interest in further developing these skills within organized medicine are eligible. The objective of the award program is to encourage involvement in organized medicine and continue leadership development among the country's brightest and most energetic medical students and residents. Twenty-five medical students will be selected. Travel expenses for award winners, including airfare and 3 night's hotel, will be paid for directly by the AMA Foundation to attend the 2001 AMA National Leadership Development Conference. For applications, call 1-800-AMA-3211, ext. 4751 or 4746.

American Medical Student Association (AMSA)

International Health Opportunities.
www.amsa.org/global/ih/ihopps.cfm

AMA-MSS Councils

The medical student section of the AMA (AMA-MSS) has several councils for which it seeks medical students. Application involves a current curriculum vitae, an essay on why you want to be a member of an AMA Council, which Council(s) you prefer, what you consider to be your major strengths and qualifications for the position, and what benefits you feel are likely to result from your participation.

- Council on Constitution and Bylaws
- Council on Ethical and Judicial Affairs
- Council on Legislation
- Council on Long-Range Planning and Development
- Council on Medical Education
- Council on Medical Service
- Council on Scientific Affairs

EDITORIAL POSITIONS WITH MEDICAL STUDENT JAMA

MS/JAMA is the 7- to 8-page medical student section of the *Journal of the American Medical Association* (JAMA) that appears in the first JAMA of every month, September through May, and is also produced each month on the MS/JAMA Web site. As a regular section of a major medical journal, produced by and for medical students, MS/JAMA represents a unique opportunity to train to become journal editors, writers, and contributors. The MS/JAMA Web site is located at *www.ama-assn.org/msjama*.

AMA-MSS Committee Application

Medical students are sought to serve on the following AMA-MSS committees:

- Committee on Computers and Technology (formerly Computer Projects Committee)
- Committee on Long-Range Planning
- Legislative Affairs Committee
- Minority Issues Committee
- Ad Hoc Committee on Community Service and Advocacy
- Ad Hoc Committee on Membership Recruitment and Retention
- Ad Hoc Committee on MSS Programs and Activities
- Ad Hoc Committee on Scientific Issues Committee (CSI)
- Ad Hoc Committee on International Health and Policy

All applications must be completed and submitted with a CV to: American Medical Association, Department of Medical Student Services, 515 North State Street, Chicago, IL 60610. Fax: 312-464-5845.

NATIONAL TAY–SACHS & ALLIED DISEASE FOUNDATION

The primary objective of these awards is to stimulate interest in the field of lysosomal storage diseases. The research may be basic, applied, or clinical and should be performed under the direction of an investigator experienced in the field. Stipend: $1,500.

New York Academy of Medicine:

The Glorney–Raisbeck Medical Student Grants in Cardiovascular Research Program

Three grants of $3,000 will be provided to support projects in either clinical or basic research initiated during the summer. Competition is open to MD candidates in a metropolitan area medical school in New York City, Long Island, Westchester County, or New Jersey. The award will be paid directly to the sponsoring medical school for distribution to the recipient. The deadline for submission of applications is March. *Contact:* Fellowship Program Coordinator, New York Academy of Medicine, 1216 Fifth Avenue, Room 612, New York, NY 10029. Phone: 212-822-7204; Fax: 212-996-7826.

New York Academy of Medicine: The Louis L. Seaman Medical Student Research Grants in Microbiology

Four grants of $2,500 will be provided to support summer research projects in the field of microbiology. Competition is open to MD students in a metropolitan area medical school in New York City, Long Island, Westchester County, or New Jersey. The award will be paid directly to the student, but is contingent on the submission of a written report on the project. *Contact:* Fellowship Program Coordinator, New York Academy of Medicine, 1216 Fifth Avenue, Room 612, New York, NY 10029. Phone: 212-822-7204; Fax: 212-996-7826.

American Medical Association Education and Research Foundation Seed Research Grants

Up to $2,500 support for medical students for small research projects, or in some instances, to provide interim funding prior to large grant approvals from other sources. Grants will be awarded in two cycles during the school year: (1) September through November and (2) January through March. *Contact:* American Medical Association Education and Research Foundation, 515 North State Street, Chicago, IL 60610. Phone: 312-464-5357; Fax: 312-464-5973; *www.ama-assn.org/med-sci/erf/toc.htm*.

WEIS CENTER FOR RESEARCH GEISINGER CLINIC

Three-month program designed to expose medical students to career opportunities in research. Primary emphasis is at the cellular/molecular level of cardiovascular function. Stipend: $800/month.

John A. Hartford/AFAR Medical Student Geriatric Scholars Program

To encourage medical students, particularly budding researchers, to consider geriatrics as a career, the Medical Student Geriatric Scholars Program awards short-term scholarships through a national competition. The program provides an opportunity for these students to train at an acclaimed center of excellence in geriatrics. Each scholar receives a $3,000 stipend. Students in the New York Metropolitan area can apply for funding through the Farr Fox and Leslie R. Samuels Foundation/AFAR Medical Student Geriatric Scholars Program. Contact American Federation for Aging Research (AFAR), 1414 Avenue of the Americas, 18th Floor, New York, NY 10019. Phone: 212-752-2327; Fax: 212-832-2298; E-mail: *amfedaging@aol.com*.

Glenn Foundation/AFAR Scholarships for Research in the Biology of Aging

Inaugurated in 1994, this scholarship program was designed to attract potential scientists and clinicians to aging research. Provides PhD and MD students the opportunity to conduct a 3-month research project. Students will work in an area of biomedical research in aging under the auspices of a mentor. Each scholarship carries an award of $5,000. *Contact:* American Federation for Aging Research (AFAR), 1414 Avenue of the Americas, 18th Floor, New York, NY 10019. Phone: 212-752-2327; Fax: 212-832-2298; E-mail: *amfedaging@aol.com*.

MERCK/AFAR RESEARCH SCHOLARSHIPS IN GERIATRIC PHARMACOLOGY FOR MEDICAL STUDENTS

To develop a corps of physicians with an understanding of medication use in the elderly, the Merck Company Foundation and AFAR created the Merck/AFAR Research Scholarships in Geriatric Pharmacology. Medical students will have the opportunity to undertake a 2- to 3-month full-time research project in geriatric pharmacology. Up to nine $4,000 scholarships will be awarded in 2001. *Contact:* American Federation for Aging Research (AFAR), 1414 Avenue of the Americas, 18th Floor, New York, NY 10019. Phone: 212-752-2327; Fax: 212-832-2298; E-mail: *amfedaging@aol.com*.

American Oil Chemists' Society

Graduate students in any area of science dealing with fats and lipids who are doing research toward an advanced degree, and who are interested in the area of science and technology fostered by this Society, are eligible. Must be a graduate student who has not yet received his or her degree or begun employment prior to the AOCS meeting he/she is to attend. The award will provide funds equal to travel costs, hotel accommodations and stipend to permit attendance at the National Meeting of the AOCS held in the spring.

Biomedical Synergistics Institute—Ninth International Conference

Award for those individuals in training who submit the best original paper dealing with the Institute enhancement of human functioning. Papers published previously are not eligible for awards. Four student award categories with each receiving a prize of $250. The All Functioning Categories winner will receive a $1,000 prize.

AAA PRESLEY–CARL ZEISS YOUNG INVESTIGATOR AWARD

Recognizes excellence in research using light and/or electron microscopy. Must be a graduate student, medical student, postdoc (within 5 years of receiving PhD), or medical resident. $500 prize and certificate. Contact the Advisory Committee of Young Anatomists (ACYA) at 301-571-8314 or *exec@anatomy.org*.

AAA Zeiss Student Research Award

Recognizes excellence in research using state-of-the-art imaging methods, such as confocal and/or electron microscopy. Must be a graduate student or medical student. $500 prize and certificate. Contact the Advisory Committee of Young Anatomists (ACYA) at 301-571-8314 or *exec@anatomy.org*.

AAA/Genentech Student Research Award

Recognizes excellence in research using molecular biological techniques in the study of morphological changes at the cellular and/or whole animal level. Must be a graduate student, medical student, postdoc (within 5 years of receiving PhD), or medical resident. $500 prize and certificate. Contact the Advisory Committee of Young Anatomists (ACYA) at 301-571-8314 or *exec@anatomy.org*.

HELLENIC UNIVERSITY CLUB OF NEW YORK DR. FRED VALERGAKIS GRANT

Research grants to graduate students of Hellenic ancestry enrolled in an accredited university engaged in research. Minimum grants of $1,000.

Alpha Omega Alpha Research Fellowships

The purpose of the fellowships is to stimulate interest in research among medical students. Areas of research may include clinical investigation, basic research, epidemiology, and the social sciences, as related to medicine. The program is designed to stimulate students who have not had prior research experience. Fellowship is for $2,000.

American Medical Association Education and Research Foundation

Open to third- and fourth-year medical students who have completed the required clerkships in medicine, surgery, and pediatrics. The program consists of 4- to 6-week clerkships in general, pediatric, and surgical nutrition. Scholarships are only for students who do not have clinical nutrition clerkships available at their own schools. Students accepted into the program will receive a $700 award to defray living and traveling costs.

AMERICAN COLLEGE OF SPORTS MEDICINE NATIONAL STUDENT RESEARCH AWARD

The National Student Research Award recognizes the most outstanding research project of the year at the graduate/professional student level. An important consideration for the award is the extent of the student's participation in the project. Each applicant must be enrolled in a graduate or professional program in the areas of clinical or basic exercise science or sports medicine at an accredited university; be principal author of a submitted and accepted abstract for presentation at the ACSM Annual Meeting; and be a member of ACSM or one of its regional chapters at the time of application and at the time the award is presented. The New Investigator and National Student Research awards provide support for the recipients to attend the annual meeting and present their research. Registration fees, travel expenses, lodging, banquet tickets, and framed certificates (presented at the annual awards banquet) are awarded to the recipients. *Contact:* American College of Sports Medicine, Graduate Scholarships for Minorities and Women, 401 W. Michigan St., Indianapolis, IN 46202-3233. Phone: 317-637-9200; Fax: 317-634-7817; *www.acsm.org/*.

American Academy of Allergy Asthma and Immunology Summer Fellowship Grant

Summer fellowship grants of $2,000 will be awarded to outstanding medical students who wish to pursue research in the following areas: physiology of allergic diseases, pharmacology of allergy and inflammation, basic cellular and molecular immunology, AIDS, and other topics pertinent to the understanding of allergic and immune mechanisms of disease. Elgibility: Full-time medical students residing in the United States or Canada who have successfully completed at least 8 months of medical school by the time the fellowship starts. Past Summer Fellowship Grant recipients are not eligible. *Contact:* American Academy of Allergy Asthma and Immunology, 611 East Wells Street, Milwaukee, WI 53202-3889. Phone: 414-272-6071; Fax: 414-272-6070; *www.aaaai.org/*.

► SUMMER EXTERNSHIPS

Africa with Crossroads

Sponsoring Agency: Operation Crossroads Africa

For senior medical school students who would like to work on a 5- to 7-week project in Africa that might focus on one of the following themes: (1) the community health approach, (2) diagnosis and treatment of tropical diseases, (3) preventive approaches to tropical diseases, and (4) the use of paramedics. Each project will also involve some labor. No stipend. The sponsoring agency will assist students in finding funds for transportation.

AMERICAN LIVER FOUNDATION STUDENT RESEARCH FELLOWSHIPS

To gain exposure in the research laboratory and possibly consider liver research a career option. Award is $2,500 per month for 3 months. *Contact:* American Liver Foundation, 1425 Pompton Avenue, Cedar Grove, NJ 07009. Phone: 201-857-2626; *www.liverfoundation.org/*.

Mucopolysaccharidosis Society Summer Fellowship

Eight-week summer fellowship for study of mucopolysaccharide diseases Stipend: $1,500.

Utica College of Syracuse Summer Clerkships

Both of the following programs offer students clinical experience augment their classroom university instruction, reinforce clinical skills, and create interest in their future choice of both medical specialty and geographic area of practice: The summer clerkships (2 to 8 weeks) are designed for students who have completed either 1 or 2 years of training. Preference is given to second-year students. Stipend is $250/2 weeks. The clinical electives are credit courses offered on a year-round basis in 22 specialties for third- and fourth-year medical students.

MEMORIAL SLOAN–KETTERING CANCER CENTER SUMMER FELLOWSHIP

Sponsored by National Cancer Institute and Eugene W. Kettering Education Fund

Eight-week summer fellowship offered to medical students in their first 2 years. Objective of program is the educational enrichment of medical students by offering experience in research and clinical oncology and enhancement of their knowledge of cancer and promotion of future interest in the field. *Contact:* Chuck Ferrero, Box 187, Memorial Sloan–Kettering Cancer Center, 1275 York Ave., NY 10012 (212) 639-8457

Paul Alexander Memorial Fellowship

To provide an international public health opportunity to a medical student after the third year to work with a Management Sciences for Health team for 2 to 3 months.

American Medical Student Association/Adolescent Substance Abuse Prevention

Six- to 8-week summer internships in homeless and runaway shelters to help develop programs in self-esteem, decision-making skills, health education relating to substance abuse, and abuse prevention. $250/week.

ALLEGHENY GENERAL HOSPITAL EXTERNSHIPS

For students who have completed at least 1 year of medical school. This is an 8-week summer clerkship. Stipend of $1,000 is available through the hospital. A peformance evaluation is submitted by Allegheny General Hospital to the student's medical school. (Second-year students preferred.)

Bertram Low–Beer, V.A. Memorial Fellowship for Radiation Oncology

Sponsored by University of California in San Francisco, this summer fellowship will support a medical student to spend 10 weeks in the Department of Radiation Oncology at the University of California, San Francisco. Student must have completed 2 years of medical school. During the 10-week experience, the student will spend time interviewing patients, learning and participating in physical examinations, and learning the natural history, psychosocial impact, and cancer treatment techniques. Student will participate in a small research project the findings of which will be presented to the staff and other students. Stipend is $1,000.

MAP–Reader's Digest Missionary Medicine Fellowship

The purpose of this program is to provide selected senior medical students with firsthand exposure to missionary medicine and inform them of the cultural, social, and health-related problems characteristic of developing countries. Students serve for a minimum of 8 weeks. MAP will provide 75% of least expensive round-trip air fare.

J.M. FOUNDATION SCHOLARSHIPS

One to 3-week scholarships covering tuition, room and board, travel at selected summer schools of alcohol studies.

Simon Kramer Externship in Radiation Oncology

Sponsored by the Thomas Jefferson Hospital, Philadelphia, this fellowship provides a unique opportunity for the medical student to obtain a 6-week experience in the Department of Radiation Therapy and Nuclear Medicine at Jefferson. Flexible beginning date; stipend of $1,200.

NEW YORK STATE LEGISLATIVE FELLOW

Fellows work as regular legislative staff members of the offices to which they are assigned. The work is full time, demanding, and is intended to use and develop the expertise of Fellows while offering an exclusive view of legislative procedures.

Education and Research Foundation of the Society of Nuclear Medicine Awards

The purpose of the Student Fellowship Program is to provide financial support for students wishing to spend time in clinical or basic research activities in a nuclear medicine division for a 3-month period with a stipend of $3,000.

Student Fellowship Award Foundation of the Society of Nuclear Medicine

This fellowship provides financial support for students to spend elective quarters and/or summers in departments of nuclear medicine assisting in clinical and basic research activities.

Upjohn Summer Extern Program

Students are assigned to a unit in either the Medical Affairs or Research Division to give them an opportunity to acquire first-hand experience within the pharmaceutical industry. There is also a biweekly lecture series to provide exposure to key scientists and a more comprehensive view of pharmaceutical operations.

ARTHRITIS FOUNDATION, NY CHAPTER, ALBERT GROEKOEST PRIZE

Eight-week summer research fellowship in rheumatic diseases and/or skeletal diseases. May be used at any American institution. Stipend of $3,000.

Harbor Branch Oceanographic Institute Internship

Ten-week internship for students interested in ocean engineering, marine sciences, biomedical marine research, and related fields. Aquaculture, computer science, marine biology, tumor biology, virology, microbiology, molecular biology, etc. Stipend: $260/wk.

Roswell Park Memorial Research Institute (Buffalo, NY) Summer Oncology Program

Provides direct support for students in the health professions engaged in research during the summer. Fellowships are awarded for an 8-week period. Research is restricted to topics in oncology. Participation in this program is limited to students completing their first or second year of study.

RUTGERS UNIVERSITY SUMMER SCHOLARSHIPS

Ten scholarships are available for this year's Summer School of Alcohol Studies to medical students. Award covers university fees, tuition, room, and meals ($975); weekend meals and travel are not included. However, a $200 stipend for related expenses will also be given to each scholarship recipient.

New York Academy of Medicine HIV Professional Development Project

Two-month internship in HIV-focused health care and social service settings. 35 hours/week, $10/hr.

Case Western Reserve University—Pathology

For those who have completed their sophomore year in medical school. This is a 12-month fellowship with a $12,000 stipend. The time will be divided between diagnostic pathology on the autopsy service and research related to the immunological and biochemical characterization of human cancer.

Clendening, Logan Traveling Fellowship

Sponsoring Agency: University of Kansas Medical Center

This fellowship is open to registered medical students of any recognized medical or school in the United States or Canada.

The fellowship is of the value of $1,500. Applicants may elect to travel anywhere in the world for the purpose of studying any aspect of medical history of interest to them.

COSTEP OF THE U.S. PUBLIC HEALTH SERVICE

U.S. Public Health Service offers opportunities in Indian Health Services, Health Resources, and Services Administration, NIH, Food and Drug Administration, CDC, Alcohol, Drug Abuse and Mental Health Administration, etc. U.S. citizenship and at least one year of medical school required. Positions are available all year round. $2,000/month plus travel costs. Information is available in Student Affairs; for application, call 1-800-279-1605 or 301-594-2633.

NIH Predoctoral Fellowship Awards for Medical Students

All branches of the NIH have grants for medical student summer research. *Contact: www.nih.gov.*

Cystic Fibrosis Foundation Student Traineeships

The Cystic Fibrosis Foundation announces student traineeships which are offered to introduce students to research related to CF. Applicants must be students in or about to enter a doctoral program (MD, PhD, or MD/PhD). Each applicant must work with a faculty sponsor on a research project related to CF. The award is $1,500, of which $1,200 is designated as a stipend for the trainee, and the remainder $300 may be used for laboratory expenses. For an application, write to: Office of Grants Management, Cystic Fibrosis Foundation, 6931 Arlington Road, Bethesda, MD 20814, or call 1-800-FLIGHT CF.

AMA-MSS GOVERNMENT RELATIONS INTERSHIP PROGRAM APPLICATION

The Department of Medical Student Services, in conjunction with the Washington office of the American Medical Association, is pleased to offer assistance to students seeking to increase their involvement and education in national health policy and in the national legislative activities of organized medicine.

Through the Government Relations Internship Program, stipends of $2,500 are available to assist selected students who are completing health policy internships in the Washington, DC area. To be eligible for the Program, students must be AMA members who have secured a policy internship in the Washington, DC, area. Through the program, students may also apply for an internship at the AMA's Washington office (two positions available), or at the Health Care Financing Administration in Baltimore, Maryland (one position available). Students participating in the program generally arrange their internships with Congressional offices, specialty societies, or federal agencies in the DC area. A list of possible internship contacts is available.

The Betty Ford Center Summer Institute for Medical Students

Provides experiential education in chemical dependency and its treatment, primarily by student participation in the patient and family rehabilitation process. Five groups of 12 students will participate in the 5-day summer school program. Each session four Family Program participants follow the weekly schedule of family members, and eight students selected for the Inpatient Program are assigned to one of four inpatient treatment units. Program activities include lectures, meals, group therapy sessions, peer groups, exercise sessions, meditation, medallion ceremonies and Alcoholics and Narcotics Anonymous meetings. Students are asked to maintain a focused journal. A basic set of books and a reference manual is provided to each student. Scholarships to this very special program include the cost of all materials, lodging and meals. A travel stipend is also included. A total of 60 scholarships will be awarded. Students may apply to attend one of four summer sessions. For application information, write: Betty Ford Center Training Department, 39000 Bob Hope Drive, Rancho Mirage, CA 92270. Phone: 619-773-4108; Toll free: 1-800-854-9211, ext. 4108; Fax: 619-773-1697.

The Albert Schweitzer Fellowship

Provides complete funding for medical students who will work in Lambaréné, Gabon, as junior physicians, supervised by Schweitzer Hospital medical staff. Prior completion of clerkships in medicine, pediatrics, and surgery are required; some background or coursework in tropical medicine or parasitology is important but not a prerequisite. Because all patient encounters occur in French, a working knowledge of that language is absolutely essential. For more information, contact: The Albert Schweitzer Foundation, 330 Brookline Avenue, Boston, MA 02215.

▶ YEAR-LONG FELLOWSHIPS

HOWARD HUGHES MEDICAL INSTITUTE RESEARCH SCHOLARS TRAINING

Students in good standing in a medical school in the United States who have completed the second year but have not yet received the MD are eligible. The program is for at least 9 months and usually 1 year at NIH. Salary program $16,800, and other benefits are included. *Contact:* 1-800-424-9924.

American Diabetes Association, Inc. Medical Scholars Program Awards

The goal of the program is to produce new leaders in diabetes research by supplying physicians-in-training the opportunity to contribute to the process of discovery in basic or clinical research laboratories. Award is $30,000 for 1 year. Eligibility: Students must have completed at least two years of medical school. *Contact:* American Diabetes Association, Inc. Research Department, 1701 North Beauregard Street, Alexandria, VA 22311. Phone: 703-549-1500, ext. 2376; Fax: 703-549-1715. *www.diabetes.org/research/*

Pew Charitable Trust/Rockefeller University Fellowships in Human Nutrition

One-year program designed to give hands-on laboratory experience and mastering of new methods in biomedical science for application to problems in human nutrition. Students should have completed their third year by July 1. Stipend: $14,700. Pierce, Chester Research Symposium.

UNIVERSITY OF PITTSBURGH PATHOLOGY FELLOWSHIP

One-year fellowship for medical students who have completed their second year and wish to spend an additional year of in-depth study of pathology in research (pathology, molecular biology, genetics, etc.) and practice before going on to the third year. The stipend is $11,000, and a scholarship for the next year of medical school (up to the state tuition rate at Pittsburgh) will be provided.

Association of Pathology Chairman Student Fellowship

Year-long full-time fellowship in participating schools for students after the second year of medical school. Intended to give students an in-depth research and/or clinical experience in pathology between the basic science and clinical years. Support varies by school, as do openings for students not from that school.

New York City Health Research Training Program

This is a practicum in public health research. The student participates in a project under the direct supervision of a preceptor. The projects are submitted by preceptors from within the Health Department or from outside agencies such as hospitals, medical schools, or other health-related institutions. A seminar series is part of the program. Work–study students are preferred. However, some alternative support is available for those not eligible for work–study. Full time in summer, part time during school year. Hourly wage of $5–$8.40.

NEW YORK CITY URBAN FELLOWS PROGRAM

Year-long program offering the opportunity and challenge of an intensive field experience in urban government. Fellows work closely with City officials on long- and short-term projects and attend weekly seminars to gain an academic perspective on the workings and problems of local government. $17,000 stipend and insurance.

National Institutes of Health Summer Research Fellowship*

With the guidance of a preceptor from one of the Institutes, students conduct research in a selected area of laboratory investigation. Program offers practical experience in research procedures and lectures and seminars designed to enhance education and investigative skills. Program runs a minimum of 8 weeks.

National Institutes of Health Clinical Electives Program

Medical students are invited to apply for clinical electives of 8 weeks with opportunities research and clinical experience with physician–scientists in Bethesda.

OSLER LIBRARY FELLOWSHIP PROGRAM

A fellowship program for historians, physicians, and students conducting research in the history of medicine. Intended to serve those who need to establish temporary residence in order to undertake research in the Osler Library.

Henry Luce Foundation Scholars Program

This program provides an intensive year-long experience in Asia designed to broaden the scholar's professional perspectives and to sharpen their perceptions of Asia, America, and themselves. The support consists of airfare, stipend, medical insurance, etc.

Echoing Green Foundation Fellowship

One-year fellowship providing entrepreneurial people with the opportunity to develop and implement an innovative public service project (health, environment, youth service, international development, etc.). Students must develop a proposal. Stipend is $25,000 per year.

HEALTH RESEARCH GROUP MEDICAL STUDENT FELLOWSHIP

One-year fellowship in Washington researching and monitoring federal health agencies, congressional lobbying, publication of consumer-oriented educational manuals, etc.

Rosalie B. Hite Cancer Center Research Fellowship

Sponsoring Agency: University of Texas System

Fellowship open to graduate students or research workers in the area of cancer research. Selection of Fellows is on the basis of academic excellence of the candidate and applicability of the proposed program to the problems of cancer research. Graduate work is to be under the supervision of a faculty member of a component of the University of Texas at Houston, affiliated with the Graduate School of Biomedical Sciences Sciences degree-granting program.

Charles A. Dana Foundation Clinical Research Training Program

Sponsoring Agency: University of Pennsylvania School of Medicine

Opportunity for medical students to participate in a year-long in-depth clinical research training experience under the guidance of selected faculty who are accomplished investigators in the fields of epidemiology, clinical research methodology and the delivery of health care services. Training will be provided in clinical research methods, clinical epidemiology, biostatistics, and scientific communication. Stipend of $11,000 plus expenses.

CHARLES A. AND ANNE MORROW LINDBERGH FOUNDATION

A foundation dedicated to furthering Charles and Anne Morrow Lindbergh's shared vision of a balance between technological advancement and environmental preservation. Lindbergh grants are made in the following categories: agriculture; aviation/aerospace; conservation of natural resources—including animals, plants, water, and general conservation (land, air, energy, etc.); education—including humanities/education, the arts, and intercultural communication; exploration; health—including biomedical research, health and population sciences, and adaptive technology; and waste minimization and management. A Jonathan Lindbergh Brown Grant may be given to a project to support adaptive technology or biomedical research which seeks to redress imbalance between an individual and his or her human environment. Grants are made to individuals as well as educational and publication programs. *Contact: www.lindbergh-foundation.org.*

▶ FOR MINORITY STUDENTS

National Medical Fellowship—Commonwealth Fund

This program is designed to encourage academically gifted minority medical students to pursue careers in academic medicine and biomedical research. Open to those students who have completed their junior year. Duration is 8 to 12 weeks. Students have the option to participate in the summer or during the academic year. Fellowship award is for $5,000 with $2,000 earmarked for mentor to offset expenses during the research period.

National Institute of Arthritis and Musculoskeletal and Skin Diseases (NIAMS)

The Minority Travel Award Program provides travel funds for minority students and faculty members from minority institutions for attendance at national scientific meetings. *Contact: www.nih.gov/niams.*

NIH PREDOCTORAL FELLOWSHIP AWARDS FOR MINORITY STUDENTS

The National Research Service Award Predoctoral Fellowship for Minority Students will provide up to 5 years of support for research training leading to the PhD or equivalent research degree; the combined MD/PhD degree; or other combined professional degree and research doctoral degree in biomedical, behavioral sciences, or health services research. These fellowships are designed to enhance the racial and ethnic diversity of the biomedical, behavioral, and health services research labor force in the United States. Accordingly, academic institutions are encouraged to identify and recruit students from underrepresented racial and ethnic groups who can apply for this fellowship. Support is *not* available for individuals enrolled in medical or other professional schools *unless* they are also enrolled in a combined professional doctorate/PhD degree program in biomedical, behavioral, or health services research. *Contact: www.nih.gov.*

National Medical Fellowships, Inc.

NMF offers awards and fellowships to American Blacks, mainland Puerto Ricans, Mexican Americans, and American Indians who are U.S. Citizens enrolled in accredited schools of allopathic or osteopathic medicine in the United States. Funding is variable, yearly, and renewable. *Contact:* National Medical Fellowships, Inc., 254 West 31st Street, 7th Floor, New York, NY 10001. Phone: 212-714-1007.

Metropolitan Life Award Program for Academic Excellence in Medicine

This program recognizes and rewards third-year minority medical students for outstanding academic achievement and demonstrated leadership. $2,500 need-based awards to underrepresented minorities. Nominated by dean's office.

AMERICAN COLLEGE OF SPORTS MEDICINE MINORITY SCHOLARSHIP

The American College of Sports Medicine annually awards graduate scholarships for minorities and females of up to $1,500 each to be used to cover college or university tuition and/or fees. The purpose of these scholarships is to provide partial support toward the education of graduate and/or medical students with outstanding promise and a strong interest in research and scholarly activities as they pursue a career in sports medicine or exercise science. Scholarships are renewable for up to 4 years based on their research and professional activities and satisfactory academic progress in full-time study toward a graduate degree. Students who are not currently ACSM members are eligible to apply. Free student membership in the American College of Sports Medicine is also provided each year of an awardee's graduate scholarship. *Contact:* American College of Sports Medicine, Graduate Scholarships for Minorities and Women, 401 W. Michigan St., Indianapolis, IN 46202-3233. Phone: 317-637-9200; Fax: 317-634-7817; *www.acsm.org/*.

Congressional Black Caucus Foundation, Inc. Scholarships

Offers grant money for doctoral study to minority students. *Contact:* Congressional Black Caucus Foundation, Inc., 1004 Pennsylvania Avenue SE, Washington, DC 20003. Phone: 1-800-784-2577 or 202-675-6730; Fax: 202-547-3806.

AMERICAN INDIAN GRADUATE CENTER GRANTS

Grants of $250–$10,000 are available for American Indian students who are members of a federally recognized American Indian tribe or Alaska Native group, or possess one-fourth degree federally recognized Indian blood with financial need after exhausting available aid at their school financial aid office. *Contact:* American Indian Graduate Center, 4520 Montgomery Blvd. NE, Suite 1-B, Albuquerque, New Mexico 87109. Phone: 505-881-4584.

▶ ETHNIC

Dr. Anthony Bagatelos Memorial Scholarship

Grant money available for Greek descent/Greek Orthodox faith with intentions to practice medicine within the nine-county area surrounding San Francisco Bay. Applications may be obtained by contacting: Annunciation Greek Orthodox Cathedral, 245 Valencia St., San Francisco CA 94103.

Chinese American Physicians Society (CAPS)

CAPS is offering eight to ten scholarships of $1,000 to $2,000 each annually to two categories of medical students. The first is the Dr. Lester Chen Memorial Scholarships to students of Asian descent from the San Francisco Bay area. The other is the CAPS Scholarships to all medical students in need of financial aid regardless of their hometown, sex, race, or color. The applicants are judged according to their academic achievements, financial needs, community service records, and essays. Special credit is also given to those who are willing to serve the Chinese communities after their graduation. The deadline for submitting the completed application is usually the first Friday in October. Due to the huge number of requests for applications and our shortage of manpower, we can no longer send out the application by mail unless a self-addressed stamped envelope is enclosed with the request. Please obtain the applications from the student financial aid office of your medical school starting from April 1 each year. You can also print a copy of the published scholarship application from our Web site. The 2000 program hasclosed. The 2001 program will start in spring. If you need more information about scholarship program, please contact Chinese American Physicians Society, Lawrence M. Ng, M.D., Executive Director, 345 Ninth Street, Suite 204, Oakland, CA 94607-4206. Phone: 510-895-5539 (voice and fax); E-mail: *scholarship@caps-ca.org*.

JAPANESE MEDICAL SOCIETY SCHOLARSHIP AWARD

$1,500–$5,000 grants to students of Japanese ancestry who are enrolled or accepted in a U.S. medical school. Applications may be obtained by contacting: Japanese Medical Society of America, Inc. Scholarship Committee, One Henry Street, Englewood Cliffs, NJ 07632.

Hellenic Medical Society of New York—Leonidas Lantzounis Research Grant

This fellowship is open to premed or medical students or science majors of Hellenic descent. Ten-week summer projects are intended to encourage, support, and assist young Greek Americans in their preparation for a scientific career in the biomedical sciences. Stipend: $2,000.

Jewish Vocational Service Academic Scholarship

For Jewish medical students living in Chicago. Applications are accepted December 1 through March 1. *Contact:* Jewish Vocational Service, One South Franklin Street, Chicago, Illinois 60606. Phone: 312-346-6700, ext. 2214.

NATIONAL HISPANIC SCHOLARSHIP FUND

$500–$1,000 awards based on academic achievement, personal strengths, leadership, and financial need for students of Mexican American, Puerto Rican, Cuban, Caribbean, Central or South American heritage. Application period is from April 1 through June 15.

Hellenic Medical Society Scholarship

Awards for medical students of Hellenic heritage from New York, New Jersey, Pennsylvania, Connecticut; Must be a second-year student enrolled at accredited U.S. school. *Contact:* Hellenic Medical Society of New York, 401 East 34th Street, New York NY 10016.

► FOR WOMEN

Business & Professional Women's Clubs Grace Legendre Fellowships

For women who are residents of New York State and citizens of the United States and within 2 years of completing studies in an advanced graduate degree program. Must show evidence of scholastic ability and need for financial assistance. Scholarships are for $1,000.

AAUW EDUCATIONAL FOUNDATION INTERNATIONAL FELLOWSHIP

This is a grant for foreign students to pursue graduate studies in the United States. *Contact:* American Association of University Women, 1111 Sixteenth St. NW, Washington, DC 20036. Phone: 1-800-326-AAUW; Fax: 202-872-1425; E-mail: *info@aauw.org*.

AMWA Carroll L. Birch Award

Sponsored by the Chicago Branch of the American Medical Women's Association, the award is presented for the best original research paper written by a Student Life Member of AMWA. Women must be enrolled in an accredited U.S. medical or osteopathic medical school to apply. The recipient of the award receives a cash prize of $500 and a plaque presented at AMWA's Annual Meeting. An article noting the award winner will appear in one of the Association's publications and an abstract may be published in AMWA's journal. Contact your school's financial aid office for more info.

AMWA Bed and Breakfast Program

The program assists students who are traveling for a residency or job interview or physician members attending an out-of-town conference. Our members contact the national office with details of the trip. The national office responds by sending the traveler a listing of volunteers in the destination area. There is an administrative fee of $10.00 for students and $15.00 for physicians.

BPW Career Advancement Scholarship for Women

$500 to $1,000 grants for women over 25 in their third or fourth year of studies with critical need for assistance. *Contact:* Scholarships/Loans Business and Professional Woman's Foundation, 2012 Mass Ave. NW, Washington, DC 20036. Phone: 202-293-1200, ext. 169.

www.acponline.org/journals/ebm/ebmmenu.htm: Reviews the evidence for current medical practice.

www.ebem.org: Evidence-based emergency medicine home page.

cebm.jr2.ox.ac.uk: NHS Research and Development Centre of Evidence Based Medicine.

www.update-software.com/cochrane.htm: Web site for the Cochrane Library, the most well-known site for critically appraised topics or evidence-based reviews.

www.ebando.com: Bandolier: online publication on evidence-based health care.

www.shef.ac.uk/~scharr/ir/netting.html: Netting the evidence: A ScHARR introduction to evidence-based practice on the Internet.

www.ti.ubc.ca/pages/letter.html: Therapeutics Letter: Evidence-based review of pharmaceutical products.

www.ncbi.nlm.nih.gov/PubMed: Pub Med, a MEDLINE search engine through the National Library of Medicine.

igm.nlm.nih.gov: Grateful Med, a MEDLINE search engine through the National Library of Medicine.

www.cdc.gov: The Centers for Disease Control and Prevention: Contains full text issues of *Morbidity and Mortality Weekly Report*.

www.nejm.org: *New England Journal of Medicine*.

www.jwatch.org: Journal Watch.

www.bmj.com/index.shtml: British Medical Journal.

jama.ama-assm.org: Journal of the American Medical Association.

Index

A

Abdominal aortic aneurysm (AAA), 103
Abdominal pain, 101–103
  causes, 101–102
  in the elderly, 102–103
  types, 101
ABG. *See* Arterial blood gas
ACE inhibitors. *See* Angiotensin-converting enzyme inhibitors
Achalasia, 106–107, 108
Acid–base disorders, 221–225
  general laboratory studies, 221–222
    anion gap, 222
    arterial blood gas, 221
    serum electrolytes, 221
  metabolic acidosis, 221, 222–223, 225
  metabolic alkalosis, 221, 224, 225
  respiratory acidosis, 221, 223, 225
  respiratory alkalosis, 221, 223–224, 225
Acinetobacter baumanii, 191
Acne vulgaris, 357–358
Acquired immune deficiency syndrome, 197–210
  CD4 counts in, 201
  definition, 197
  disease, 200
  epidemiology, 200
  major AIDS-defining clinical conditions, 198
  opportunistic infections and, 202–210
    fungal infections, 206–207
    Mycobacterium avium complex, 205
    Pneumocystis carinii pneumonia, 202–204
    protozoal diarrhea, 205
    toxoplasmosis, 204–205
    tuberculosis, 206
    viral infections, 207–209
Acromegaly, 74–75, 233
ACTH (Cortrosyn) test, 91
Actinomyces, 144
Activated partial thromboplastin time (aPTT), 160
Acute coronary syndromes, 19–24
  determining the type of, 20
  initial evaluation of, 20
  initial treatment for, 22
  medications at discharg for patients with, 23
  postinfarction complications, 24
  risk stratification, 22
  secondary prevention, 24
  treatment for ST-elevation MI, 23
  treatment for unstable angina and non-ST-elevation MI, 22–23
Acute lymphocytic leukemia, 167
Acute myelocytic leukemia, 166
Acute renal failure, 237–239
  serologic testing, 238
  tubulointerstitial diseases, 238–239
    acute interstitial nephritis, 239
    acute tubular necrosis, 238–239
  urinary sediment, 238
  urinary sodium, 237–238
Acute interstitial nephritis, 239
Acute tubular necrosis, 238–239
Adenovirus, 191
Addison's disease, 90, 233
Adrenal disorders, 89–95
  adenoma, 93
  adrenal excess (Cushing's syndrome), 92–93
  adrenal insufficiency, 89–91
  pheochromocytoma, 94–95
Advance directives, 377
Adult respiratory distress syndrome, 270
Adult vaccinations, 366–367
AIDS. *See* Acquired immune deficiency syndrome
Alcohol abuse, 369–370
Aldosterone, 90–91
ALL. *See* Acute lymphocytic leukemia
Allergic rhinitis, 268
Alpha-glucosidase inhibitors, 66
α-Thalassemia, 153–154
Alzheimer's disease, 324–325
AML. *See* Acute myelocytic leukemia
Anaphylaxis, 333
Anemia, 149–153, 253
  aplastic, 152
  of chronic disease, 152–153
  cold hemlytic, 156
  Cooley's, 154
  folate deficiency, 149
  G6PD deficiency, 151–152
  immune-mediated hemolytic, 156
  iron deficiency, 149
  macrocytosis, 149
  pernicious, 150–151
  sickle cell, 155
  vitamin B_{12} (cobalamin) deficiency, 150
  warm hemolytic, 156
Angina, 17, 24, 30, 38
  Prinzmetal's, 24–25
  stable, 24–25
  unstable, 24–25
Angioedema, 333
Angiotensin-converting enzyme inhibitors, 26
Angiotensin receptor blockers (ARBs), 26
Angular cheilosis, 149
Ankylosing spondylitis, 293–294
Annual exams, 365–366
Anthrax, 210–211
Antidiuretic hormone disorders, 76
  diabetes insipidus, 76–77
Antihypertensive agents, 58
Antinuclear antibody, 280
Antiplatelet agents, 59
Aortic dissection, 17, 18, 49–50
Aortic regurgitation, 38–39
Aortic stenosis, 37–38
Aphthous ulcers, 133
Aplastic anemia, 152
Apnea, 266
ARDS. *See* Adult respiratory distress syndrome
Argyll Robertson pupil, 185
Arterial blood gas, 221
  interpreting, 224–225
Arthritis, 280
  gonococcal septic, 296
  nongonococcal septic, 300–301
  reactive, 294–295
Asbestosis, 276
Aspergillus, 195, 196, 258
Aspergillus fumigatus, 207
Asthma, 263–265
Astrocytoma, 317
Atrial fibrillation, 42–43
Autonomy, 377
Avascular necrosis (AVN) of the hip, 301
Awards and opportunities for students interested in medicine, 381–398
  ethnic, 396–397
  evidence-based medicine links, 398
  general awards, 382–386
  for minority students, 395–396
  research awards, 387–389
  summer externships, 389–393
  for women, 397
  year-long fellowships, 393–395

B

Babesia, 196
Babesiosis, 215
Bacillus cereus, 140
Bacteremia, 181
Bacterial endocarditis, 50–53, 331
Bacterial vaginosis, 184
Bacteriuria, 181
Balanitis, 186
Balloon valvuloplasty, 36
Barium swallow, 107
Barrett's esophagus, 110
Basal cell carcinoma, 358–359
Basic natriuretic peptide (BNP), 26
Beck's triad, 34
Behçet's syndrome, 295
Beta blockers, 26, 30, 49, 57
β-Thalassemia, 154
Biguanides, 66
Bile acid sequestrants, 56
Biliary tree disorders, 117–120
  acalculous cholecystitis, 119
  ascending cholangitis, 119
  bile storage and release, 117
  cholelithiasis, 117–118
  primary sclerosing cholangitis, 120
Bioterrorism agents, 210–214
  anthrax, 210–211
  botulism, 211
  pneumonic plague, 211–212
  smallpox, 212–213
  tularemia, 213–214
Boerhaave's syndrome, 105
Bone disorders, 95–98
  osteomalacia, 95–96
  osteoporosis, 96–97
  Paget's disease of bone, 97–98
Bone metastasis, 176
Bone mineral density scoring, 97
Bordetella pertussis, 269
Borrelia burgdorferi, 214–215
Botulism, 211, 315
Bouchard's nodes, 283, 284
Brain death, features of, 327
Brain herniation, 312
Brain metastasis, 176
Brain neoplasms, 316–318
Breast cancer, 171–172
Bronchiectasis, 270–271
Bronchitis, chronic, 262
Burkitt's lymphoma, 171
Byssinosis, 276

C

Calcium channel blockers, 57
Campylobacter, 294
Campylobacter jejuni, 319
Cancer
  breast, 171–172
  cervical, 174
  colorectal, 134–136
  esophageal, 110
  lung, 276–278
  ovarian, 173
  prostate, 174–175
  skin, 358–361
    basal cell carcinoma, 358–359
    malignant melanoma, 359–361
    squamous cell carcinoma, 359
  testicular, 175–176
  thyroid, 87
Candida, 105, 195, 196, 206
Candida albicans, 186
Candidiasis, 206
Carbon monoxide poisoning, 253
Carcinoid tumor, 128–129
Cardiac catheterization, 18–19, 23
Cardiac medications, common, 57–59
Cardiac testing, 17–19
Cardiomyopathy
  dilated, 27
  hypertrophic, 30
  restrictive, 29
Carpal tunnel syndrome, 302–303
Case control study, 377
Catecholamine, 70
Cauda equina syndrome, 282–283
Celiac sprue, 142
Cellulitis, 348–349
Central pontine myelinolysis, 228
Central retinal artery occlusion, 323
Cervical cancer, 174
Charcot's triad, 119
CHF. *See* Congestive heart failure
Chickenpox, 346. *See also* Varicella-zoster virus
Chlamydia pneumoniae, 189, 190
Chlamydia psittaci, 190
Chlamydia trachomatis, 183–184
Cholangitis
  ascending, 119
  primary sclerosing, 120
Cholecystitis, 118–119
  acalculous, 119
Choledocholelithiasis, 119
Cholelithiasis, 117–118
Christmas disease, 165. *See also* Hemophilia B
Chronic ambulatory peritoneal dialysis, 244
Chronic bronchitis, 262
Chronic lymphocytic leukemia, 168–169
Chronic myeloid leukemia, 167–168
Chronic obstructive pulmonary disease, 262–263
Chronic renal failure, 242–245
  dialysis, 244
  polycystic kidney disease, 245
  uremic syndrome, 245
Chronotropic agents, 58
Churg–Strauss disease, 297
Chylomicrons, 54
Cirrhosis, 121–122
CLL. *See* Chronic lymphocytic leukemia
Clostridium botulinum, 315
Clostridium difficile, 131, 139
Clostridium perfringens, 140
Cluster headache, 322
CML. *See* Chronic myeloid leukemia
CMV. *See* Cytomegalovirus
CNS infections, 312–315
  bacterial meningitis, 313–314
  botulism, 315
  rabies, 312–313
  viral meningitis, 314–315
Coagulation, 159–161
  activated partial thromboplastin time, 160
  bleeding time, 161
  coagulation cascade, 159
  direct Coombs', 161
  heparin, 159
  indirect Coombs', 161
  prothrombin time, 160
  thrombin time (TT), 161
  warfarin, 159
Coal workers' pneumoconiosis, 276
Coccidioides, 195
"Coffee ground" emesis, 137
Cohort study, 377
Collagen vascular disorders, 241
Colon, disorders of, 128—136
  carcinoid tumor, 128–129
  colorectal cancer, 134–136
  diverticulitis, 129–131
  diverticulosis, 129
  hereditary colon cancer syndromes, 136
  inflammatory bowel disease, 132–134
  irritable bowel syndrome, 131–132
  pseudomembranous colitis, 131
Colorectal cancer, 134–136
Common variable hypogammaglobulinemia, 195
Condylomata lata, 185
Congenital heart disease, 18, 19
Congestive heart failure, 25–26
Connective tissue disorders, 284–293
  drug-induced lupus, 288
  polymyositis and dermatomyositis, 292–293
  rheumatoid arthritis, 284–286
  sarcoidosis, 289–290
  scleroderma, 289
  Sjögren's syndrome, 291–292
  systemic lupus erythematosus, 286–288
Conn's syndrome, 93–94. *See also* Hyperaldosteronism
Constipation, 146
Cooley's anemia, 154
COPD. *See* Chronic obstructive pulmonary disease
Coronary artery disease, 17–31
  causes of chest pain, 17
  risk factors for, 17
"Corrigan" pulse, 38
Corticosteroids, 134
Cortisol, 71
Corynebacterium diphtheriae, 192
Costochondritis, 17, 302
Cough
  acute, 266, 267
  chronic, 266–267
Craniopharyngiomas, 73
Creatine kinase, 19
Crohn's disease, 132–134
Cryptococcus, 195
Cryptococcus neoformans, 258
Cryptosporidium, 104, 140, 195
Cushing's disease, 90, 92
Cushing's syndrome, 92–93. *See also* Adrenal disorders
Cutaneous fungal infections, 355
Cystitis, 102, 181–183
Cystometry, 182, 250
Cystoscopy, 182, 250
Cytomegalovirus, 31, 104, 195, 207, 258

D

Dawn phenomenon, 64
DeBakey classification, 49
Decubitus ulcers, 344–345
Delirium tremens, 370
Dementia, 324
De Musset's sign, 38
Depression, 368
Dermatitis, 336–338
  allergic contact, 337
  atopic, 336–337
  irritant contact, 337–338
Dermatitis herpetiformis, 142
Dermatomyositis, 292–293

Diabetes insipidus (DI), 76–77
Diabetes mellitus, 63–72
complications of, 64
counterregulatory hormones, 70–71
diabetic ketoacidosis, 67–68
hypoglycemia, 69–70
insulin preparations, 64
metabolic syndrome, 71–72
nonketotic hyperosmolar coma, 68
type 1, 63–65
dawn phenomenon, 64
Somogyi effect, 65
type 2, 65
Diabetic ketoacidosis, 67–68
Dialysis, 244
Diarrhea, 138, 139–141
acute, 139–140
chronic, 140–141
distinguishing types of, 141
protozoal, 205
Diascopy, 332
Diastolic dysfunction, 25
DIC. *See* Disseminated intravascular coagulation
Diffuse large cell lymphoma, 171
Dilated cardiomyopathy, 27–29
Direct Coombs, 161
Disseminated gonococcal infection, 331
Disseminated intravascular coagulation, 163
Distributive justice, 377
Diverticulitis, 129–131
Diverticulosis, 129
DM. *See* Diabetes mellitus
Domestic violence, 367–368
Drug-induced lupus (DIL), 288
Duke's criteria, 51
Duodenal ulcer (DU), 111–113
Duroziez sign, 38
Dysbetalipoproteinemia, 55
Dyslipidemia, 54–56
Dysrhythmias, 19, 41–46
atrial fibrillation, 42–43
heart block, 44–45
pulseless ventricular tachycardia, 41
sinus bradycardia, 45–46
torsades de pointes, 42
ventricular fibrillation, 41
Wolfe–Parkinson–White syndrome, 41, 43–44

E

Eaton–Lambert syndrome, 277
Echocardiography, 19
Ectopic pregnancy, 102
Eczema, 336–338
Egophony, 254
Ehlers–Danlos, 38, 49
Electrolyte disorders, 226–237
body fluids, 226
general principles of management, 236–237
hypercalcemia, 233–234
hyperkalemia, 231–232
hypermagnesemia, 236
hypernatremia, 229–230
hyperparathyroidism, 234–235
hyperphosphatemia, 236
hypocalcemia, 232–233
hypokalemia, 230
hypomagnesemia, 236
hyponatremia, 226–228
hypophosphatemia, 236
renal osteodystrophy, 235
Emphysema, 262
Endocrinopathies, 233
Entamoeba histolytica, 140
Enterobacter, 181, 191
Enterobacteriaceae, 258
Ependymoma, 317
Epidural abscess, 216
Epididymitis, 102
Epstein–Barr virus, 31, 191–192
Erysipelas, 346–348
Erythema chronicum migrans, 215, 356
Erythema infectiosum, 347
Erythema multiforme, 341–342
Erythema nodosum, 331, 340–341
Escherichia coli, 140, 181, 182, 191
Esophageal cancer, 110
Esophageal perforation or rupture, 105–106
Esophageal spasm, 106–107
Esophageal variceal bleeding, 123
Esophagitis, 104, 110
infectious, 104
Evidence-based medicine, principles of, 376–377
Exercise stress testing, 17–18

F

Falls, 372–373
Familial polyposis coli, 136
Farmer's lung, 276
Febrile neutropenia, 177
Fibrinates, 56
Fifth disease, 347. *See also*Erythema infectiosum
FIGO staging of ovarian cancer, 173
Focal glomerulosclerosis, 240
Folate deficiency, 149–150
Foreign body ingestion, 105
Francisella tularensis, 213, 216
Frostbite, 375–376

G

Gallstones, 117–118. *See also* Cholelithiasis
Gardner's syndrome, 136
Gastric outlet obstruction, 111
Gastric ulcer (GU), 113
Gastritis, 114
Gastroesophageal reflux disease, 109, 266
Gastrointestinal bleeds, 136—138
general approach to, 136–137
determining the source of, 137
resuscitation, 136–137
lower GI bleeds, 138
upper GI bleeds, 137–138
General preventive care, 365–367
Genital herpes, 186
Genitourinary procedures, common, 250
GERD. *See* Gastroesophageal reflux disease
GI webs and rings, 107–108
Plummer–Vinson syndrome, 107
Schatzki's ring, 107, 109
Giardia lamblia, 140, 195
Glomerular disorders, 240–242
glomerulonephritis, 241–242
nephrotic syndrome, 240
Glomerulonephritis, 241–242
IgA nephropathy, 241
membranoproliferative, 241
poststreptococcal, 241
rapidly progressive, 242
Glossitis, 149
Glucagon, 70
Glucose-lowering drugs, 66
Gonococcal septic arthritis, 296
Gout, 298–299
Graves' disease, 80–81
Growth hormone, 71
G6PD deficiency, 151–152
Guillain–Barré syndrome, 319–320
Gummas, 185

H

Haemophilus influenzae, 155, 189, 190, 191, 196, 258, 313, 348
Hammon's crunch, 106
Hashimoto's thyroiditis, 82, 85, 86
Headache, 320–323
cluster, 322
migraine, 320
of temporal (giant cell) arteritis, 322–323
tension, 321
Health maintenance and evidence-based medicine, 363–379
cold-related illness, 375–376
environmental exposures, 375
general preventive care, 365–367
health promotion in women, 367–368
injury prevention, 372–373
nutritional disorders, 373–374
substance abuse, 369–372
Heart block, 44–45
first degree, 44
second-degree, 44
Mobitz I (Wenckebach), 44
Mobitz II, 45
third-degree (complete heart block), 45
Heart failure, 18, 25–31
acute pulmonary edema, 27
dilated cardiomyopathy, 27–29
hypertrophic cardiomyopathy, 30
paroxysmal nocturnal dyspnea, 27
restrictive cardiomyopathy, 29
Heart murmur, 18
Heat exhaustion, 375
Heatstroke, 375
Heberden's nodes, 283, 284
Helicobacter pylori, 111, 112, 113
Hematemesis, 137
Hematochezia, 137
Hematuria, 181
Hemodialysis, 244
Hemoglobin, 153
Hemolysis, 151–152
Hemophilia
A, 164–165
B (Christmas disease), 165
Hemoptysis, 271
Henoch–Schönlein purpura, 335
Heparin, 159
Hepatic encephalopathy, 123
Hepatitis, 124–127, 209
hepatitis A virus, 125
hepatitis B virus, 125–126, 196
vaccination, 366
hepatitis C virus, 126–127, 196
hepatitis D virus ("delta" agent), 127
hepatitis E virus, 127
Hepatorenal syndrome, 124
Hereditary nonpolyposis colon cancer (HNPCC), 136
Herpes simplex virus, 104, 196, 207–208, 354
Herpes zoster, 353–355
Herpetic whitlow, 354

Hiatal hernia, 109
Hill's sign, 38
Histoplasma, 195
Histoplasma capsulatum, 258
HIV. *See* Human immunodeficiency virus
Hives, 333
Hodgkin's lymphoma, 169–170
Hormone replacement therapy (HRT), 367
Hormones, counterregulatory, 70–71
Horner's syndrome, 277
Howell–Jolly bodies, 155
HPV. *See* Human papillomavirus
Human immunodeficiency virus, 31, 197–210
  acute HIV syndrome, 200–201
  life cycle of, 198
  neoplastic disease and, 209–210
    Kaposi's sarcoma, 209
    lymphomas, 209–210
  treatment of, 201–202
  transmission of, 198–199
Human papillomavirus, 187
Humoral immunity, 193–194
Hyperaldosteronism, 93–94
Hypercalcemia, 177, 233–234
  malignancy and, 234
Hypercholesterolemia
  familial, 55
  isolated, 54
  polygenic, 55
  treatment of, 56
Hyperkalemia, 231–232
Hypermagnesemia, 236
Hypernatremia, 229–230
Hyperparathyroidism, 87–88, 233
  primary, 234–235
  secondary, 235
Hyperphosphatemia, 236
Hypertension, 46–50
  aortic dissection, 49–50
    DeBakey classification, 49
    Stanford classification, 49
  definition of (JNC-7), 47
  hypertensive emergency, 48
Hyperthyroidism, 78, 233
Hypertriglyceridemia
  familial, 55
  isolated, 54
Hypocalcemia, 232–233
Hypoglycemia, 69–70
Hypokalemia, 230
Hypomagnesemia, 236
Hyponatremia, 226–228
Hypoparathyroidism, 88–89
Hypophosphatemia, 236
Hypopnea, 266
Hypopituitarism, 75–76
Hypothermia, 376
Hypothyroidism, 81–83
  subclinical, 83
Hypoxia, 253

I

Idiopathic thrombocytopenic purpura (ITP), 162
IgA nephropathy, 241
Immunodeficiency, 195–197
  cell-mediated, 195
  general principles of evaluation and management, 197
  humoral immune deficiency disorders, 195–196
  major causes of fever in the immunocompromised, 196
  pulmonary infiltrate in the immunocompromised patient, 197
Immunoglobulins, 194
Immunomodulators, 134
Immunity
  cellular, 194
  humoral, 193–194
Indirect Coombs, 161
Inflammatory bowel disease, 132–136
Influenza virus, 192
  vaccine, 366
Injury prevention, 371–373
Inotropic agents, 58
Interstitial lung disease, 275–276
Intravenous pyelography, 182, 250
Irritable bowel syndrome, 131–132

J

Janeway lesions, 51, 52
Joint disorders, 298–303
  avascular necrosis of the hip, 301
  carpal tunnel syndrome, 302–303
  costochondritis, 17, 302
  gout, 298–299
  nongonococcal septic arthritis, 300–301
  pseudogout, 300
Jones criteria, 53
Jugular venous distention (JVD), 34, 40

K

Kaposi's sarcoma, 209
Kawasaki's disease, 31, 331
Keratomalacia, 374
Kerley B lines, 35
Klebsiella, 181, 182
Klebsiella pneumoniae, 190, 191, 196, 258
KOH preparation, 332
Koilonychia, 149
Korsakoff's syndrome, 374
Kussmaul respirations, 67
Kussmaul's sign, 35

L

Lactase deficiency, 143–144
Lactate dehydrogenase, 19
Lactobacillus, 104
Leading causes of death in the United States, 365
Legionnaire's disease, 191
Legionella, 189, 195
Legionella pneumophila, 190–191, 258
Leukemia
  acute, 165–166
  acute lymphocytic, 167
  acute myelocytic, 166
  chronic lymphocytic, 168–169
  chronic myeloid, 167–168
Light's criteria, 254
Lipoproteins, 54
Listeria, 195
Listeria monocytogenes, 313
Lithotripsy, 118
Liver disorders, 120–128
  cirrhosis, 121–122
    alcoholic, 121
    primary biliary, 122
  esophageal variceal bleeding, 123
  hepatic encephalopathy, 1123
  hepatorenal syndrome, 124
  normal function, 120
  portal hypertension, 122–123
  spontaneous bacterial peritonitis, 124
Liver metastasis, 176
Liver transplantation, 127–128
Lower back pain, 280–284
  leading causes, 280–281
  lumbar disk herniation, 281
  osteoarthritis (OA), 283–284
  spinal metastasis and cauda equina syndrome, 282–283
  vertebral compression fracture, 281–282
Lower GI bleeds, 138
Lumbar disk herniation, 281
Lung auscultation, 254
Lung cancer, 276–278
Lung physical exam, 253–254
Lyme disease, 214–215, 356–357
Lymphoblastic lymphoma, 171
Lymphoma, 169–171, 209–210
  Burkitt's, 171
  central nervous system, 317
  diffuse large cell, 171
  Hodgkin's, 169–170
  lymphoblastic, 171
  non-Hodgkin's, 170–171

M

Macrocytosis, 149
Macroglossia, 78
Malabsorption, major types of, 142–146
  celiac sprue, 142
  constipation, 146
  lactase deficiency, 143–144
  Ménétrier's disease, 145–146
  protein-losing enteropathy, 145
  tropical sprue, 142–143
  Whipple's disease, 144–145
Malaria, 196, 216–217
Malignant melanoma, 359–361
Mallory–Weiss syndrome, 105
Mallory–Weiss tears, 137, 138
Malnutrition, 373
Marfan's syndrome, 38, 49
Measles, 331, 346
Measles, mumps, rubella (MMR) vaccine, 367
Mediastinitis, 275
Mediastinum, 274–275
Medical ethics, principles of, 376, 377
Medicine clerkship, how to succeed in the, 1–12
Melena, 137, 138
Membranous glomerulonephritis, 240
Ménétrier's disease, 145–146
Meningiomas, 317
Meningitis
  bacterial, 313–314
  viral, 314–315
Meningococcemia, 331, 350–351
Meningococcus, 31
Meningoencephalitis, 206–207
Mesalamine, 134
Mesenteric ischemia, 102, 104
Meta-analysis, 377
Metabolic acidosis, 221, 221–223, 225
Metabolic alkalosis, 221, 224, 225
Metabolic syndrome, 71–72
Migraine headache, 320–321
Mitral regurgitation, 36–37
Mitral stenosis, 35–36
Mitral valve prolapse, 37
Mononucleosis, 347
Moraxella catarrhalis, 190
Motor vehicle injuries, 372
Motorcycle collisions, 372
Multiple myeloma, 169, 233, 240

Murphy's sign, 118
Myasthenia gravis, 318–319
Mycobacterium avium complex (MAC), 203, 205, 258
Mycobacterium tuberculosis, 104, 195, 258
Mycoplasma pneumoniae, 31, 189, 190
Myocardial infarction, 17, 18, 19
  serum markers for, 19
Myocarditis, 31
Myoglobin, 19
Myxedema coma, 84

N

Neisseria gonorrhoeae, 183–184
Neisseria meningitidis, 196, 313, 314
Nephritic syndrome, 241. *See also* Glomerulonephritis
Nephrolithiasis, 102
Nephrotic syndrome, 240
Neurological disorders, 324–327
  Alzheimer's disease, 324–325
  dementia, 324
  normal pressure hydrocephalus, 326–327
  Parkinson's disease, 325–326
Neuropathies, 318–320
  Guillain–Barré syndrome, 319–320
  myasthenia gravis, 318–319
Neurosyphilis, 185
Nicotinic acid, 56
Nitroglycerin, 22
Nocardia, 195, 258
NOMAD, 27
Nongonococcal septic arthritis, 300–301
Non-Hodgkin's lymphoma, 170–171
Nonketotic hyperosmolar coma (NKHC), 68
Nonmalfeasance, 377
Normal pressure hydrocephalus (NPH), 326–327
Norwalk virus, 140

O

Obesity, 373–374
Obstructive sleep apnea (OSA), 266
Oligodendrogliomas, 317
Onychomycosis, 355
Opioid use, 371
Optic neuritis, 323
Osler's nodes, 51
Osteoarthritis (OA), 283–284
Osteomalacia, 95–96
Osteoporosis, 96–97
Ovarian cancer, 173
Ovarian torsion, 102

P

Paget's disease of bone, 97–98, 233
Pancoast's syndrome, 277
Pancreas, disorders of, 114–117
  acute pancreatitis, 114–116
  chronic pancreatitis, 116–117
Pancreatitis
  acute, 114–116
  chronic, 116–117
Parathyroid disorders, 87–89
  hyperparathyroidism, 87–88
  hypoparathyroidism, 88–89
Parkinson's disease, 325–326
Paroxysmal cold hemoglobinuria, 156
Paroxysmal nocturnal dyspnea, 27
Parvovirus B19, 152, 192
Patch testing, 332
Patent foramen ovale, 18
PCP. *See Pneumocystis carinii* pneumonia
Pellagra, 374
Pelvic inflammatory disease, 102, 187–188
Peptic stricture, 110
Peptic ulcer disease (PUD), 110
Pericardial effusion, 18
Pericardial tamponade, 34
Pericarditis, 17, 32—33
  constrictive, 34–35
Pertussis, 269
Peutz–Jeghers syndrome, 136
Phalen's sign, 302
Pheochromocytoma, 94–95
Pica, 149
PID. *See* Pelvic inflammatory disease
Pituitary hormones, 73
Pituitary tumors, 72–76, 317
  acromegaly, 74–75
  adenomas, 72, 93
  craniopharyngiomas, 73
  hypopituitarism, 75–76
Pityriasis rosea, 338–339
Pleural effusion, 254–255
Plummer–Vinson syndrome, 107
Pneumococcal vaccine, 366
Pneumocystis carinii, 104, 195, 196, 197, 258
Pneumocystis carinii pneumonia, 197, 202–204
Pneumomediastinum, 275
Pneumonia, 189–191, 257–259
  aspiration, 191
  community-acquired, 189–190
    atypical, 190–191
    typical, 189–190
  hospital-acquired, 191
Pneumonic plague, 211–212
Pneumothorax, 273–274
Podagra, 299
Polyarteritis nodosa (PAN), 296–297
Polycystic kidney disease, 245
Polycythemia vera, 158–159
Polymyositis, 292–293
Polyps, 135
Polysomnography, 266
Portal hypertension, 122–123
Postnasal drip syndrome, 267–268
Poststreptococcal glomerulonephritis, 193
Prinzmetal's angina, 24–25
Prostate cancer, 174
Prostatitis, 102, 188–189
  bacterial, 188
  nonbacterial, 189
Protein-losing enteropathy, 145
Proteus mirabilis, 181, 182
Prothrombin time (PT), 160
Pseudogout, 300
Pseudohyponatremia, 227–228
Pseudomembranous colitis, 131
Pseudomonas, 181, 182, 191
Pseudomonas aeruginosa, 191, 258
Psoriasis, 339–340
Pulmonary embolism, 17, 18, 272–273
Pulmonary function tests, 255–256
Pulseless ventricular tachycardia, 41
Pulsus paradoxus, 34
PV. *See* Polycythemia vera
Pyelonephritis, 102, 181–183
Pyuria, 181

Q

Quincke's sign, 38

R

Rabies, 312–313
Ramsay Hunt syndrome, 354
Randomized controlled clinical trial, 377
Ranson's criteria, 115, 116
Raynaud's phenomenon, 289
Reactive arthritis, 294–295
Reiter's syndrome, 186, 294–295
Renal failure
  acute, 237–239
  chronic, 242—245
Renal osteodystrophy, 235
Renal tubular acidosis, 246
Renal ultrasound, 182, 250
Respiratory acidosis, 221, 223, 225
Respiratory alkalosis, 221, 223–224, 225
Retinal detachment, 323
Reynolds' pentad, 119
Rheumatic fever, 53–54, 347
Rheumatoid arthritis (RA), 284–286
Rheumatoid factor, 280, 285
Rhinovirus, 192
Rickets, 95. *See also* Osteomalacia
Rickettsia rickettsii, 214, 351
Riedel's thyroiditis, 85, 86
Rocky Mountain spotted fever, 214, 331, 351–353
Rotavirus, 140
Roth's spots, 51
Rubella, 331, 348

S

Salmonella, 140, 195, 196, 294, 300
Salpingitis, 102
Sarcoidosis, 289–290
Scalded skin syndrome, 193
Scarlet fever, 193, 331, 347
Schatzki's ring, 107, 109
Schilling test, 151
Schistosomiasis, 122
Schwannomas, 317
Sclerodactyly, 289
Scleroderma, 289
Scurvy, 374
Seatbelt use, 372
Selective IgA deficiency, 196
Seizure disorders, 316
Sepsis, 181
Septic shock, 181
Seronegative arthritides, 293–296
  ankylosing spondylitis, 293–294
  Behçet's syndrome, 295
  gonococcal septic arthritis, 296
  Reiter's syndrome and reactive arthritis, 294–295
Serratia, 181
Serum chemistries, 227, 228
Serum osmolarity, 226
Sexually transmitted diseases, 185–189
  balanitis, 186
  genital herpes, 186
  human papillomavirus, 187
  pelvic inflammatory disease, 187–188
  syphilis, 185–186
Sheehan's syndrome, 75, 82
Shigella, 140, 294
SIADH. *See* Syndrome of inappropriate antidiuretic hormone secretion
Sickle cell anemia, 155, 240, 300
Sigmoid volvulus, 102
Silicosis, 276

Sinus bradycardia, 45–46
Sinusitis, 268–269
SIRS. *See* Systemic inflammatory response syndrome
Sjögren's syndrome, 291–292
Skin cancers, 358–361
  basal cell carcinoma, 358–359
  malignant melanoma, 359–361
  squamous cell carcinoma, 359
Skin infections, 193
Skin lesions, 331–332
Skip lesions, 133
SLE. *See* Systemic lupus erythematosus
Smallpox, 212–213
Smoking cessation
  counseling, 370
  pharmacotherapy, 371
Sodium channel blockers, 57
Spinal cord compression, 178
Spinal metastasis, 282–283
Splinter hemorrhages, 51, 52
Spontaneous bacterial peritonitis, 124
Squamous cell carcinoma, 359
Stanford classification, 49
Staphylococcal scalded syndrome, 331
Staphylococcus aureus, 140, 189, 191, 193, 258, 300, 348
Statins, 56
Statistical concepts, 378
Stevens–Johnson syndrome, 343
Stomach disorders, 110–114
  duodenal ulcer, 111–113
  gastric ulcer, 113
  gastritis, 114
  peptic ulcer disease, 110
Strangulated hernia, 102
Streptococcus, 104
Streptococcus pneumoniae, 189, 196, 313, 314
Streptococcus pyogenes, 193, 348
Stress myocardial perfusion imaging, 18
Strongyloides stercoralis, 195
Stroke, 306–311
  neurological deficits in, 307–308
  risk factors, 308
Sulfonylureas, 66
Superior vena cava (SVC) syndrome, 177–178, 277
Sympathomimetics, 371–372
Syndrome of inappropriate antidiuretic hormone secretion, 77–78, 277
Syphilis, 185–186
Systemic inflammatory response syndrome, 181
Systemic lupus erythematosus, 31, 286–288
Systemic sclerosis. *See* Scleroderma

T

Tactile fremitus, 253
Takayasu's arteritis, 298
Temporal (giant cell) arteritis, 298, 323
  headache of, 322–323
Tension headache, 321
Testicular cancer, 175–176
Testicular torsion, 102
Tetanus vaccination, 366
Thiazolidinediones, 66
Thrombin time (TT), 161
Thrombocytopenia, 161–163
  disseminated intravascular coagulation, 163
  idiopathic thrombocytopenic purpura, 162
  thrombotic thrombocytopenic purpura, 162–163
Thrombolytics, 23, 59
Thrombotic thrombocytopenic purpura (TTP), 162–163
Thrush, 206
Thyroid disorders, 78–87
  Graves' disease, 80–81
  hyperthyroidism, 78
  hypothyroidism, 81–83
    subclinical, 83
  myxedema coma, 84
  thyroid cancer, 87
  thyroid nodule, evaluation of, 86
  thyroid storm, 79–80
  thyroiditis, 85
Thyroid storm, 79–80
Thyroiditis, 85
TIA. *See* Transient ischemic attack
Tick-borne diseases, 214–216
  babesiosis, 215
  Borrelia burgdorferi, 214–215
  Rickettsia rickettsii, 214
  tularemia, 216
TIMI Risk Score, 22
Tinea corporis, 355
Tinea cruris, 355
Tinea pedis, 355
Tinel's sign, 302
Tobacco-related disease, 370
Tobacco use, 370–371
Tophi, 299
Torsades de pointes, 42
Toxic shock syndrome, 193, 331, 349–350
Toxic epidermal necrolysis, 343–344
Toxoplasma, 195, 196
Toxoplasmosis, 203, 204–205
Transfusion reactions, 156–158
  acute hemolytic, 156–157
  allergic reactions to plasma, 158
  delayed hemolytic, 157
  febrile nonhemolytic, 157–158
  transfusion-related acute lung injury (TRALI), 158
Transient ischemic attack, 306, 310
Treponema pallidum, 185
Trichomonas vaginalis, 184
Tricuspid regurgitation, 40
Tricuspid stenosis, 39–40
Tropheryma whippelii, 144
Troponin T/I, 19
Trousseau's syndrome, 277
Trypanosoma cruzi, 31
Tuberculosis, 203, 206, 259–262
Tubo-ovarian abscess, 102
Tubulointerstitial diseases, 238–239
  acute interstitial nephritis, 239
  acute tubular necrosis, 238–239
Tubulovillous polyps, 135
Tularemia, 213–214, 216
Turner's syndrome, 38, 49

U

Ulcerative colitis, 132–134
Upper GI bleeds, 137–138
Upper respiratory tract infections, 189–192
Ureaplasma urealyticum, 181
Uremic syndrome, 245
Urethritis, 183–184
URI. *See* Upper respiratory tract infections
Urinalysis, 248–249
Urinary sediment, 238
Urinary sodium, 237–238
Urinary tract infection, 181–183
Urolithiasis, 246–250
Urticaria, 333
UTI. *See* Urinary tract infection

V

Vaccinations, adult, 366–367
Vaginitis, 184
Valvular heart disease, 19, 35–40
  aortic regurgitation, 38–39
  aortic stenosis, 37–38
  mitral regurgitation, 36–37
  mitral stenosis, 35–36
  mitral valve prolapse, 37
  tricuspid regurgitation, 40
  tricuspid stenosis, 39–40
Varicella-zoster virus, 104, 195, 208, 346, 353
Vasculitis, 296–298
  Churg–Strauss disease, 297
  hypersensitivity, 331, 334
  polyarteritis nodosa, 296–297
  Takayasu's arteritis, 298
  temporal arteritis, 298
  Wegener's granulomatosis, 297
Venous/coronary dilators, 58
Ventricular fibrillation, 41
Vertebral compression fracture, 281–282
Vibrio cholerae, 140
Villous polyps, 134
Vision loss, acute, 323
Vitamin B_{12} (cobalamin) deficiency, 150
Vitamin D deficiency, 95–96
Vitaminoses, 374
Vitreous hemorrhage, 323
Voiding cystourethrogram, 182, 250
von Willebrand's disease, 164

W

Waterhouse–Friderichsen syndrome, 90
Wegener's granulomatosis, 297
Wernicke's encephalopathy, 374
Whipple's disease, 144–145
Whooping cough. *See* Pertussis
Wolfe–Parkinson–White syndrome, 41, 43–44
Wood's lamp, 332, 355

X–Z

Xanthelasma, 54
Xanthoma, 54
Yersinia, 294
Zenker's diverticulum, 106
Zollinger–Ellison syndrome, 111, 233
Zona fasciculata, 90
Zona glomerulosa, 90
Zona reticularis, 90